Frontiers of Cord Blood Science

Niranjan Bhattacharya · Phillip Stubblefield
Editors

Frontiers of Cord Blood Science

Foreword by Eliane Gluckman

Springer

Editors
Niranjan Bhattacharya
Advanced Medical Research Institute
Vidyasagore Hospital
Calcutta
India
sanjuktaniranjan@gmail.com

Phillip Stubblefield
Boston University Medical Centre
Boston, MA
USA
phillip.stubblefield@bmc.org

ISBN: 978-1-84996-742-6 e-ISBN: 978-1-84800-167-1
DOI 10.1007/978-1-84800-167-1

British Library Cataloguing in Publication Data
A catalogue record for this book is available from the British Library

Printed on acid-free paper

springer.com

Foreword

Evidence supporting the efficacy of umbilical cord blood hematopoietic stem cells for allogeneic transplantation has significantly increased over the past years, as it now becomes a standard alternative to bone marrow transplantation in many centers. Since the first cord blood transplant successfully performed in a child with Fanconi anemia with his HLA-identical sibling, the number of allogeneic unrelated and related transplants performed for various hematological disorders is increasing steadily. To perform these transplants, cord blood banks are dedicated for collecting, cryopreserving, and performing searches for international exchanges. More than 8000 unrelated cord blood transplants have been performed worldwide; the transplants have been provided by cord blood banks that have collected more than 200,000 cord blood units. Cord blood cells have proliferative advantage and decreased immune reactivity when they are compared to adult bone marrow cells. These properties give a clear advantage for engraftment and diminution of graft-versus-host disease. In consequence, several studies have shown that cell dose and HLA are important factors for survival after transplant. The best units should contain more than 2×10^7 nucleated cells per kilogram and more than 2×10^5 $CD34^+$ cells per kilogram, the number of HLA mismatches should not be superior to 2. The advantages of cord blood compared to bone marrow transplants are the absence of risk to the donor, the direct availability of the cells, and the absence of infectious disease at birth. Further research are currently undertaken to improve the results of allogeneic hematopoietic stem cell transplants: they include the use of double cord blood transplants, the preparative regimen with non-myeloablative drugs, and the *in vitro* expansion of progenitor cells.

In addition to the presence of hematopoietic progenitors, it is now known when cord blood contains stem cells that have retained embryonic properties, they can be isolated, and, when cultured in appropriate conditions, give rise to cell lines that can be used for tissue engineering and regeneration of non-hematopoietic organs or tissues. Already, various cell lines have been generated from cord blood, including mesenchymal cells, endothelial cells, hepatocytes, muscle, cardiac myoblasts, pancreatic islets, keratinocytes, and neuronal cells. These results are very promising, but more research is needed before large-scale production for clinical use. Comparison with adult and embryonic stem cells will determine the best source for each indication. Considering the availability of cord blood and the absence of ethical problems, cord blood will probably become the best source for cell therapy.

Hematology Bone Marrow
Transplantation Department, Hospital
Saint Louis, Paris, France

Professor Eliane Gluckman, MD, RFSP

Preface

Francis Bacon once wrote that science progresses by a succession of small steps through a fog through which even the keen sighted explorer can seldom see more than few paces ahead; occasionally, the fog lifts and an eminence is gained, and scientific truth gets kaleidoscopically rearranged into fact and fiction. In the year 1988, a 6-year-old boy from North Carolina with Fanconi anemia was transplanted with HLA-matched umbilical cord blood from his baby sister by Prof. Elaine Gluckman in Paris. Nobody at that time dreamt of the enormous possibilities of such an experimentation (Gluckman E, et al. Hematopoietic reconstitution in a patient with Fanconi's anemia by means of umbilical cord blood from a HLA-identical sibling. *N. Engl. J. Med.* 1989;321:1174–1178). Most scientists and physicians were highly skeptical, doubting that a few ounces of cord blood contained sufficient stem and progenitor cells to rescue bone marrow after myeloablative therapy. However, this child engrafted without incident, and his blood, bone marrow, and immune system were fully regenerated with donor cells. He remains well and durably engrafted with donor cells 17 years following the original transplant.

Since the first successful transplantation of umbilical cord blood in 1988, cord blood has become an important source of hematopoietic stem and progenitor cells for the treatment of blood and genetic disorders. Significant progress has been accompanied by challenges for scientists, ethicists, and health policy makers. With the recent recognition of the need for a national system for the collection, banking, distribution, and use of cord blood and the increasing focus on cord blood as an alternative to embryos as a source of tissue for regenerative medicine, cord blood has garnered significant attention. Cells from cord blood have been shown to trans-differentiate into non-hematopoietic cells, including those of the brain, heart, liver, pancreas, bone, and cartilage, in tissue culture, and in animal systems (Porada GA, Porada C, Zanjani ED. The fetal sheep: a unique model system for assessing the full differentiative potential of human stem cells. *Yonsei Med. J.* 2004;45(Suppl):7–14). Recently, it has been demonstrated that both cardiac and glial cell differentiation of cord blood donor cells occurred in recipients of unrelated donor cord blood transplantation as part of a treatment regime for Krabbe disease and Sanfilippo syndrome (Hall J, Crapnell KB, Staba S, Kurtzberg J. Isolation of oligodendrocyte precursors from umbilical cord blood [abstract] *Biol. Blood Marrow Transplant.* 2004;10**:**67.; Crapnell KB, Turner K, Hall JG, Staba SL, Kurtzberg J. Umbilical cord blood cells engraft and differentiate in cardiac tissues after human transplantation [abstract] *Blood.* 2003;102:153b). These observations raise the possibility that cord blood may serve as a source of cells to facilitate tissue repair and regeneration in the future. While this is purely speculative at this time, developments over the next decade are expected to clarify the potential role of both allogeneic and autologous cord blood in this emerging field.

Most of the work is this field has been with cord blood stem cells, which constitute only 0.01% of the nucleated cells in umbilical cord blood. The utility of the other cells which constitute 99.9% of umbilical cord whole blood has not been properly studied. Cord blood is a rich source of fetal hemoglobin, growth factor, cytokine-rich plasma as well as other nucleated cells, of which stem cells are an important constituent.

Transfusion of blood and other blood products has made possible many of the advances of modern surgery. Without the ability to safely give blood during many of the complex surgical procedures that have saved countless lives, these procedures would not have succeeded. For the last 70 years since the publication of the report of Amberson, there have been global attempts to find a genuine blood substitute. In a report of the World Health Organization, it was revealed that there are about 500,000 pregnancy-related deaths globally, of which at least 25% maternal deaths are due to the loss of blood. An estimated 13 million units of blood worldwide are not tested against human immunodeficiency viruses or hepatitis viruses, and in some developing countries 80% of the blood supply comes from paid donors or replacement donors (family, friends, or acquaintances) even when the infected population is high.

The current generation of blood substitutes can transport oxygen to tissues, and there are agents to replace platelets, plasma coagulation factors, and its various combinations. However, none of the attempts to provide a hemoglobin-based oxygen carrier, be it from a human or a bovine source of hemoglobin, has passed through the Phase III clinical trials in the United States. Apart from this, there are other issues of forbidding costs and complications.

It is a known fact that asceptically collected and properly screened human cord blood is pure, that is, free from bacteria, virus, protozoal contamination, in case of healthy newborn babies, as the cord blood passes through the finest biological sieve, i.e., the placenta. This blood has a much higher hemoglobin, platelet, and leukocyte content than adult whole blood. Additionally, it has a high concentration of cytokine/growth factors in its plasma, which eventually helps in the gene-switching mechanism after the birth of the baby. This blood also has a much higher oxygen-carrying capacity, and hence, the transfusion of fetal hemoglobin-rich cord blood may lead to better tissue perfusion of oxygen (vol/vol) to the recipient's tissue than an identical volume of adult whole blood. Patients with severe anemia, renal failure, and other conditions of low cardio-respiratory reserve or tissue hypoxic condition in any age group might benefit from cord blood transfusion. This is especially important in high-risk cases with varying degrees of bone marrow senescence or failure due to any etiology. Here, CD34 stem cell-rich umbilical cord whole blood transfusion has the potential to have an immediate benefit of better tissue oxygenation with an additional delayed benefit of possible engraftment of umbilical cord stem cells. These stem cells may prove capable of the rejuvenation of the bone marrow in case of structural or functional immunodeficiency as is the experience of transfusion in certain advanced cancers. Finally, another interesting aspect is the possibility of augmentation of surgical wound healing by the growth factor/cytokine-rich umbilical cord blood plasma, and use of cells from cord blood to coat synthetic grafts for reconstructive surgery, allowing their better adhesion.

There is a famous saying which is also very practical, "All that glitters is not gold". Only time will prove whether these are mere hype or a true reality. With over 100 million births globally each year, more than 40 million units (250 ml) of human umbilical cord blood are produced, the vast majority of which is totally discarded as trash. With the ethical constraints surrounding the use of embryonic and fetal-derived stem cell sources, human umbilical cord blood represents the world's greatest untapped resource for interventional therapy.

Acknowledgments

The editors give profuse thanks to Prof. S. Arulkumaran of London University, and currently the Secretary General of FIGO, and Dr. Himangsu Basu, former executive board member of the Royal College of the Obstetricians and Gynaecologists, UK, for their keen interest, advice, and support.

The editors are particularly grateful to Mr. John Harrison for his suggestion and guidance. Suggestions for improvement and advice from colleagues around the world, just to name a few, like Prof. Elaine Gluckman of Paris who is extremely kind to write the foreword of this book, Prof. Terry Storm of Harvard University, Prof. Linda Heffner, Prof. Anderson Deborah of Boston University, Prof. Hal Broxmeyer of the University of Indiana School of Medicine, and Prof. Ian McNiece of Johns Hopkins University. The editors also gratefully acknowledge the contributions of all the authors who took precious time from their busy schedules in order to help us to complete the book in time. The editors are also grateful to their wives (Prof. Sanjukta Bhattacharya for Dr. Niranjan Bhattacharya, and Linda Stubblefield, MSW, for Prof. Phillip Stubblefield) for their encouragement, understanding, and forbearance. With their own commitment in their respective fields, it is no surprise that their affection for the book would be less than that of ours but they tolerated and indulged in spite of the time subtracted from family activities. There are also innumerable patients, students, friends who have facilitated our work immeasurably. May God bless all of them for their support of cord blood science.

Dr. Niranjan Bhattacharya
Prof. Phillip Stubblefield

Contents

Contributors

Thangavel Ayyappan, MCh, DNB
Department of Surgery, The Chinese University of Hong Kong, Prince of Wales Hospital, Hong Kong SAR, China

Karen K. Ballen, MD
Department of Haematology and Oncology, Massachusetts General Hospital, Boston, MA, USA

Debabrata Basu, PhD
Department of Bio-Ceramics and Coating Division, Central Glass and Ceramic Research Institute, Kolkata, India

Himansu Kumar Basu
Department of Gynaecology, Oakfield Clinic, Gravesend, Kent, UK

Niranjan Bhattacharya, DSc, MBBS, MD, MS, FACS(USA)
Advanced Medical Research Institute (AMRI) Hospitals, B.P. Poddar Hospital, Apollo Gleneagles Hospital and Vidyasagore Hospital, Calcutta, India

Karen Bieback, PhD
Department of Stem Cell Laboratory, Institute of Transfusion Medicine and Immunology and Medical Faculty Mannheim, University of Heidelberg, Mannheim, Germany

Pablo Bosch, Ph.D.
Instituto Technológico de Chascomús (IIB-INTECH), CONICET-Universidad Nacional de General San Martín, Chascomús, Buenos Aires, Argentina

Andrew Burd, MD, FRCS, MBChB
Department of Surgery, The Chinese University of Hong Kong, Prince of Wales Hospital, Hong Kong SAR, China

Raquel L. Canabarro, M.Sc.
Department of Transplant Immunology, Santa Casa De Porto Alegre Porto Alegre, Rio Grande do Sul, Brazil

Curtis L. Cetrulo, MD.
Department of Maternal Fetal Medicine, Tufts University School of Medicine, Boston, MA, USA

Kyle Cetrulo
International Cord Blood Society, Brighton, MA, USA

Jui Chakraborty, MSc, PhD
Department of Bio-Ceramics and Coating Division, Central Glass and Ceramic Research Institute, Kolkata, India

Ranes Chakravorty, MD, Med, FRCS, FACS
Department of Surgery, University of Virginia, Salem, Virginia, USA

Abhijit Chaudhuri, DM, MD, PhD, FACP, FRCP
Department of Neurology, Queen's Hospital, London, UK

Peter Hollands, Ph.D. CSci. FIBMS
Senior Lecturer in Biomedical Science, Department of Biomedical Science, University of Westminster, 115, New Cavendish Street, London W1W 6UW, UK

Wolfgang Holzgreve, MD, FRCOG, FACOG
Department of Obstetrics and Gynaecology, University Hospital Basel, Switzerland

Lin Huang, PhD, MBBS
Department of Surgery, The Chinese University of Hong Kong, Prince of Wales Hospital, Hong Kong SAR, China

K. Kaladhar
Biosurface Technology Division, Sree Chitra Tirunal Institute for Medical Science and Technology, Thiruvananthapuram, Kerala, India

Tatjana Kilo, MD
Department of Oncology, The Children's Hospital at Westmead, Sydney, Australia

Harald Klüter, MD
Institute of Transfusion Medicine and Immunology and Medical Faculty Mannheim, University of Heidelberg, Mannheim, Germany

Ian K. McNiece, Ph.D.
Interdisciplinary Stem Cell Institute, University of Miami, Miami, FL, USA

Anjali Mehta, MD.
Department of Obstetrics and Gynaecology, University of Chicago, Chicago, IL, USA

Patricia Pranke, Ph.D.
Department of Clinical Analysis, Federal University of Rio Grande do Sul, Porto Alegre, Rio Grande do Sul, Brazil

Karen Quillen, MD.
Department of Laboratory Medicine, Boston University Medical Center, Boston, MA, USA

Chandra P. Sharma, Ph.D, DSc
Biosurface Technology Division, Sree Chitra Tirunal Institute for Medical Science and Technology, Thiruvananthapuram, Kerala, India

Peter J. Shaw, MA, MB, BS, MRCP, FRACP
Department of Oncology, The Children's Hospital at Westmead, Sydney, Australia

Elizabeth J. Shpall
Department of Stem Cell Transplantation, M.D. Anderson Cancer Centre, Houston, TX, USA

Glyn N. Stacey, BSc, MP, PhD
Department of Cell Biology and Imaging, National Institute for Biological Standards and Control, South Mimms, UK

Steven L. Stice, Ph.D.
Department of Animal and Dairy Science, University of Georgia, Athens, GA, USA

Phillip G. Stubblefield, MD.
Department of Obstetrics and Gynaecology, Boston University School of Medicine, Boston, MA, USA

Carolyn Troeger
Department of Obstetrics and Gynaecology, University Hospital, Basel, Switzerland

Introduction

In the animal kingdom, swallowing the afterbirth by the mother is a general norm. Nature appears to have provided this precious wisdom to some of its creatures. Even herbivorous animals swallow the placenta after the birth of their babies (for example, the cow). But humans, for the most part, do not appear to know about the potential use of this precious afterbirth, which has protected and nurtured the baby for so long in the womb. In traditional Chinese medicine, however, the dried human placenta (*zi he che*) has been used for therapeutic purposes for over thousands of years. According to this system of medicine, the placental biological property has been described as being sweet and salty in flavor, warm in nature, and it has been noted that it is tropistic to the heart, lung, and kidney channels. Being sweet, salty, warm, and moist in nature and mild in action, it functions in strengthening 'Yang', reinforcing essence and Qi, and nourishing blood, and is used as an excellent tonic. The dried human placenta, combined with other herbs, serves to treat syndromes of insufficiency of Yin, Yang, Qi, and blood.

In the rest of the world, however, there is little knowledge about the therapeutic properties of the human placenta. Of late, particularly since 1989, global consciousness is increasing, not on the use of the placenta per se but on the use of umbilical cord blood stem cells as an easily available source of hematopoietic stem cells for bone marrow transplantation. The first cord blood transplantation was done in Paris by Prof. Elaine Gluckman, a dedicated scientist, who has very kindly written the foreword to the present volume. Her pioneering work marked the initiation of the clinical application of cord blood. In the years following, cord blood transplantation has been successful, particularly in children with hematological, immunological, metabolic, and neoplastic diseases. Cord blood as an alternative source for hematopoietic progenitor cells (HPC) has several advantages, including rapid availability and lower risk of graft-versus-host disease (GVHD) despite human leukocyte antigen (HLA) disparity.

In cases where there is a non-availability of bone marrow or where the cord blood cell count is very low or where there is extensive myoablation due to drug, radiation or both, problems may occur in the host undergoing the transplant procedure. In such cases, multiple cord blood units or in vivo expansion of cord blood cells can provide a solution, with sophisticated infrastructural support. For example, many older patients, or those with extensive prior therapy or serious co-morbidities, are unable to tolerate conventional myeloablative conditioning.

Currently, research is on-going all over the world, which may improve the effectiveness of cord blood transplantation for the treatment of a variety of conditions, including non-myeloblative regimens; the use of ex vivo expansion to increase the numbers of HPCs; the development of new approaches to the acceleration of immune recovery; the use of multiple units of cord blood in transplantation; and facilitation of the upregulation of homing receptors. Attempts are being also made to clarify the existing scientific confusion about the transdifferential property of mesenchymal stem cells (MSC). The primary reason for the current interest in the use of cord blood is because of the stem cells which are found in cord blood and their trans-differentiational abilities, which have clinical implications in degenerative diseases. Hence, cord blood research is related to stem cell research. These fetal stem cells (CD 34), which are inherent in cord blood, cause less graft-versus-host reactions after transplantation. Recognition of this potentiality in the scientific world has resulted in the collection and harvesting of these cord blood stem cells in many laboratories all over the world. However, these hematopoietic stem cells constitute only 0.01% of the nucleated cells of the cord blood. The rest, i.e., 99.99% of the cord blood is not used for the most part. This wasted precious gift of Mother Nature is rich in fetal hemoglobin, growth factors, and other cytokine filled plasma, and is moreover protected in the infection-free environment inside the placenta in case of a healthy newborn. It, too, has great potentials, and it has been shown that it can be used not only as a safe alternative to adult blood for transfusion, but also has the added advantage of its various properties, which actually help in the all-round development of a neonate. This is significant because for years a search has been going on for a suitable hemoglobin-based oxygen carrier, and chemically or genetically modified bovine RBC or hemoglobin extracted from sea creatures like the sea worm (*Arenicola merina*) have been tried out for the purpose.

As a new human grows and develops inside its mother, blood is made to circulate to all the vital organs bringing nutrients from the mother to the fetus and carrying waste products back to the mother. Fetal blood in the placenta exchanges waste products from the baby for nutrients and oxygen from the mother and carries the ‘good stuff’ from the mother back to the fetus through one large vessel, the umbilical vein. Roughly one-third to 40% of all blood that the fetus makes is outside the fetus at any point of time, flowing to the mother or coming back from the mother. In pregnancy, there are dramatic and continuous molecular and biochemical changes with the progression of the gestation both for the fetus and the mother because there are two distinct separate genomes operating under the same organism (the mother). There are two distinct lines of blood supply with a unique interface (trophoblast) which have the specific functions of anchoring, controlling, transporting and metabolizing the specific need for the growth and maturation of the fetus, for that gestational state of growth and maturation. There are direct and indirect interactions between the mother, the embryo or the fetus, the placenta, the extra-amniotic membrane and the amniotic fluid. And the cord blood carries all the nutrition to meet the growth requirements of the organism at that specific gestational age.

The major emphasis of research internationally, however, is not on the transfusion of cord blood, but on the use of umbilical cord blood stem cells. These have a different set of microenvironmental exposures compared to those of adult marrow or peripheral blood stem cells. The placenta is a complex organ that regulates feto-maternal interactions. Many cytokines that can influence lympho-hematopoietic development, i.e., granulocyte colony stimulating factor (G-CSF), c-kit ligand (stem cell factor), granulocyte macrophage colony-stimulating factor (GM-CSF), interleukin-15 (IL-15), all are produced by the placenta. The red cell collected from cord blood of the new born differs from the adult RBC in many ways. For example, there is an increase in the immunoreactive myosin of the red cell membrane [1], and the total value of the lipid, phospholipid, and cholesterol are more in proportion than the red cells of the adult [2].

Even the antigen expression of cord blood RBC differs from the adult RBC, viz., the A, B, S and Lutheran antigens are expressed in lesser amounts in cord blood than in adult RBC and there is a complete absence of Lewis antigens in cord blood [3]. Of greater interest, however, is the fact that there are fundamental metabolic differences between adult and cord blood RBCs, for example, the activities of phosphoglycerate kinase, enolase, glyceraldehydes-3- phosphate dehydrogenase, glucose phosphate isomerase, etc., which are the essential enzymes of the Embden-Meyerhof pathway, are definitely increased for the cell age in case of cord blood when compared with the adult RBC activities of those enzymes [4]. Apart from the enzymes mentioned above, the activity of a number of non-glycolytic enzymes is different in cord blood, viz., carbonic anhydrase, and acetylcholine esterase, only to name the essential few [5].

The full potential for the use of placental umbilical cord blood is as yet unknown. This volume is a compilation of the work of distinguished investigators who are currently engaged in discovering the latent possibilities of cord blood in the treatment of various diseases. The contributors summarize the current state of research in the field and discuss the potential future applications of cord blood both for research and for the treatment of different diseases and conditions. There are four chapters which are mainly hypothetical, one of which is a preview of the clinical uses of cord blood (Part III, Chapter 13). One is on the use of cord blood in strokes and other neurological disorders (Part III, Chapter 11), another is on the bioengineering applications of cord blood to improve the biofriendliness of a mechanical prosthesis or implant (Part V, Chapter 16), and the fourth one is also on how to increase the biofriendliness of a ceramic prosthesis with the use of cord blood MSCs and other cells (Part V, Chapter 17). There is one chapter on umbilical cord whole blood transfusion, based on actual clinical human trials in chronic anemias of several diseases to combat anemia, which is a co-morbidity in many chronic serious diseases (Part III, Chapter 10). There are 13 chapters dealing with the basic science and transplantation, preservation, in vivo expansion, and other aspects of cord blood stem cell application. And finally, one investigator has explored the ethics of cord blood research (Part VI).

Perspectives on Cord Blood Banking and Cord Blood Stem Cell Transplantation

There are several interesting observations on the transplantation of cord blood stem cells in this volume from different parts of the world like the USA, the UK,

Australia, Germany, Hong Kong, etc. Dr Anjali Mehta and colleagues noted that the placenta may prove to be a non-controversial source of hematopoietic and MSCs as well as endothelial progenitor cells (Part I, Chapter 1). A 'cocktail' of these three elements might be used in the future to treat hypoxic ischemic encephalopathy (HIE) in the peripartum period for neuroregeneration, and a combination of these cells might also be used to treat one of the more than 80 diseases that have responded to stem cell transplantation. Furthermore, these cells have the potential to treat degenerative diseases, such as heart disease, endocrine disorders like diabetes, and neurodegenerative diseases such as stroke, Alzheimer's disease, Parkinson's disease, and spinal cord injuries. These cells may also be useful in the treatment of orthopedic problems.

Further insight into the subject was has been provided by Dr. Peter Hollands of the UK Cord Blood Bank (Part I, Chapter 2) who has the experience of more than two decades in this field. He presents the advantages and disadvantages of cord blood as a source of stem cells.

The advantages in the use of cord blood as a source of stem cells for transplant are:

- Ease of procurement, processing, and storage
- No risk to donors
- Reduced risk of transmitting infection
- Immediate availability of cryopreserved units
- Acceptable partial HLA mismatches (4/6 HLA match)

Holland notes an added advantage that cord blood stem cells do not carry any of the legal, moral, ethical or religious objections associated with the use of embryonic stem cells.

The current disadvantages in the use of cord blood stem cells as a source of stem cells for transplant are:

- The limited number of hematopoietic stem cells in a cord blood unit which may lead to failed or delayed hematopoietic reconstitution or restricted use in adults
- Possible abnormalities in cord blood stem cells, e.g., early malignant mutations, which may have an effect on recipients
- It is not possible to collect additional donor stem cells, or donor lymphocytes, for those recipients who relapse following cord blood stem cell transplant.

For the purpose of easy availability of cord blood stem cells, cord blood banks have sprung up in different parts of the world. There are problems and controversies associated with cord blood banking. Dr. G.N. Stacey, the director of the UK Stem Cell Bank, has discussed the problems and advantages of different stem cell lines as practiced in UK Stem Cell Bank and mentions how others can use the facilities provided by the bank (Part V, Chapter 16). Prof. Stacey points out that the embryonic stem cell lines established in the UK are required, under the licence for derivation from the Human Fertilization and Embryology Authority, to be deposited in the UK Stem Cell Bank. Other groups working on the derivation of adult and non-UK hES cells are also very welcome to use the UK Stem Cell Bank facility.

Donation of cell lines into the bank is initiated by submission of information on the lines to the bank's Steering Committee using the forms available on the bank and Medical Research Council websites. Confirmation by the Steering Committee that the cells meet ethical requirements for the UK and other scientific and technical criteria then activates the depositing process with the bank and establishment of the transfer agreements between depositor and the bank. There is also a generic agreement between the depositor and any institution receiving cells from the bank, to protect the depositor's intellectual property in the cells.

In another chapter on cord blood banking and the controversies involved therein by Dr. Carolyn Troeger and colleagues, Switzerland (Part V, Chapter 17). According to them, cord blood stem cells are increasingly being used to repopulate bone marrow in the treatment of malignant and non-malignant diseases in children and adults. This development, however, is also related to a continuing debate on the role of public versus private cord blood banks. Public cord blood banks store HSC for allogeneic, usually unrelated, transplantations. Currently between 175,000 and 200,000 units are stored frozen worldwide. The infant and its parents donate the cord blood to the bank and therewith to the public. Unlike private cord blood banks, public banks do not charge for collection and storage. Most of the transplants are used for the allogeneic treatment of leukemia, about a quarter for the treatment of genetic diseases. Similarly, a related allogeneic HSC transplantation using the stored cord blood from a sibling is well established in public banks. Public cord blood banks have the opportunity to provide HSC also for ethnic minorities that are under-represented in bone marrow registries.

There are several chapters on the clinical applications of cord blood transplantation. Prof. Patricia Pranke and Dr. Raquel Canabarro from Brazil have suggested that umbilical cord blood stem cells are an efficient alternative for the transplantation of HPCs (Part I, Chapter 3). Parameters commonly used to evaluate an umbilical cord blood unit and predict transplant outcomes have been total nucleated cells and $CD34^{+}$cells counts. Lack of CD38, HLA-DR and lineage committed antigens, as well as the co-expression of Thy-1 (CDw90), c-kit receptor (CD117), among others surface markers, have been shown to identify the hematopoietic stem cells in umbilical cord blood. A number of factors can influence the volume and amount of $CD34^{+}$cells, which are considered as immature and capable of proliferation. Quantification of $CD34^{+}$as well as correlations of such factors as maternal age, gestational age, newborn sex and weight, umbilical cord length, placental weight with increased volume and concentration of immature cells, among others, are important issues that can influence the success of umbilical cord blood cells transplantation. According to the authors, ex vivo culture is a crucial component of several clinical applications currently in development including gene therapy, and stem/progenitor cell expansion.

Dr. Karen Quillen, Director of the Boston University Blood Bank, has done a retrospective comparison of 113 cord blood transplants and 2052 marrow transplants in children (15 years of age or younger), for the period 1990–1997 (Part II, Chapter 8). Over half the patients were transplanted for malignancy, most commonly acute leukemia. The recipients of cord blood were younger (median age of 5 years versus 8 years) and smaller (median weight of 17 kg versus 26 kg) than the recipients of bone marrow. The median cell dose was 4.7 × 10E7 cells/kg for cord blood as compared to 3.5 × 10E8 cells/g for marrow. Despite less intense GVHD prophylaxis (with the omission of methotrexate in 72% of cord blood recipients), cord blood transplants had a lower risk of acute GVHD (14% versus 24%) and chronic GVHD (5% versus 14%). Hematopoietic recovery in terms of neutrophil (26 versus 18 days) and platelet (44 days versus 24 days) engraftment was significantly slower for cord blood transplantation compared to marrow. Interestingly, the three-year survival rate in patients transplanted for malignancy was similar in the two groups (46% for cord blood recipients, 55% for marrow recipients).

Prof. Karen K. Ballen of Harvard University comments in her review that over the last 17 years, there has been a dramatic growth in the use of cord blood as an alternative stem cell source for patients without matched related or unrelated bone marrow donors (Part II, Chapter 9). Initially, the majority of transplants were performed in children. Recently, the results in adult cord blood transplantation, according to her, appeared promising. She has discussed the outcome data for adult cord blood transplantation, with an emphasis on new techniques using double or sequential cord blood transplantation in her article. She has noted that cord blood $CD34^+$ cells in culture increase in cell number every 7–10 days, several hundred-fold greater than the increase in cultures of similar cells from adult bone marrow, thereby allowing a 10-fold lower $CD34^+$ cell dose to be used for successful cord blood transplantation. Moreover, cord blood cells have greater proliferative capacity and longer telomere length has been proposed as a possible explanation. Ballen further mentions that decreased GVHD following cord blood transplantation with preservation of a graft-versus-leukemia effect may be because the immunologic properties of cord blood differ from mature bone marrow or peripheral blood stem cells. Cord blood contains a high proportion of 'naive' phenotype T cells that are $CD45RA^+/CD45RO^-$, $CD62L^+$. The chemokine receptor CCR5, expressed by TH1 T cells, is less abundant among cord blood T cells than adult T cells. She notes that cord blood T cell receptors when compared to adult blood T cell receptors, have a less complex repertoire. Cord blood cells express T cells with less clonal diversity than expressed by adult peripheral blood.

Prof. Shaw and his group from Australia state that the majority of hematopoietic stem cells transplants (HSCT) are done for patients with malignant diseases (Part II, Chapter 7). But, at the same time, it should be remembered that a high proportion of paediatric transplants are done for non-malignant disease, particularly true for unrelated transplants. HSCT is a curative option for many inherited and acquired non-malignant diseases that show abnormalities of the blood or bone marrow-derived cells. Current experience shows that unrelated CBT is a feasible procedure for children with bone marrow failure with the background of inborn errors, immunodeficiencies, hemoglobinopathy, etc.

Key researchers in the field such as Prof. Ian K. McNiece and Dr. Elizabeth J. Shpall of Johns Hopkins University, Baltimore, USA, have noted that cord blood products contain similar cell populations to bone marrow and mobilized peripheral blood progenitor cell products (PBPC), including hematopoietic stem cells (HSC), primitive progenitor cells, mature progenitor cells, and mature functional cells (Part I, Chapter 4). However, the total cell number and progenitor cells are much lower in cord blood compared to bone marrow and PBPC. For example, bone marrow and PBPC contain approx 10^8 $CD34^+$ cells while cord blood contains approximately 5×10^6 $CD34^+$ cells. In contrast, the frequency of HSC, as determined by NOD/SCID engraftment, is enriched in the $CD34^+$ cell population of cord blood compared to bone marrow or PBPC. As few as 100,000 cord blood $CD34^+$ cells can engraft NOD/SCID mice, while approx 1 million bone marrow $CD34^+$ cells and 5 million PBPC $CD34^+$ cells are required for engraftment of human cells. McNiece and colleagues noted that these numbers suggest that cord blood contains similar levels of HSC to bone marrow and PBPC, but significantly lower levels of committed progenitor cells.

Dr. Karen Bieback of the University of Heidelberg, Germany, has commented that: for allogeneic use, the primitive umbilical cord blood derived non-hematopoietic stem cell population provides perhaps the most readily accessible and at the same time, underutilized stem cell source, with little ethical conflict and a number of advantages (Part I, Chapter 6) However, the question as to whether cord blood progenitor cells will prove to be superior or more practical in terms of an alleviating allogeneic use when compared to other adult tissue derived progenitor cells, remains open at this time. Nevertheless, efficient and reproducible methods to isolate, expand and differentiate cord blood progenitor cells are required. When extrapolated to the developments in hematopoietic stem cell transplantation, where within 10 years cord blood has become an increasingly accepted alternative source for HSC, Bieback is of the opinion that probably as many years will go by before the eventual use of cord blood-derived non-hematopoietic stem cells in clinical therapy.

In addition to hematopoietic stem cells, on which the investigators mentioned so far have written, it has been long recognized that the post-natal bone marrow in mammals is populated by a distinct stem cell population known as MSCs, also referred as marrow somatic cells or colony forming unit fibroblastic cells. In vivo, MSCs and other non-hematopoietic cells (e.g. macrophages, reticular cells, endothelial cells, smooth muscle cells, adipocytes) in combination with the extra cellular matrix, form what is known as a "hematopoietic inductive microenvironment". This complex bone marrow microenvironment provides support for hematopoiesis, i.e., the process of formation of new blood cells, through cell-to-cell interactions and soluble clues. However, MSCs are not exclusively located in the bone marrow and are found in various other tissues, including the cord blood, fetal blood and liver, amniotic fluid and, in some circumstances, in adult peripheral blood.

Prof Steve Stice and Dr Pablo Bosch, from the University of Georgia, USA, report that MSCs can be isolated from several tissues (Part I, Chapter 6). MSCs are a fairly rare and unique cell type, and form, at most, 0.01% of adult human bone marrow. This is true for cord blood as well. However, more MSC cells exists within the umbilical vein endothelial/subendothelial layer. MSCs are considered pluripotent cells with a capacity to differentiate into mesodermal lineages, such as adipocytes, osteoblasts and chondrocytes both in vivo and in vitro. Several studies have demonstrated that these pluripotent stem cells derived from the marrow stroma, can be easily isolated from bone marrow specimens, proliferate extensively ex vivo to originate relatively homogeneous cell populations and are endowed with the capacity to differentiate into mesodermal and non-mesodermal cell types. Due to their multipotentiality and extensive self-renewal capacity, MSCs hold great promise as a source of cells for many cell-based strategies for the treatment of human diseases. This chapter presents an in-depth description of the biology, isolation, characterization and potential therapeutic applications of MSCs.

Prof. Andrew Burd, Dr. T. Ayyappan, Dr. Lin Huang, representing the Chinese University of Hong Kong, China, are currently working on the problem of chronic wound healing (Part III, Chapter 12). They opine that the chronic wound becomes more vascular and can then be definitively closed with a skin graft. They cite a report on the use of allogenic bone marrow MSCs for the treatment of a patient with deep skin burns. Burd et al. feel that it is in such cases that there is a great potential for topical application of cord blood as a biological wound healing modulator. They further note that amniotic membranes have been used in the past as biological dressings for wounds but comment that concerns about risks of disease transmission have severely limited this practice in many parts of the world. Similarly, the question of potential risk of disease transmission when using cord blood may also be raised. However, they feel that there are already well defined screening processes to reduce and/or eliminate such risks as applied in routine blood banking. They assert that as the understanding of the range and nature of the stem cell composition in cord blood becomes more clear, it may be possible to apply more selective fractions onto wounds, both chronic and acute, to modulate the biological healing mechanisms, and an additional benefit is that it will be cost effective.

Perspectives on Cord Blood Transfusion

In a report of the World Health Organization, it was revealed that there are about 500,000 pregnancy related deaths globally, of which at least 25% maternal deaths are due to the loss of blood [6]. One of the most important advances in surgery has been the availability of blood and other blood products. Without the ability to safely give blood during many of the complex surgical procedures that have saved countless lives, these procedures would not have succeeded. However, an estimated 13 million units of blood worldwide are not tested against human immunodeficiency viruses or hepatitis viruses, and in some developing countries 80% of the blood supply comes from paid or replacement donors (family friends or acquaintances) even when the rate of infection in the population is high [7]. For the last 70 years since the publication of a report by Amberson et al. [8] there have been global attempts to find a genuine blood substitute. A reliable supply of safe blood is essential to improve health standards at several levels, especially among women and children, and particularly in the poorer sections of society anywhere in the world. Apart from mortality related to complications of pregnancy and childbirth among women, malnutrition, thalassaemia, and severe anemia are prevalent diseases in children which require blood transfusion, apart from other complicated diseases.

Over 80 million units of blood are collected every year, but the tragedy is that only 39% of this is collected in the developing world which contains 82% of the global population. On the other hand, with over 100 million births globally each year, more than 10 billion milliliters of human umbilical cord blood (HUCB) are produced, the vast majority of which is totally discarded as trash. In one chapter, Dr. Niranjan Bhattacharya, Calcutta, India, discusses the transfusion perspective of freshly collected and properly screened cord blood. The author is of the opinion that the transfusion of cord blood is safe in case of anemia of any etiology, i.e., from thalassemia, HIV, leprosy, uncontrolled diabetes with albuminuria, advanced cancer, arthritis, tuberculosis, malaria and emergency condition necessitating blood transfusion support. What is interesting is the observation that there is a transient peripheral rise of CD34 in the peripheral blood without clinical graft-versus-host reaction, in HLA randomized transfusion without the support of immunosuppressive or growth factor on the host system. This hitherto unreported phenomenon could indicate a potential for immunotherapy from cells in cord blood that might improve prognosis. This observation, if verified in other institutions, may have enormous clinical significance. This phenomenon could also help in the understanding of the etiology of any advanced disease on the basis of a local or regional or selective structural or functional immunosuppression affecting different organs or its subsystem level. The question asked by Bhattacharya is whether immunosuppression is a mosaic like phenomenon. He observes that only time will prove or reject this clinical work based hypothesis (Part III, Chapter 10).

H.K. Basu, a senior consultant in Ob/Gyn, UK, has given an overview of the use of cord blood and has noted that the yield of cord blood varies from a volume of 67–134 ml mean 88 + 14 ml SD and mean hemoglobin 17.6 gm% (Part III, Chapter 13). This blood has a much higher hemoglobin (mostly fetal hemoglobin), platelet, and leukocyte content than adult whole blood. Additionally, it has a high concentration of cytokine/growth factors in its plasma, which eventually helps in the gene-switching mechanism after the birth of the baby. This blood has a much higher oxygen-carrying capacity than that of adult whole blood, and hence, the transfusion of fetal hemoglobin rich cord blood has the potential for better tissue perfusion of oxygen (vol/vol) to the recipient's tissue than an identical volume of adult whole blood.

The futuristic potential of the use of cord blood in medicine and engineering has been touched upon by different distinguished authors, concentrating in this field of cord blood stem cells. Dr. A. Chaudhuri, a senior consultant neurologist of the Essex Neuroscience Centre (Part III, Chapter 11), UK, and Dr. Niranjan Bhattacharya from the Advanced Medical Research Center Hospital, Calcutta, India, described neurological diseases as responsible for significant disability all over the world. Based on the epidemiological data presented in the Global Burden of Disease 2000 study of the World Health Organization, it was calculated that in Europe, brain diseases account for a third of all disabilities and this is likely to increase in the coming years especially in the absence of any effective and established therapy for neuronal regeneration and repair. It is therefore imperative that potential strategies to minimize the burden of brain disease are rapidly developed and tested by ethical research and clinical trials. The authors cited many animal studies involving umbilical cord blood in brain cell repair. In an animal study, twenty-four hours after traumatic brain injury, umbilical cord blood was administered intravenously in the rats. Treated animals showed significant improvement in the neurological deficit compared with the control animals by 4th week. In another experimental mouse model (G 93A) of motor neuron disease (amyotrophic lateral sclerosis), intravenous administration of umbilical cord blood in pre-symptomatic animals resulted in a delay of the disease progression by 2–3 weeks and increased life span in the diseased mice. The transplanted cells survived for 10–12 weeks after administration and entered in the areas of motor neuron degeneration in the brain and spinal cord where they were found to express neural markers. In addition, the transplanted cells were widely distributed in the peripheral circulation and in the spleen. High volumes of HUCB mononuclear cell infusion in a mice model of Huntington's disease (B6CBA-TgN 62 Gpb mice) reduced the rate of weight loss, which appears before the onset of chorea, and total duration of survival. These workers also found improved survival of mice overexpressing amyloid precursor protein (a model of Alzheimer's disease) with high dose cell therapy.

Bioengineering Application of Cord Blood

Cord blood stem cells also have application in the field of bioengineering. According to Dr. D. Basu and his associates, a globally renowned scientist group from India working on the ceramic biofriendly interface, the main cause of premature failure of an orthopedic implant in vivo is due to various biological reactions with the surrounding tissues/environment (Part V, Chapter17). To combat this situation, continuous efforts have been concentrated on the improvement of the biocompatibility of the implant material by adopting different strategies. MSCs are one of the adult stem cell types that can be made to develop a limited number of different kinds of tissues, with bone, cartilage, muscle and skin, being the most important types. They are found primarily in the bone marrow, but are also available elsewhere in the body such as in umbilical blood or fatty tissue. One possible application for these versatile cells is to aid in the production of optimized materials for bone implants, such as those used in artificial hip joints.

Another internationally renowned bioengineering group from India, Dr. K. Kaladhar, and Dr. Chandra P. Sharma have also commented on the futuristic potential use of cord blood stem cells in making a healthy long lasting biofriendly interface in case of different orthopedic and neurosurgical implants (Part V, Chapter 16). They propose that the major problem associated with medical devices implanted inside the body is performance failure due to biological reactions, regulated by the adsorbed proteins and the pathological cells on the material surface. The surface of the material is being modified to make the material biocompatible. Introducing specific surface groups, immobilizing proteins with certain conformations, or by immobilizing certain cell lines, often does this. Strategies have also been adopted to modify the material/biology interface. Basically this type of cell-mediated therapy is being done to improve the device integration by augmenting the tissue regeneration, e.g., endothelialization of the vascular grafts to improve the blood compatibility; utilizing platelet rich plasma for improving tissue regeneration in periodontitis, etc. Cord blood stem cell, the investigators feel, could potentially be a very useful material in such diverse applications.

Ethics and Cord Blood

In our final chapter, Prof. Ranesh Chakraborty (Part VI), former Chairman Surgical Sciences, University of Virginia, USA, considers the ethical aspects on stem cell biology specially involving the cord blood stem cells. He notes that the English word 'ethics' has some equivalence with the Sanskrit term 'dharma,' Dharma means the principles that 'support' or guide an individual in the passage through life. As he states, the major ethical controversy is the source of stem cells, whether from embryonic tissue or not. Since ethical opinions on this issue vary widely in the diverse belief systems of our world, one possible solution to reducing conflict may be to explicitly identify the source of stem cells lines. As one example, this would allow those to benefit who can accept stems cells from embryos donated by infertile couples but not from embryos specifically obtained for treatment of disease.

Today, if there is any problem in medicine not amenable to conventional treatment, the application of stem cell technology may offer new hope, but we must not sacrifice our objectivity in proper assessment of the situation. In this connection, the famous teaching of the legendary scientist Prof. J.B.S. Haldane is appropriate: "Science is vastly more stimulating to the imagination than are the classics"(Daedalus) [J.B.S. Haldane, *Daedalus* (in Henry Davidoff, ed., *The Pocket Book of Quotations* (Pocket Books, New York, 1952), p.329].

References

Matovcik LM, Groschel-Stewart U, Schrier SL. Myosin in adult and human erythrocyte membranes. Blood 1986;67:1668.

Tuan D, Feingold E, Newman M, Weissman SM, Forget BG. Different 3′ end points of deletions causing delta beta-thalassemia and hereditary persistence of fetal hemoglobin: implications for the control of gamma-globin gene expression in man. Proc Natl Acad Sci U S A 1983 Nov;80(22):6937–41.

Marsh WL, Erythrocytes blood groups in human. In: Hematology of Infancy and Childhood, 3rd ed, DG Nathan, FA Oski (ed), Philadelphia:WB Saunders,1987.

Travis SF, Kumar SP, Paez PC, Delivoria-Papadopoulos M. Red cell metabolic alterations in postnatal life in term infants: glycolytic enzymes and glucose-6-phosphate dehydrogenase. Pediatr Res 1980 Dec;14(12):1349–52.

Stevenson SS. Carbonic anhydrase in newborn infants. J Clin Invest 1943;22:403.

World Health Organization, International Federation of Red Cross and Red Crescent Societies, "Safe blood starts with me", Geneva:World Health Organization 2000:12.

Sloane EM, Pitt E, Klein HG. Safety of blood supply. JAMA 1995;274:1368–73.

Amberson WR, Mulder AG, Steggerda FR, et al. Mammalian life without red blood corpuscles. Science 1933;78:106–7.

Section I
Umbilical Cord Blood Stem Cell
(Basic Science)

Chapter 1
Placental and Pregnancy Stem Cells

Anjali Mehta, Curtis Cetrulo, Phillip Stubblefield, and Kyle Cetrulo

The placenta may prove to be a non-controversial source of hematopoietic and mesenchymal stem cells (MSCs) as well as endothelial progenitor cells. A "cocktail" of these three elements might be used in future to treat hypoxic ischemic encephalopathy (HIE) in the peripartum period for neuroregeneration, and a combination of these cells might also be used to treat one of the more than 80 diseases that have responded to stem cell transplantation (Table 1.1). Furthermore, these cells have the potential to treat degenerative diseases (e.g., heart disease), endocrine disorders (e.g., diabetes), and neurodegenerative diseases (e.g., stroke, Alzheimer's disease, Parkinson's disease, and spinal cord injuries). These cells may also be useful in the treatment of orthopedic problems.

Hematopoietic Stem Cells

Hematopoietic stem cells (HSCs), present in umbilical cord blood, have been used in over 6000 umbilical cord blood transplants since the initial report in the *New England Journal of Medicine* in 1989 showed a successful treatment of Fanconi's anemia. Two thousand umbilical cord blood transplants occurred last year.

Mesenchymal Stem Cells

MSCs have been found in the Wharton's jelly of the umbilical cord (matrix cells) as well as in the first and third trimester chorion, first trimester amnion, villous stroma (placental chorionic villi), and amniotic epithelial cells and surrounding fluid [1, 2, 3]. MSCs from Wharton's jelly and the other sources listed above have broader plasticity than previously thought, and can differentiate into neuronal cells, adipocytes chondroblasts, osteoblasts, and myocytes.

A. Mehta (✉)
Department of Obstetrics and Gynaecology, University of Chicago, Chicago, IL, USA
e-mail: amehta@babies.bsd.uchicago.edu

N. Bhattacharya, P. Stubblefield (eds.), *Frontiers of Cord Blood Science*,
DOI 10.1007/978-1-84800-167-1_1,

Table 1.1 Diseases treatable by stem cell transplantation

Stem cell disorders	Inherited erythrocyte abnormalities	Congenital immune system disorders
Aplastic anemia (severe)	Beta thalassemia major	Ataxia-telangiectasia
Fanconi anemia	Pure red cell aplasia	Kostmann syndrome
Paroxysmal nocturnal hemoglobinuria (PNH)	Sickle cell disease	Leukocyte adhesion deficiency
		DiGeorge syndrome
Acute leukemias	**Liposomal storage diseases**	Bare lymphocyte syndrome
Acute lymphoblastic leukemia (ALL)	Mucopolysaccharidoses (MPS)	Omenn's syndrome
Acute myelogenous leukemia (AML)	Hurler's syndrome (MPS-IH)	Severe combined immunodeficiency (SCID)
Acute biphenotypic leukemia	Scheie syndrome (MPS-IS)	SCID with adenosine deaminase
Acute undifferentiated leukemia	Hunter's syndrome (MPS-II)	Deficiency
Chronic leukemias	Sanfilippo syndrome (MPS-III)	Absence of T & B Cells SCID
Chronic myelogenous leukemia (CML)	Morquio syndrome (MPS-IV)	Absence of T Cells, Normal B Cell
Chronic lymphocytic leukemia (CLL)	Maroteaux–Lamy syndrome (MPS-VI)	SCID
Juvenile chronic myelogenous leukemia (JCML)	Sly syndrome, beta-glucuronidase	Common variable immunodeficiency
Juvenile myelomonocytic leukemia (JMML)	Deficiency (MPS-VII)	Wiskott–Aldrich syndrome
	Adrenoleukodystrophy	X-linked lymphoproliferative
Myeloproliferative disorders	Mucolipidosis 11(1-cell disease)	Disorder
Acute myeloflbrosis	Krabbe disease	
Agnogenic myeloid metaplasia (myelofibrosis)	Gaucher's disease	**Inherited platelet abnormalities**
Polycythemia vera	Niemann-Pick disease	Amegakaryocytosis I congenital
Essential thrombocythemia	Wolman disease	Thrombocytopenia
	Metachromatic leukodystrophy	
Myelodysplastic syndromes		**Plasma cell disorders**
Refractory anemia (RA)	**Histiocytic disorders**	Multiple myeloma
Refractory anemia with ringed sideroblasts (RARS)	Familial erythrophagocytic	Plasma cell leukemia
	Lymphohistiocytosis	Waldenstrom's macroglobulinemia
Refractory anemia with excess blasts	Histiocytosis-X	
Refractory anemia with excess blasts in	Hemophagocytosis	**Other inherited disorders**
Transformation (RAEB-T)		Lesch–Nyhan syndrome
Chronic myelomonocytic leukemia (CMML)	**Phagocyte disorders**	Cartilage-hair hypoplasia
	Chediak–Higashi syndrome	Glanzmann thrombasthenia

Table 1.1 (continued)

Lymphoproliferative disorders	Chronic granulomatous disease	Osteopetrosis
Non-Hodgkin's lymphoma	Neutrophil actin deficiency	**Other malignancies**
Hodgkin's disease	Reticular dysgenesis	Breast cancer
Prolymphocytic leukemia		Ewing sarcoma
		Neuroblastoma
		Renal cell carcinoma

Source: National Marrow Donor Program, 2002

Endothelial Progenitor Cells

Endothelial progenitor cells have been isolated from the umbilical vein as well as from the umbilical cord blood. These cells, also called angioblasts, are capable of neovascularization in response to hypoxia and ischemia [4, 5]. The fetal cells found in maternal circulation, even years after the pregnancy has ended, possibly contain the potential to protect the mother from hypoxia and ischemia [6].

Plasticity

Plasticity is the ability of stem cells to give rise to progeny of different cell types. Embryonic stem (ES) cell differentiation reduces the potential that stem cells might give rise to cells of other tissue types. ES cells are totipotent, meaning that they are able to give rise to all other fetal or adult cell types. Post-embryonic stem cells are multi- or pluripotent – that is, they only give rise to many, but not all, cell types. Stem cells in adult tissues generally only possess the ability to give rise to a limited number of cell types, usually one or two.

Another alternative to inherent plasticity is cell fusion, where a stem cell fuses with a somatic cell, and the nuclear material of two cells is combined in one. Cell fusion has made it possible for tissue stem cells to give rise to cells of other tissue types, such as epithelial cells, neurons, or endothelial cells. Therefore, it appears that stem cells present in the tissue of one type may give rise to cells of a different cell lineage by either inherent plasticity or cell fusion. In 1999, an article in *The New England Journal of Medicine* titled "Blood to brain and brain to blood" demonstrated that, when neural stem cells (NSCs) are placed in bone marrow environments they become hematopoietic stem cells, and when HSCs are placed in the central nervous system they become neural stem cells [7].

Embryology of the Placenta/Amnion, Amniotic Fluid, and the Umbilical Cord

In mammals, the allantois forms the umbilical cord and the mesodermal components of the fetal placenta. The amnion and chorion are derived from the embryo. The chorion is derived from the trophoblast and the amnion from the epiblast as early

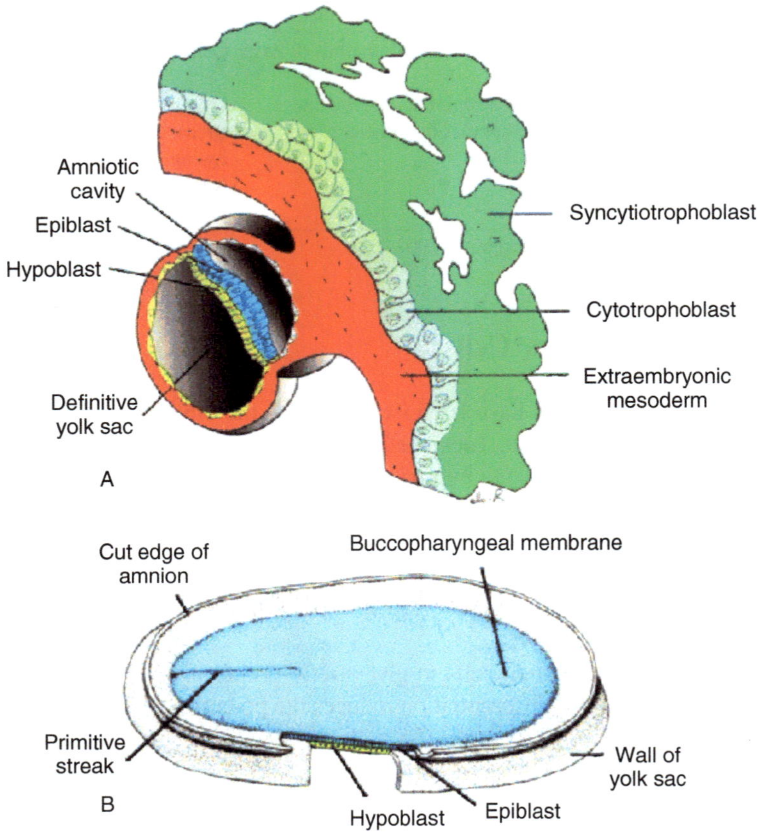

Fig. 1.1 At 8 weeks, the chorion derived from the trophoblast and the amnion derived from the epiblast

as 8 days after fertilization (Fig. 1.1). Gastrulation occurs during the third week of gestation, and the process establishes all three germ layers, including the ectoderm, the mesoderm, and endoderm. Gastrulation begins on the surface of the epiblast and is responsible for the differentiation and specification of cell fate.

At the end of the second month of gestation, the yolk sac is in the chorionic cavity between the amnion and the chorion. By the end of the third month, the amnion and chorion would fuse, and the uterine cavity is obliterated (Fig. 1.2). The amnion continues to enlarge at the expense of the chorion and forms a primitive umbilical cord. Amniotic fluid is produced by the cells lining the amniotic cavity (the amniotic epithelial cells – AE) and from maternal blood. The fluid increases from approximately 30 ml at 10 weeks gestation to 450 ml at 20 weeks gestate, and reaches 800–1000 ml at term (38–41 weeks). Excess amniotic fluid (1500–2000 ml) is termed polyhydramnios (amniotic fluid index of 25 or more or a single pocket of >8 cm on ultrasound). Oligohydramnios or decreased fluid is when there is less than 400 ml of amniotic fluid (amniotic fluid index of 5 or less). The volume of

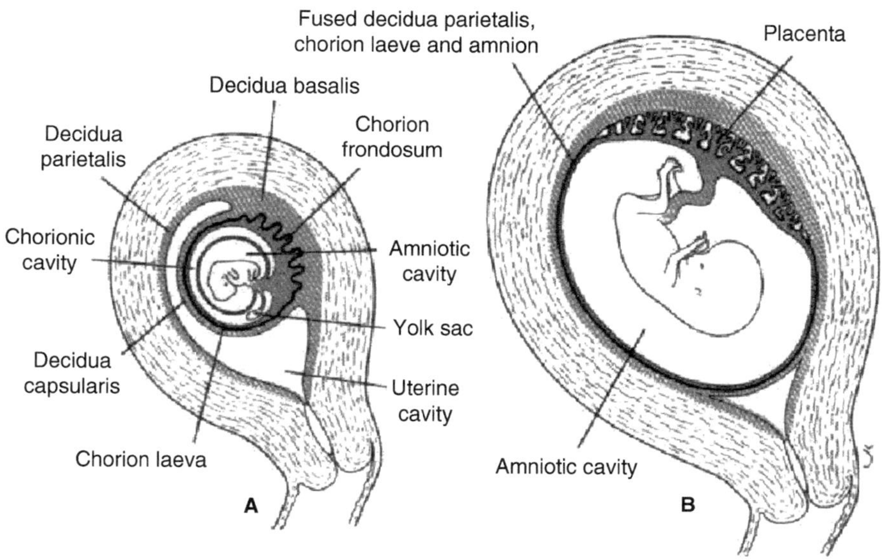

Fig. 1.2 (A) At 8 weeks, the amniotic cavity and the uterine cavity are separate. (B) The fusion of amnion and chorion and eradication

amniotic fluid is replaced every 3 h, with the fetus swallowing amniotic fluid beginning as early as the fifth month and adding fetal urine daily. The amniotic fluid serves as a cushion for the fetus within the uterine cavity, allowing the fetus to move about freely. The amnion also covers the umbilical cord that contains two arteries and a vein surrounded by Wharton's jelly, which is rich in proteoglycans and protects the umbilical cord blood vessels. The umbilical cord develops from the primitive allantois and from the mesoderm components of the fetal placenta in conjunction with hematopoietic cell development. Hematopoietic stem cells are first seen in the yolk sac, then in the aortic-gonadotropin-mesonephric (AGM) region in the hindgut of the developing embryo (Fig. 1.2). As the placenta is developing, HSCs migrate to the fetal liver through the umbilical cord vessels and then return through the umbilical cord vessels to seed the fetal bone marrow. Because of the simultaneous development of HSCs with the development of placenta, the umbilical cord, the amnion, and fetal vessels, HSCs appear to retain some of the pluripotent properties of the epiblast. These primitive cells get trapped in Wharton's jelly or the matrix of the umbilical cord during their journey through the primitive umbilical cord and are present within the Wharton's jelly of the umbilical cord, umbilical cord blood, the umbilical vein, amniotic epithelial cells, various placental tissues, and amniotic fluid. These cells, including the matrix cells of the Wharton's jelly, the amniotic epithelial cells, the MSCs from various placental tissues, and the amniotic fluid, retain the pluripotent/multipotent properties of early stem cells. The abundance of HSCs in various fetal/placental areas is of great interest (Fig. 1.3).

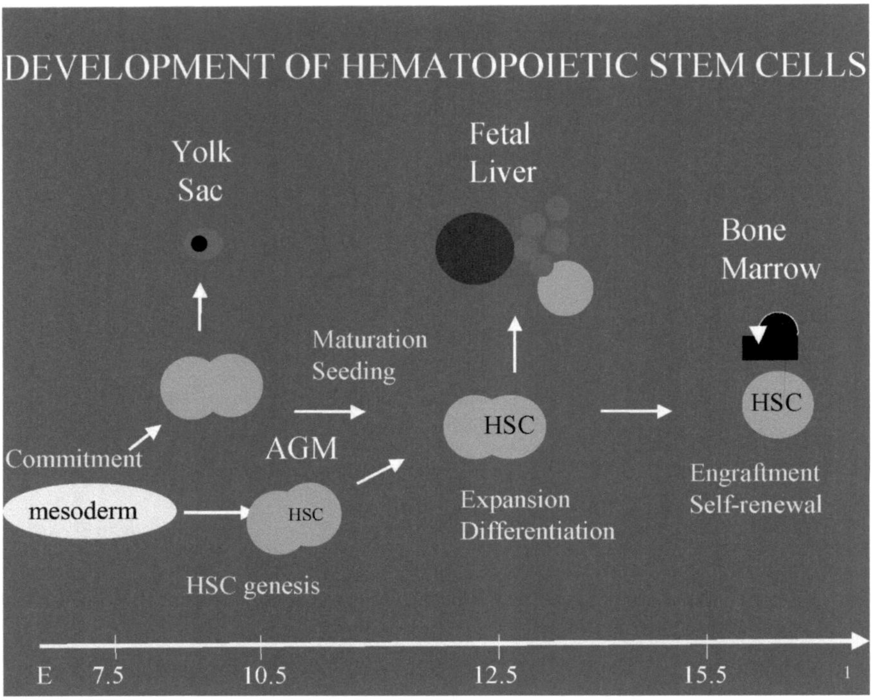

Fig. 1.3 Development of hématopoietic stem cells

The Ontogeny of Stem Cells

Totipotent human ES cells, the ancestors of all the somatic and germ cells of the entire organism, are found soon after the cleavage of the zygote. Stem cells retain this totipotency in the pre-implantation embryo (E.3.5), but shortly before implantation, at the blastocyst stage, stem cells become committed to certain types of tissues. Stem cells at the blastocyst stage are considered to be pluripotent, capable of differentiating into three cell types. The trophectoderm is committed to forming the trophoblast of the placenta. The primitive endoderm is committed to forming the parietal and visceral endoderm. In the placenta, the primitive endoderm forms all cells in the embryo proper and some internal extra-embryonic membranes, such as the allantois, the amnion, and the yolk sac mesoderm. After implantation (E5–6), these stem cells undergo further commitment in the embryo proper as the embryonic ectoderm, mesoderm, and endoderm form, producing the final cellular diversity consisting of approximately 260 distinguishable cell types and an estimated total cell number of one trillion in an adult human. If the cell retains the potential to form multiple differentiated cells, then the cell is considered multipotent.

Primordial germ cells (PGCs) are present proximal to the epiblast and migrate to and colonize the genital ridges (E6.5) (Fig. 1.1). The first “blood islands” or sites of hematopoiesis are the extra-embryonic yolk sac followed by the intrayonic

AGM region. The AGM region generates the adult hematopoietic system, harbors migrating PGCs, and perhaps produces populations of MSCs, vascular progenitors, and hemangioblasts.

From the AGM region, a common unrestricted precursor migrates to the fetal liver through the allantois. The onset of placental HSC activity coincides with AGM and yolk sac and precedes fetal liver and circulating blood. During or shortly after this migration (E10.5–E11) and before the liver is involved (E12.5–12.5), these multipotent progenitors are trapped in the Wharton's jelly or matrix of the developing placenta and umbilical cord [8, 9]. It remains possible that the placenta forms a niche for HSC maturation and expansion and for HSC mobilization and intra-embryonic colonization. The placenta HSCs pool expands during mid-gestation with greater than a 15-fold increase of HSCs as compared to the AGM and the yolk sac (Fig. 1.3).

The multipotent progenitors that are trapped or imbedded in the Wharton's jelly or matrix of the umbilical cord can be extracted at delivery and form a unique source of stem cells [10]. These "jell cells" (JCs) have been shown to survive xenotransplantation and to respond to local signals to differentiate along a neural lineage. Because these JCs "get stuck" in the Wharton's jelly at approximately day E9.5 of embryonic life, they are probably immunologically different than the hematopoietic stem cell found in umbilical cord blood and are a rich source of very primitive cells. Immunogenicity of a stem cell depends on the expression of the major histocompatibility complex (MHC) genes. Human ES cells have been found to express only low levels of MHC-1 proteins inhibitory effect on NK cells [11, 12]. The fact that these cells seem not to be recognized by NK cells suggests that these cells may not be readily rejected by NK cells [13, 14, 15].

The human fetus develops immunological competence around 9–15 weeks of gestation. Fetal cell-mediated and humoral immunity begin to develop by 9–15 weeks (63–105 days) [16]. Cells destined to become B cells differentiate from hematopoietic precursors in the fetal liver by 8 weeks of gestation and in the fetal bone marrow by 12 weeks. Mature plasma cells expressing IgM appear at 15 weeks of gestation while those secreting IgG and IgM are present by 20–30 weeks gestation. The migration of a common unrestricted precursor to the fetal liver through the allantois and trapping in the matrix of the umbilical cord occurs well before the fetus develops immunological competence. These cells are relatively non-immunogenic and engraft without stimulating significant immune rejection, perhaps the reason why male fetal progenitor cells can survive in their mothers as long as 27 years postpartum [6, 17]. When placed in the microenvironment of the brain, they differentiate along a neural lineage [3].

Hematopoietic Stem Cells

In 1974, Hal Broxmeyer first described HSCs in human umbilical cord blood. He suggested using HSCs for transplantation in 1982, and was involved in the first transplant performed in 1988 in a patient with Fanconi's anemia [18, 19]. Fifteen years later that patient was reported as free of the manifestations of the disease. As reported in the *New England Journal of Medicine* in 2004, there have been over 6000 transplants so far using umbilical cord blood as the source of stem cells. The journal also reported and reinforced the concept of the role of umbilical cord blood stem cells for transplantation in adults [20]. The use of umbilical cord blood stem cells is now state-of-the-art, and the standard of care compares favorably with the gold standard of stem cells derived from bone marrow.

Among the problems with umbilical cord blood stem cells, however, are low cell dose and delayed engraftment. The nucleated cell dose is the most important determinant along with HLA typing to determine the success and speed of engraftment. A nucleated cell dose of less than 2.5×10^7 shows poor success of engraftment. In one study, only 25% of samples collected met this critical level [21]. For this reason, novel approaches to the use of cord blood transplantation have been suggested, including using double unit transplants, expanding stem cells, and combining the stem cells with mesenchymal (MSCs) components. Wagner and Barker have successfully used double cord blood transplants [22]. The expansion of stem cells *in vitro* has not proven to be successful. The potent combination of MSCs and HSCs from umbilical cord blood could address these problems and make transplantation and engraftment more successful.

Another important determinant regarding successful engraftment relates to the way the cord blood itself is collected. There is mounting evidence that collecting and storing the whole blood rather than a fractionated component results in more successful engraftment because less of the important cells is lost [23].

Mesenchymal Stem Cells

In human bone marrow transplants, both MSCs and HSCs are collected and transplanted. In a fractionated or separated cord blood sample, many cells are lost, often including the MSC component. A combination of MSCs and HSCs could potentially lead to more successful transplants. The placenta and umbilical cord are potential sources for MSCs.

MSCs have been isolated from the Wharton's jelly of the umbilical cord (umbilical cord matrix cells, or UCM), from first and third trimester chorion, first trimester amnion as well as from villous stroma (placental chorionic villi) [1]. Weiss has attempted to characterize the cells from Wharton's jelly as well as to show that they can differentiate into neuronal cells [3]. These matrix cells expressed markers common to MSCs, including CD 166, CD 105, CD 90, CD 73, CD 49e, CD 44, CD 29, CD 13, as well as MHC class I, but they are negative for CD 14, CD 34, CD 45, and MHC class II markers. Portman-Lang has shown similar cells isolated from first and third trimester chorion, first trimester amnion, and villous stroma (placental chorionic villi). Recently, Kathy Mitchell reported that the matrix cells from Wharton's jelly also expressed Oct-4 and nanog [24].

MSCs have been isolated from the Wharton's jelly, also known as the human UCM. These cells proliferate in culture and express markers found in other stem cells. Specifically, UCM cells express the transcription factors Oct 4 and nanog, which are important for maintaining the undifferentiated, pluripotent state of ES cells. Oct-4 and nanog have previously been reported to be restricted to pluripotent cells [25, 26]. These Oct-4-expressing cells are found in the perivascular region of the umbilical cord. They can differentiate into multiple cell types, including neuronal, endothelial, and epithelial cells, and are, therefore, candidates for cell-based therapies. In contrast to ES cells, but like umbilical cord blood cells, UCM cells display more immune tolerance and have been shown not to form tumors when injected into immunocompromised mice. These cells are more easily accessible than bone marrow MSCs, are more abundant than MSCs found in cord blood but lack the ethical considerations of ES cells

Recent reports have described the identification of pluripotent or multipotent stem cells from human placental cord blood and amniotic fluid. The pluripotent stem cells have been identified in cord blood, whereas multipotent MSCs have been detected in various placental tissues [27, 28, 29]. MSCs have also been isolated from amniotic fluid.

The latest issue of *Stem Cells* carried an exciting report about the isolation of stem cells from amniotic epithelial cells [30]. Miki has shown that amniotic epithelial cells isolated from human term placenta express surface markers normally present in embryonic and germ cells. Amniotic epithelial cells also express the pluripotent stem cell-specific transcription factor octamer-binding proteins (Oct-4). These cells do not express telomerase, are non-tumorigenic, and have the potential to differentiate into all three germ layers:

- Endoderm (liver, pancreas)
- Mesoderm (cardio myocyte)
- Ectoderm (neural cells)

The author's conclusion was that, "amnio derived from term placenta after birth may be useful as a non-controversial source of stem cells for cell transplantation and regenerative medicine."

Pluripotent stem cells have also been isolated from amniotic fluid. This heterogeneous cell population expresses markers for all three germ layers [2]. These cells also show a high cell renewal capacity with >300 population doublings [31].

Endothelial Progenitor Cells

Human Umbilical Vein Endothelial Cells

The human umbilical cord is one of the most important sources of endothelial cells. The availability of these cells has played a major role in the development of the field of vascular biology [32, 33, 34, 35]. Perfusion of the human umbilical vein with collagenase results in a pure preparation of the single layer of endothelial cells that line this vessel [36]. Initial passages of these cells, which are grown in the presence of heparin and pituitary extract, maintain nearly all the features of native endothelial cells, including the expression of endothelial cell-specific markers such as von WilleBrand factor and CD31; expression of receptors for growth factors, cytokines, and vasoactive ligands; and specific signaling pathways for vascular endothelial growth factor (VEGF), fibroblast growth factor (FGF), transforming growth factor β (TGFβ), tumor necrosis factor α (TNFα), and angiotensin II [37, 38, 39, 40]. Human umbilical vein endothelial cells (HUVECs) have provided a critical *in vitro* model for major breakthroughs in molecular medicine, including seminal insights into cellular and molecular events in the pathophysiology of atherosclerosis and plaque formation. They have also provided a mechanism for the control of ischemic tissue in embryogenesis [41, 42, 43].

Monolayers of HUVECs have been used for the study of the interaction of leukocytes and macrophages with the endothelial cell layer resulting in the discovery of adhesion molecules, chemokines, and kinases that medicate the interaction of inflammatory cells with the endothelial surface and their migration into the media [44]. Monolayers of HUVECs have been generated on deformable surfaces or in chambers, which allow the study of the effects of shear stress and pulsatile flow on cell signaling in order to reproduce the effects of blood flow on endothelial cell function *in vivo*. These monolayers have been used to identify transcription factors, such as KLF2, that regulate endothelial adhesion molecule E-selection in response to stress and proinflammatory cytokines, such as TNFα, that mediate changes in cell adhesion and migration, which play a role in the early changes of atherosclerosis [45, 46, 47].

Angiogenesis plays a role in the pathophysiology of atherosclerosis, rheumatoid arthritis, diabetic retinopathy, psoriasis, and tumor growth [48]. Angiogenesis involves the replication, migration, and remodeling of endothelial cells in the process of tube formation. HUVECs have offered an important *in vitro* model for the study of all three processes. A culture of HUVECs on Matragel, an extract of endothelial basement membrane, results in the formation of honeycomb-like structures that simulate tube TGFβ. Inhibitors of angiogenesis on the formation and organization of honeycombs by HUVECs have helped elucidate the mechanisms by which these factors regulate both these processes [49]. An important example has been the demonstration that HMG-CoA reductase inhibitors, the cholesterol-lowering drugs referred to as statins, exert a dose-dependent effect on honeycomb formation and signaling pathways, suggesting that statins might decrease the progression of atherosclerosis and stimulate the revascularization of ischemic tissues via an effect on angiogenesis [50, 51].

HUVECs continue to play a major role as tools in the study of mechanism, pathogenesis, and therapeutics in the vascular system.

Endothelial progenitor cells, also called angioblasts, have been isolated not only from umbilical cord blood but also from the umbilical vein [5]. "Endothelial progenitor cells have been shown to functionally contribute to neoangiogenesis during wound healing, vascularization after myocardial ischemia and limb ischemia, endothelialization of vascular grafts, atherosclerosis, and retinal neovascularization" [15]. "Administration of cord blood CD 34 positive, peripheral blood mononuclear cells (PB-MNCs) accelerated epithelial progenitor cell (EPC) functions and increased incorporation into newly formed vessels twofold" [5, 52].

Fetal Cells in Maternal Circulation

Fetal cells can be detected in maternal circulation as early as 6 weeks of gestation, and by 37 weeks of gestation, 100% women have fetal cells circulating in maternal blood [53]. The discovery of fetal cells that persist in maternal blood decades after delivery may provide a new paradigm that facilitates the understanding of the many possibilities of fetal cells [17]. A new field that emerges is the study of fetal cell microchimerism, where fetal cells persist in maternal circulation and tissues. Findings suggest that the fetal cells may contain stem cell properties that are transferred to maternal blood. These cells, termed pregnancy-associated progenitor cells, persist after delivery and may aid in a response to injury in the maternal system.

One case study of a woman with hepatitis C showed a convincing evidence that fetal male cells were aiding the maternal system to control her disease. The patient stopped treatment with interferon and ribavarin against medical advice. DNA analysis suggested that the male cells were derived from a pregnancy with a male fetus that was terminated more than 15 years ago. The male cells from liver biopsy were similar in morphology to the surrounding liver cells, therefore making it likely that the male cells were derived from hepatocytes [54].

The discovery of fetal cells in the blood of women who have been pregnant suggests that fetal stem cells have a protective effect in women, even years after pregnancy. In a recent *JAMA* publication, Diana Bianchi reported on this remarkable finding [6]. The study examined the tissue of 10 women, ranging in age from 34 to 37 years, who suffered from a variety of diseases and who had had male offspring. Biopsies were taken from the thyroid, cervix, gallbladder, intestine, liver, spleen, and lymph node. The tissue samples were evaluated for morphology, cell surface, and intracellular phenotype of fetal cells in maternal organs. Seven hundred one male XY+ microchimeric cells were identified in the tissue sections from the 10 women; 14–60% of the XY+ cells in epithelial tissues (thyroid, cervix, gallbladder, and intestine) expressed cytokeratin, a marker of epithelial differentiation. In the epithelial cell samples, CD45, a common leukocyte antigen, was expressed in the microchimeric cells associated with areas of inflammation or with the healthy tissue surrounding the diseased tissue. In hematopoietic tissues, such as lymph nodes and spleen, CD45 was found in 90% of the XY+ microchimeric cells. In a sample of liver tissue of one woman, 4% of the XY+ cells were consistent with hepatocytes. This study suggests that fetal cells found in women years after pregnancy not only persist, but may have multi-lineage capacity with the potential for a variety of protective functions.

By one estimate, if the umbilical cord blood and/or matrix cells were saved at birth, the probability of usage would be approximately 1 in 415 if degenerative diseases were included in the list of diseases that might be treated [55].

The treatment of chronic diseases with stem cells has been referred to as a new field in medicine called regenerative medicine. The National Academy Committee report titled “Stem cells and the future of regenerative medicine” provides a thorough review of the subject [56].

Three of the most prominent areas of future treatment with stem cells include addressing neurological diseases, heart disease, and diabetes. A summary of the extensive literature on these three subjects is given below.

Endogenous NSCs have poor regenerative ability. Neural stem cells, therefore, are ideally suited for molecular and cellular therapy required by extensive, diffuse, and even global degeneration processes. Neurodegenerative conditions, such as myelin disorders; storage diseases; motor neuron degeneration; dementing conditions, such as Alzheimer’s disease; and ischemic and traumatic pathology, such as stroke, would be amenable to such treatment. Parkinson’s disease, Huntington’s disease, spinal cord injuries as well as cerebellar degeneration to the hindbrain appear to be more restricted in their involvement. These disorders, however, would be amenable to multiple neuronal cell type replacement by a migratory, responsive, multipotent neural progenitor because they require cell replacement [57, 58, 59, 60, 61].

It is clear that cardiomyocytes can be transplanted into normal or injured adult hearts [62]. Cardiomyocyte transplantation is a paradigm for treating diseased heart and has emerged as a potential therapeutic intervention, enhancing angiogenesis, providing structural support, and restoring lost myocardial mass in damaged or infracted heart. The sources of these cardiomyocytes have included angioblasts and vascular precursors, bone marrow and MSCs, skeletal myoblasts, and fetal cell-derived cardiomyocytes [63, 64]. Fetal cardiomyocytes have been demonstrated to directly participate in the functional syncytium, and the transplantation is not associated with any anomalies in intracellular calcium handling [65, 66, 67, 68].

The introduction of the Edmonton protocol in 2000 has provided encouraging results regarding the transplantation of pancreatic islet cells for the treatment of diabetes [69]. The success of this approach, which has now been used in over 100 patients worldwide, has allowed for much better glycemic control [70]. The search continues to find a new source of insulin-producing cells that can be used for transplantation.

Although there is much debate about the mechanism of plasticity, there is no debate that adult stem cells offer enormous potential to treat disease across all systems in the human body [71, 72]. There have been many studies with promising results focused on the nervous system [73]. Cells from cord blood and bone marrow have shown the ability to repair the liver and the heart [74]. These cells may become standard of care in many cancer therapy treatments. The phenomenon of cells adopting the behaviors of another system may take place secondary to cell fusion, plasticity, or yet an undiscovered term. Regardless of how we define this process, these cells are changing medicine and the way we will approach disease treatments in future.

> “Through a careful and circumspect series of experiments and trials we may learn whether we, indeed, have found within nature’s own tool box, a powerful and versatile therapeutic tool.”
>
> –Rodolfo Gonzalez, p. 698, *Handbook of Stem Cells*, Vol. 1.

References

1. Portman-Lanz CB, Huber A, Sager R. et al. Placental mesenchymal stem cells as potential autologous graft for pre- and perinatal neuroregeneration. American Journal of Obstetrics and Gynecology. 2005;193(6)S 24.
2. Cremer M. Schachner M. Cremer T. Schmidt W. Voigtlander T. Demonstration of astrocytes in cultured amniotic fluid cells of three cases with neural-tube defect. Human Genetics. 1981;002056(3):365-70.
3. Weiss ML. Mitchell KE. Hix JE. Medicetty S. El-Zarkouny SZ. Grieger D. Troyer DL. Transplantation of porcine umbilical cord matrix cells into the rat brain. Experimental Neurology. 2003;182(2):288–99.
4. Pelosi E. Valtieri M. Coppola S. et al. Identification of the hemangioblast in postnatal life. Blood. 2002;100(9):3203–8.
5. Murohara T. Ikeda H. Duan J. et al. Transplanted cord blood-derived endothelial precursor cells augment postnatal neovascularization. Journal of Clinical Investigation. 2000;105(11):1527–36.
6. Khosrotehrani K. Johnson KL. Cha DH. Salomon RN. Bianchi DW. Transfer of fetal cells with multilineage potential to maternal tissue. JAMA. 2004;292(1):75–80.
7. Moore MA. Turning brain into blood – clinical applications of stem-cell research in neurobiology and hematology. New England Journal of Medicine. 1999;341(8):605–7.
8. Melchers F. Murine embryonic B lymphocyte development in the placenta. Nature. 1979;277(5693):219–21.
9. Alvarez-Silva M. Belo-Diabangouaya P. Salaun J. Dieterlen-Lievre F. Mouse placenta is a major hematopoietic organ. Development. 2003;130(22):5437–44.
10. Mitchell KE. Weiss ML. Mitchell BM. et al. Matrix cells from Wharton's jelly form neurons and glia. Stem Cells. 2003;21(1):50–60.
11. Moretta L. Bottino C. Cantoni C. Mingari MC. Moretta A. Human natural killer cell function and receptors. Current Opinion in Pharmacology. 2001;1(4):387–91.
12. Drukker M. Katz G. Urbach A. et al. Characterization of the expression of MHC proteins in human embryonic stem cells. Proceedings of the National Academy of Sciences of the United States of America. 2002;99(15):9864–9.
13. Dorshkind K. Pollack SB. Bosma MJ. Phillips RA. Natural killer (NK) cells are present in mice with severe combined immunodeficiency (scid). Journal of Immunology. 1985;134(6):3798–801.
14. Lee N. Goodlett DR. Ishitani A. Marquardt H. Geraghty DE. HLA-E surface expression depends on binding of TAP-dependent peptides derived from certain HLA class I signal sequences. Journal of Immunology. 1998;160(10):4951–60.
15. Lanza R. ed. Handbook of Stem Cells Vol 2. Boston, MA. Elsevier Academic Press. 2004:667.
16. Stirrat G. In: Hytten F. ed. Clinical Physiology in Obstetrics. London. Blackwell Scientific Pub. 1991:101.
17. Bianchi DW. Zickwolf GK. Weil GJ. Sylvester S. DeMaria MA. Male fetal progenitor cells persist in maternal blood for as long as 27 years postpartum. Proceedings of the National Academy of Sciences of the United States of America. 1996;93(2):705–8.
18. Gluckman E. Broxmeyer HA. Auerbach AD. et al. Hematopoietic reconstitution in a patient with Fanconi's anemia by means of umbilical-cord blood from an HLA-identical sibling. New England Journal of Medicine. 1989;321(17):1174–8.
19. Broxmeyer HE. Douglas GW. Hangoc G. et al. Human umbilical cord blood as a potential source of transplantable hematopoietic stem/progenitor cells. Proceedings of the National Academy of Sciences of the United States of America. 1989;86(10):3828–32.
20. Laughlin MJ. Eapen M. Rubinstein P. Wagner JE. et al.. Outcomes after transplantation of cord blood or bone marrow from unrelated donors in adults with leukemia. New England Journal of Medicine. 2004;351(22):2265–75

21. Kogler G. Somville T. Gobel U. Hakenberg P. Knipper A. Fischer J. et al. Haematopoietic transplant potential of unrelated and related cord blood: the first six years of the EUROCORD/NETCORD Bank Germany. Klinische Padiatrie. 1999;211(4):224–32.
22. Barker JN. Weisdorf DJ. DeFor TE. Blazar BR. McGlave PB. Miller JS. et al.. Transplantation of 2 partially HLA-matched umbilical cord blood units to enhance engraftment in adults with hematologic malignancy. Blood. 2005;105(3):1343–7.
23. Robert C. et al. Stem Cyte data Presented at Ash and Clinical Outcome of Hematopoietic Stem Cell Transplantation (HSCT) Using Plasmo-Depleted Umbilical Cord Blood Units (UCB) That Were Not Depleted of Red Blood Cells Prior to Cryopreservation. Session Type: Poster Session 249-II.
24. Kathy M. Expressing Cells Isolated from Umbilical Cord Matrix are Multipotential Stem Cells. University of Kansas, http://www.healthtech.com/2005/stm/day2.asp 2:35 October 4.
25. Niwa H. Masui S. Chambers I. Smith AG. Miyazaki J. Phenotypic complementation establishes requirements for specific POU domain and generic transactivation function of October-3/4 in embryonic stem cells. Molecular and Cellular Biology. 2002;22(5):1526-36.
26. Chambers I. Colby D. Robertson M. Nichols J. Lee S. Tweedie S. Smith A. Functional expression cloning of Nanog, a pluripotency sustaining factor in embryonic stem cells. [see comment]. Cell. 2003;113(5):643-55.
27. Kogler G. Sensken S. Airey JA. et al. A new human somatic stem cell from placental cord blood with intrinsic pluripotent differentiation potential. Journal of Experimental Medicine. 2004;200(2):123–35.
28. Tsai MS. Lee JL. Chang YJ. Hwang SM. (2004) Isolation of human multipotent mesenchymal stem cells from second-trimester amniotic fluid using a novel two-stage culture protocol. Human Reproduction. 2004;19(6):1450–6.
29. In 't Anker PS. Scherjon SA. Kleijburg-van der Keur C. et al. Amniotic fluid as a novel source of mesenchymal stem cells for therapeutic transplantation. Blood. 2003;102(4): 1548–9.
30. Miki T. Lehmann T. Cai H. Stolz DB. Strom SC. Stem cell characteristics of amniotic epithelial cells. Stem Cells. 2005;23(10):1549–59.
31. Siddiqui MM. Amniotic Fluid Derived Pluripotent cells. In: Lanza R. ed. Handbook of Stem Cells Vol 2. Boston, MA. Elsevier Academic Press. 2004:175.
32. Yamada T, Fan J, Shimokama T. et al. Induction of fatty streak-like lesions in vitro using a culture model system simulating arterial intima. The American Journal of Pathology. 1992;141(6):1435–44.
33. Bevilacqua MP, Gimbrone MA, Jr. Inducible endothelial functions in inflammation and coagulation. Seminars in Thrombosis and Hemostasis. 1987;13(4):425–33.
34. Libby P. Changing concepts of atherogenesis. Journal of Internal Medicine. 2000;247(3): 349–58.
35. Davies PF. Overview: temporal and spatial relationships in shear stress-mediated endothelial signalling. Journal of Vascular Research. 1997;34(3):208–11.
36. Gimbrone MA, Jr. Culture of vascular endothelium. Progress in Hemostasis and Thrombosis 1976;3:1–28.
37. Goldberger A, Middleton KA, Oliver JA. et al. Biosynthesis and processing of the cell adhesion molecule PECAM-1 includes production of a soluble form. The Journal of Biological Chemistry. 1994;269(25):17183–91.
38. Namiki A, Brogi E, Kearney M. et al. Hypoxia induces vascular endothelial growth factor in cultured human endothelial cells. The Journal of Biological Chemistry. 1995;270(52): 31189–95.
39. Nozawa F, Hirota M, Okabe A. et al. Tumor necrosis factor alpha acts on cultured human vascular endothelial cells to increase the adhesion of pancreatic cancer cells. Pancreas. 2000;21(4):392–8.
40. Muscella A, Marsigliante S, Carluccio MA. et al. Angiotensin II AT1 receptors and Na+/K+ ATPase in human umbilical vein endothelial cells. The Journal of Endocrinology 1997;155(3):587–93.

41. Burns MP, DePaola N. Flow-conditioned HUVECs support clustered leukocyte adhesion by coexpressing ICAM-1 and E-selectin. American Journal of Physiology Heart and Circulatory Physiology. 2005;288(1):H194–204.
42. Kokura S, Wolf RE, Yoshikawa T. et al. Molecular mechanisms of neutrophil-endothelial cell adhesion induced by redox imbalance. Circulation Research 1999;84(5):516–24.
43. Zhang W, DeMattia JA, Song H. et al. Communication between malignant glioma cells and vascular endothelial cells through gap junctions. Journal of Neurosurgery. 2003;98(4):846–53.
44. Bevilacqua MP, Stengelin S, Gimbrone MA, Jr. et al. Endothelial leukocyte adhesion molecule 1: an inducible receptor for neutrophils related to complement regulatory proteins and lectins. Science. 1989;243(4895):1160–65.
45. Parmar KM, Larman HB, Dai G. et al. Integration of flow-dependent endothelial phenotypes by Kruppel-like factor 2. The Journal of Clinical Investigation 2006;116(1):49–58.
46. Parmar KM, Nambudiri V, Dai G. et al. Statins exert endothelial atheroprotective effects via the KLF2 transcription factor. The Journal of Biological Chemistry. 2005;280(29):26714–9.
47. Dai G, Kaazempur-Mofrad MR, Natarajan S. et al. Distinct endothelial phenotypes evoked by arterial waveforms derived from atherosclerosis-susceptible and -resistant regions of human vasculature. Proceedings of the National Academy of Sciences of the United States of America. 2004;101(41):14871–6.
48. Kumar S, Li C. Targeting of vasculature in cancer and other angiogenic diseases. Trends in Immunology. 2001;22(3):129.
49. Nagata D, Mogi M, Walsh K. AMP-activated protein kinase (AMPK) signaling in endothelial cells is essential for angiogenesis in response to hypoxic stress. The Journal of Biological Chemistry. 2003;278(33):31000–1006.
50. Park HJ, Kong D, Iruela-Arispe L. et al. 3-hydroxy-3-methylglutaryl coenzyme A reductase inhibitors interfere with angiogenesis by inhibiting the geranylgeranylation of RhoA. Circulation Research. 2002;91(2):143–50.
51. Weis M, Heeschen C, Glassford AJ. et al. Statins have biphasic effects on angiogenesis. Circulation. 2002;105(6):739–45.
52. Lanza R. ed. Handbook of Stem Cells Vol 2. Boston, MA. Elsevier Academic Press.2004:462.
53. Ariga H. Ohto H. Busch MP. et al. Kinetics of fetal cellular and cell-free DNA in the maternal circulation during and after pregnancy: implications for noninvasive prenatal diagnosis. Transfusion. 2001;41(12):1524–30.
54. Johnson KL. Samura O. Nelson JL. McDonnell Md WM. Bianchi DW. Significant fetal cell microchimerism in a nontransfused woman with hepatitis C: Evidence of long-term survival and expansion. Hepatology. 2002;36(5):1295–7.
55. Marcelo C. Pasquini Brent R. Logan, Frances Verter, Mary M. Horowitz, J.J. The Likelihood of Hematopoietic Stem Cell Transplantation (HCT) in the United States: Implications for Umbilical Cord Blood Storage. Session Type: Poster Session 488-I. Nietfeld Center for International Blood and Marrow Transplant Research (CIBMTR), Medical College of Wisconsin, Milwaukee, WI; Department of Pathology, University Medical Center Utrecht (UMCU), Utrecht, Netherlands. www.ParentsGuideCordBlood.org; December 10 9:15 AM, Hall B4.
56. National research council (2002). Washington D.C. National Academies Press, http://www.nap.edu/catalog/10195.html.
57. Lu D. Sanberg PR. Mahmood A. Li Y. Wang L. Sanchez-Ramos J. Chopp M. Intravenous administration of human umbilical cord blood reduces neurological deficit in the rat after traumatic brain injury. Cell Transplantation. 2002;11(3):275–81.
58. Ourednik V. Ourednik J. Flax JD. et al. Segregation of human neural stem cells in the developing primate forebrain. Science. 2001;293(5536):1820–4.
59. Villa A. Snyder EY. Vescovi A. Martinez-Serrano A. Establishment and properties of a growth factor-dependent, perpetual neural stem cell line from the human CNS. Experimental Neurology. 2000;161(1):67–84.
60. Blits B. Boer GJ. Verhaagen J. Pharmacological, cell, and gene therapy strategies to promote spinal cord regeneration. Cell Transplantation. 2002;11(6):593–13.

61. Chen J. Sanberg PR. Li Y. Wang L. Lu M. Willing AE. Sanchez-Ramos J. Chopp M. Intravenous administration of human umbilical cord blood reduces behavioral deficits after stroke in rats. Stroke. 2001;32(11):2682–8
62. Wang HS. Hung SC. Peng ST. et al. Mesenchymal stem cells in the Wharton's jelly of the human umbilical cord. Stem Cells. 2004;22(7):1330–7.
63. Dowell JD. Rubart M. Pasumarthi KB. Soonpaa MH. Field LJ. Myocyte and myogenic stem cell transplantation in the heart. Cardiovascular Research. 2003;58(2):336–50.
64. Hassink RJ. Dowell JD. Brutel de la Riviere A. Doevendans PA. Field LJ. Stem cell therapy for ischemic heart disease. Trends in Molecular Medicine. 2003;9(10):436–41.
65. Rubart M. Pasumarthi KB. Nakajima H. Soonpaa MH. Nakajima HO. Field LJ. Physiological coupling of donor and host cardiomyocytes after cellular transplantation. Circulation Research. 2003;92(11):1217–24.
66. Orlic D. Kajstura J. Chimenti S. et al. Bone marrow cells regenerate infarcted myocardium. Nature. 2001;410(6829):701–5.
67. Dengler TJ. Katus HA. Stem cell therapy for the infarcted heart ("cellular cardiomyoplasty"). Herz. 2002;27(7):598–610.
68. Laham RJ. Oettgen P. Bone marrow transplantation for the heart:fact or fiction? Lancet. 2003;361(9351):11–2.
69. Shapiro AM. Lakey JR. Ryan EA. et al. Islet transplantation in seven patients with type 1 diabetes mellitus using a glucocorticoid-free immunosuppressive regimen. New England Journal of Medicine. 2000;343(4):230–8.
70. Ryan EA. Lakey JR. Paty BW. Imes S. Korbutt GS. Kneteman NM. Bigam D. Rajotte RV. Shapiro AM. Successful islet transplantation: continued insulin reserve provides long-term glycemic control. Diabetes. 2002;51(7):2148–57.
71. Hussain MA. Theise ND. Stem-cell therapy for diabetes mellitus. Lancet. 2004;364(9429):203–5.
72. Korbling M. Estrov Z. Adult stem cells for tissue repair – a new therapeutic concept? New England Journal of Medicine. 2003;349(6):570–82.
73. Rice CM. Scolding NJ. Adult stem cells – reprogramming neurological repair? Lancet. 2004;364(9429):193–9.
74. Mathur A. Martin JF. Stem cells and repair of the heart. Lancet. 2004;364(9429):183–92.

Chapter 2
Cord Blood Stem Cells – The Basic Science

Peter Hollands

Cord blood stem cells have been transplanted since 1988 [1], and are now an acceptable source of stem cells for transplant in a range of hematological diseases [2] and in the repair of bone marrow following high-dose chemotherapy for cancer. The basis of these applications is that cord blood contains $CD34^+$ myeloid progenitor cells [3] that, upon transplantation, achieve long-term, stable bone marrow reconstitution [4]. To date, there have been over 6,000 transplants of cord blood stem cells in the treatment of 45 different diseases [5], and the future can only see an increase in the use of cord blood stem cells in the treatment of a wide range of diseases. The advantages in the use of cord blood as a source of stem cells for transplant are:

- Ease of procurement, processing, and storage
- No risk to donors
- Reduced risk of transmitting infection
- Immediate availability of cryopreserved units
- Acceptable partial HLA mismatches (4/6 HLA match)

In addition, cord blood stem cells do not carry any legal, moral, ethical or religious objections associated with the use of embryonic stem cells.

The current disadvantages in the use of cord blood stem cells as a source of stem cells for transplant are:

- The limited number of hematopoietic stem cells in a cord blood unit, which may lead to failed or delayed hematopoietic reconstitution or restricted use in adults
- Possible abnormalities in cord blood stem cells, e.g. early malignant mutations, which may have an effect on the recipients
- It may not be possible to collect additional donor stem cells, or donor lymphocytes, for recipients who relapse following a cord blood stem cell transplant

P. Hollands (✉)
Senior Lecturer in Biomedical Science, Department of Biomedical Science, University of Westminster, 115, New Cavendish Street, London W1W 6UW, UK
e-mail: peterh63@hotmail.com

N. Bhattacharya, P. Stubblefield (eds.), *Frontiers of Cord Blood Science*,
DOI 10.1007/978-1-84800-167-1_2, © Springer-Verlag London Limited 2009

Transplantation Biology

The rate of cord blood stem cell reconstitution and the kinetics of engraftment are slower when compared to bone marrow grafts [2, 6, 7]. The factors that appear to be predictive in the outcome of cord blood stem cell transplants are total nucleated cell dose and HLA matching. Minor histocompatibility differences in allogeneic transplantation may contribute to graft rejection and graft-versus-leukemia [8]. The relatively slow kinetics of cord blood stem cell engraftment may be due to varying levels of adhesion molecule expression [9], homing characteristics [10, 11] and the maturational stages of the cells. Nevertheless, it is also possible that donor lymphocytes contained in the cord blood units are capable of inhibiting or even eliminating the residual recipient immune cells capable of mounting a rejection episode [12]. This observation may help to explain those cases in which engraftment has occurred in adults and in transplants of low graft $CD34^+$ and low total nucleated cell doses.

The quantification of $CD34^+$ myeloid progenitor cells and the relationship of this count to engraftment is not consistently predictive of the outcome. There is poor correlation between engraftment kinetics and $CD34^+$ content of a given transplant, possibly due to reduced surface epitope density of the CD34 antigen on cord blood stem cells [13]. In addition, $CD34^+$ myeloid progenitor cells in cord blood have been shown *in vitro* to have less mature phenotype compared to adult marrow and peripheral blood stem cells [14]. This observation indicates that cord blood stem cells have a significantly increased proliferative potential when compared to adult bone marrow and peripheral blood stem cells [15]. Further evidence for this is provided by cobblestone area-forming cell (CAFC) assays, which show the $CD34^+$ compartment of cord blood to have a 3.6 to 10-fold increase in CAFC as compared to adult bone marrow and peripheral blood stem cells [16]. It is also interesting to note that the engraftment capacity of $CD34^+$ cord blood myeloid progenitor cells *in vivo* using the non-obese diabetic/severe combined immunodeficiency (NOD/SCID) repopulation assay is significantly increased [16]. Taking all these unique properties into account, one can explain why cord blood stem cells engraft well despite low cellular content, and also why late graft failure is rare [17].

Transplantation Immunology

HLA mismatch between donor and recipient in allogeneic transplantation is an important factor in the development of acute and chronic GVHD. Nevertheless, transplantation of cord blood stem cells with HLA class I and class II mismatch results in a decreased incidence of acute GVHD when compared to recipients on unrelated adult donor stem cells [18, 19, 20]. In this context, it may be important to note that cord blood T lymphocytes are $CD45RA^+$ and express low levels of activation markers, indicating that they are the naïve Th0 phenotype [21]. There are several possible explanations for the decreased incidence of GVHD following a cord blood stem cell transplant, including [22]:

- Reduced donor lymphocyte numbers
- Donor T cell down-regulation of recipient self-antigen recognition and APC interaction
- Limited response of naïve donor T cells to recipient alloantigen
- Limitation of the cytokine/cellular cascade needed to amplify donor alloreactivity to recipient antigens
- Enhanced immunosuppression resulting from anti-thymocyte globulin and fludarabine used to achieve myeloablation in cord blood stem cell recipients

In vitro studies have shown that alloreactive T cells in cord blood grafts lack the full expression of immunomodulatory cytokines [21, 23], and that the same cells in primary mixed lymphocyte culture show less cytotoxic effector function, less proliferation, and greater activation-induced cell death (AICD). In addition, there is altered adhesion molecule expression on donor cord blood antigen-presenting cells [24]. The presence of NK cells, capable of early recovery and activation of the granzyme/perforin lytic pathway, and Fas/Fas ligand (FasL) activity may also contribute to the low incidence of GVHD in cord blood stem cell transplantation [25]. The same properties may also contribute to delayed engraftment kinetics in cord blood stem cell recipients. Slow engraftment kinetics have been shown to correlate with increased risk of bacterial, fungal, and viral infections following an allogeneic transplantation. Despite this, it has been reported that early post-transplantation infection in adult patients with HLA mismatched allogeneic cord blood stem cells is increased when compared to later infections that are the same as those patients who received adult stem cell transplants [7]. The high incidence of early post-transplantation infection in cord blood stem cell recipients may reflect the neutropenia and lymphopoenia seen following a transplantation of relatively low numbers of nucleated cells and $CD34^+$ cells. In addition, adult recipients of cord blood stem cells tend to be in higher risk groups with extensive treatment prior to transplantation [26].

There is clearly still much to understand about the immunology of cord blood stem cells in relation to GVHD and transplantation kinetics.

Cord Blood Stem Cell Amplification

Most cord blood transplants require $1–2 \times 10^7$ nucleated cells/kg in order to achieve safe engraftment kinetics, and an average cord blood unit, after processing, contains $3–4 \times 10^8$ nucleated cells. This makes the ideal weight of a patient getting a cord blood stem cell transplant in the range of 30–40 kg, thus restricting the use of cord blood stem cell transplantation to children and small adults. In order to make cord blood stem cells available for transplant, it is necessary to amplify the number of stem cells in the cord blood unit. Extensive research is ongoing in this field.

Clonogenic cord blood progenitors, after the removal of more mature CD34− cells, have been expanded from 50- to 100-fold using cytokine cocktails, and more primitive Delta cells also show a 10–20 fold increase in similar conditions [27]. In addition, long-term culture-initiating cells (LTCIC) in the cord blood have been amplified 10-fold using low-dose cytokines and continuous perfusion technology [28]. It must be noted, however, that none of the current amplification studies have assessed NOD/SCID repopulating cells, and therefore the true extent of stem cell amplification in these studies is difficult to assess. Lewis et al. [29] have subsequently shown that, during *ex vivo* cytokine amplification of cord blood stem cells, there was a 20–25-fold increase in the colony forming cells (CFC) whilst LTCIC only increased by 40%, and NOD/SCID repopulating cells were maintained but showed no increase in number. This raises serious questions about the overall efficacy of cytokine-based cord blood stem cell amplification in clinical practice. Further research may refine the technology to the point of true stem cell amplification.

An alternative approach is to amplify stem cells using bioreactor technology such as that pioneered by Cytomatrix. In this system, stem cells are seeded onto a three-dimensional, tantalum-coated biomatrix to grow and amplify under the influence of naturally produced cytokines [30]. This technology only achieves a threefold increase in $CD34^+$ myeloid progenitor cells, but may be an alternative source of amplified cord blood stem cells for transplantation in future.

It is, of course, possible that, simply increasing the cord blood stem cell numbers available for transplant will not increase engraftment kinetics. Cord blood stem cells may require additional maturation and enhancement in the immune cells; antigen-presenting cells and mesenchymal stromal cell components of the graft may also be required. The interaction of the cord blood stem cells and the rest of the cellular compartment may possibly enhance the overall engraftment kinetics of transplantation [31].

Cord Blood Stem Cells and Regenerative Medicine

Cord blood stem cells have enormous potential in the ever expanding field of regenerative medicine. A rare population of pluripotent $CD45^-$ cells have been identified in the cord blood, which grow in adherent culture and can be amplified up to 10^{15} cells without loss in pluripotency [32]. This $CD45^-$ population has been shown to be capable of differentiating into osteoblasts, chondroblasts, adipocytes, hematopoietic cells, and neural cells. Neural cells derived from the $CD45^-$ population include astrocytes and neurons expressing neurofilament, sodium channel protein, and neurotransmitter phenotypes. Transplantation of $CD45^-$ cells into the adult rat brain shows the presence of human Tau-positive cells for up to 3 months post-transplantation and typical neuron morphology. Cord blood stem cells clearly have potential in the future therapy of neurodegenerative diseases and repair to the central nervous system following traumatic injury.

Another possible source of cells for transplant from cord blood can be obtained from the culture of $CD34^+$ endothelial precursor cells (EPC) amplified to clinically useful numbers [33]. These cells have been shown to proliferate *in vivo* to form vascular structures and to improve experimentally induced myocardial infarction. The cells migrate to the infarcted myocardium where they engraft and participate in neoangiogenesis, thus benefitting the remodeling process in post-infarction repair. Similar studies have shown that $CD34^+$ cells obtained from cord blood can significantly improve ventricular function following myocardial infarction [34]. These studies indicate a potential role for cord blood stem cells in the treatment of acute myocardial infarction and possibly cardiomyopathy.

Experimental studies have also indicated that cord blood stem cells have potential in the treatment of both type-1 and type-2 diabetes [35, 36].

In summary, cord blood stem cells represent a readily available source of stem cells for transplant for hematological malignancy and diseases and repair of the bone marrow following high-dose chemotherapy for cancer. Future applications are likely to be wide ranging and represent significant therapies in years to come.

References

1. Gluckman E, Broxmeyer HA, Auerbach AD, et al. Hematopoietic reconstitution in a patient with Fanconi's anemia by means of umbilical-cord blood from an HLA-identical sibling. N Engl J Med. 1989;321:1174–1178.
2. Laughlin MJ, Eapen M, Rubinstein P, et al. Outcomes after transplantation of cord blood or bone marrow from unrelated donors in adults with leukaemia. N Engl J Med. 2004;351: 2265–2275.
3. Ljungman P, Urbano-Ispizua A, Cavazzana-Calvo M, et al. Allogeneic and autologous transplantation for haematological diseases, solid tumours and immune disorders: definitions and current practice in Europe. Bone Marrow Transplant. 2006;37:439–449.
4. Brunstein CG, & Wagner JE. Umbilical cord blood transplantation and banking. Annu Rev Med. 2006;57:403–417.
5. Kurtzberg J, Drapkin-Lyerly A, & Sugarman, J. Untying the Gordian knot: policies, practices and ethical issues related to banking of umbilical cord blood. J Clin Invest. 2005;115: 2592–2597.
6. Rocha V, Labopin M, Sanz G, et al.; Acute Leukemia Working Party of European Blood and Marrow Transplant Group; Eurocord-Netcord Registry. Transplants of umbilical-cord blood or bone marrow from unrelated donors in adults with acute leukaemia. N Engl J Med. 2004;351:2276–2285.
7. Hamza NS, Lisgaris M, Yadavalli GK, et al. Infectious complications after unrelated HLA-mismatched hematopoietic stem cell transplantation. Blood. 1999;94:333–339.
8. Mommaas B, Steghuis-Kamp J, van Halteren AG, et al. Cord blood comprises antigen-experienced T cells specific for maternal minor histocompatibility antigen HA-1. Blood. 2005;105:1823–1827.
9. Roy V, & Verfaillie CM. Expression and function of cell adhesion molecules on fetal liver, cord blood and bone marrow hematopoietic progenitors: implications for anatomical localization and developmental stage specific regulation of hematopoiesis. Exp Hematol. 27; 1999:302–312.
10. Peled A, Kollet O, Ponomaryov T, et al. The chemokine SDF-1 activates the integrins LFA-1, VLA-4 and VLA-5 on immature human CD34(+) cells: role in transendothelial/stromal migration and engraftment of NOD/SCID mice. Blood. 2000;95:3289–3296.
11. Zheng Y, Watanabe N, Nagamura-Inoue T, et al. Ex vivo manipulation of umbilical cord blood-derived hematopoietic stem/progenitor cells with recombinant human stem cell factor can up-regulate levels of homing-essential molecules to increase their transmigratory potential. Exp Hematol. 2003;31:1237–1246.

12. Hiruma K, Nakamura H, Henkart P, et al. Clonal deletion of postthymic T cell: vetocells kill precursor cytotoxic T lumphocytes. J Exp Med. 1992;175:863–870.
13. Bender J, Unverzagt K, Walker D, et al. Phenotypic analysis and characterization of CD34+ cells from normal human bone marrow, cord blood, peripheral blood, and mobilized peripheral blood from patients undergoing autologous stem cell transplantation. Clin Immunol Immunopathol. 1994;70:10–18.
14. Gomi S, Hasegawa S, Dan K, et al. A comparative analysis of the transplant potential of umbilical cord blood versus mobilized peripheral blood stem cells. Nippon Ika Daigaku Zasshi. 1997;64:307–313.
15. Theunissen K, & Verfaillie C. A multifactorial analysis of umbilical cord blood, adult bone marrow and mobilized peripheral blood progenitors using the improved ML-IC assay. Exp Hematol. 2005;33:165–172.
16. Ng YY, van Kessel B, Lokhorst HM, et al. Gene-expression profiling of CD34+ cells from various hematopoietic stem-cell sources reveals functional differences in stem-cell activity. J Leukoc Biol. 2004;75:314–323.
17. Rubinstein P, Carrier C, Scaradavou A, et al. Outcomes among 562 recipients of placental-blood transplants from unrelated donors. N Engl J Med. 1998;339:1565–1577.
18. Wagner JE, Barker JN, DeFor TE, et al. Transplantation of unrelated donor umbilical cord blood in 102 patients with malignant and non-malignant diseases: influence of CD34 cell dose and HLS disparity on treatment-related mortality and survival. Blood. 2002;100:1611–1618.
19. Rocha V, Wagner JE, Sobocinski KA, et al.; Eurocord and International Bone Marrow Transplant Registry Working Committee on Alternative Donor and Stem Cell Sources. Graft-versus-host disease in children who have received a cord-blood or bone marrow transplant from an HLA identical sibling. N Engl J Med. 2000;342:1846–1854.
20. Michel G, Rocha V, Chevret S, et al.; the Eurocord Group. Unrelated cord blood transplantation for childhood acute myeloid leukaemia: a Eurocord Group analysis. Blood. 2003;102:4290–4297.
21. Chalmers I, Janossy G, Contreras M, et al. Intracellular cytokine profile of cord and adult blood lymphocytes. Blood 1998;92:11–18.
22. Kadereit S, Deeds LS, Haynesworth SE, et al. Expansion of LTC-ICs and maintenance of p21 and BCL-2 expression in cord blood CD34(+)/CD38(−) early progenitors cultured over human MSCs as a feeder layer. Stem Cells. 2002;20:573–582.
23. Kadereit S, Mohammad S, Miller R, et al. Reduced NFAT1 protein expression in human umbilical cord blood T lymphocytes. Blood. 1999;94:3101–3107.
24. Liu E, Law HK, & Lau YL. Tolerance associated with cord blood transplantation may depend on the state of host dendritic cells. Br J Haematol. 2004;126:517–526.
25. Brahmi Z, Hommel-Berrey G, Smith F, et al. NK cells recover early and mediate cytotoxicity via perforin/granzyme and Fas/FasL pathways in umbilical cord blood recipients. Hum Immunol. 2005;62:782–790.
26. Laughlin MJ, Barker J, Bambach B, et al. Hematopoietic engraftment and survival in adult recipients of umbilical cord blood from unrelated donors. N Engl J Med. 2001;344: 1815–1822.
27. Moore MA, & Hoskins I. Ex vivo expansion of cord blood-derived stem cells and progenitors. Blood Cells. 1994;20:468–479.
28. Van Zant G, Drubachevsky I, Rummel S, et al. Expansion of hematopoietic progenitor cells from umbilical cord blood via continuous perfusion culture. Blood Cells. 1994;20:482–491.
29. Lewis ID, Almeida-Porada G, Du J, Lemischka IR, Moore KA, Zanjani ED, et al. Umbilical cord blood cells capable of engrafting in primary, secondary, and tertiary xenogeneic hosts are preserved after ex vivo culture in a noncontact system. Blood. 2001;97:3441–3449.
30. Ehring B, Biber K, Upton TM, et al. Expansion of HPCs from cord blood in a novel 3D matrix. Cytotherapy. 2003;5:490–499.
31. Barker JN, Weisdorf DJ, DeFor TE, et al. Rapid and complete donor chimerism in adult recipients of unrelated donor umbilical cord blood transplantation after reduced-intensity conditioning. Blood. 2003;102:1915–1919.

32. Kogler G, Sensken S, Airey JA, et al. A new human somatic stem cell from placental cord blood with intrinsic pluripotent differentiation potential. J Exp Med. 2004;200:123–135.
33. Ma N, Stamm C, Kaminski A, Li W, et al. Human cord blood cells induce angiogenesis following myocardial infarction in NOD/scid-mice. Cardiovasc Res. 2005;66:45–54.
34. Hirata Y, Sata M, Motomura N, et al. Human umbilical cord blood cells improve cardiac function after myocardial infarction. Biochem Biophys Res Commun. 2005;327:609–614.
35. Ende N, Chen R, & Reddi AS. Effect of human umbilical cord blood cells on glycemia and insulitis in type 1 diabetic mice. Biochem Biophys Res Commun. 2004;325:665–669.
36. Ende N, Chen R, & Reddi AS. Transplantation of human umbilical cord blood cells improves glycemia and glomerular hypertrophy in type 2 diabetic mice. Biochem Biophys Res Commun. 2004;321:168–171.

Chapter 3
Stem Cells from Umbilical Cord Blood

Patricia Pranke and Raquel Canabarro

In the umbilical cord blood (UCB) there are several different types of stem cells (SCs), such as hematopoietic stem cells (HSCs), endothelial progenitor cells (EPCs), and mesenchymal stem cells (MSCs). UCB SCs represent an important alternative source of progenitor cells for transplantation and other therapeutic approaches. Therefore, in order for these cells to be used, their accurate identification and characterization is important. The HSCs are known to express $CD34^+$ and c-kit molecules and lack CD38, human leukocyte antigen (HLA)-DR and lineage committed antigens. EPCs and HSCs are believed to derive from common precursor cells. EPCs have a potent ability for neovascularization and that the transplantation of these cells improves ischemic tissue. MSCs are an important cell population in the bone-marrow microenvironment and are considered to be engaged mainly in the support of hematopoiesis, necessary for a successful transplant. Phenotypically, MSCs are characterized by their negativity of the hematopoietic cell markers, CD34, and CD45, and for being positive for CD90, Stro-1, and major histocompatibility complex (MHC) class I molecules, but do not express HLA-DR. Moreover, it has been shown that MSCs have a great plasticity and so have the capacity to give rise to different types of cells, widening the range of therapeutic uses of SCs from UCB. Cord blood cells, in contrast to bone marrow cells, have the advantage of being an inexhaustible source of SCs, having more immunologically immature cells, leading to a lower frequency of graft versus host disease after transplantation, lower risk of the transmission of infectious diseases and for apparently being more susceptible to gene transfer. These findings show that UCB cells are a good source of SCs and future studies will probably lead to their greater use in cellular therapy.

P. Pranke (✉)
Hematology Laboratory, Federal University of Rio Grande do Sul, Av Ipiranga, 2752 Porto Alegre, Rio Grande do Sul, CEP 90610-000, Brazil
e-mail: patriciapranke@ufrgs.br

N. Bhattacharya, P. Stubblefield (eds.), *Frontiers of Cord Blood Science*,
DOI 10.1007/978-1-84800-167-1_3, © Springer-Verlag London Limited 2009

Introduction

Over the last years, UCB has been clinically investigated as an alternative source of hematopoietic tissue for allogeneic transplantation of patients lacking a human leukocyte antigen (HLA)-matched marrow donor [1]. It is an attractive alternative source of HSCs to bone marrow (BM) or mobilized peripheral blood (MPB) and is being used increasingly to restore the formation of blood cells not only in patients with hematologic disorders and malignancies, but also those with inherited immunodeficiencies, metabolic diseases [2, 3], and solid tumors [3].

As compared to other sources of HSCs, like peripheral blood and BM, the UCB offers numerous logistic and clinical advantages such as: (1) pratically unlimited offer, (2) immediate availability of cryopreserved units in public UCB banks, and which decrease an average 25–36 days the wait for transplantation as compared to BM, (3) extension of the pool of donors due to the tolerance of up to two mismatches in the HLA system, (4) lower frequency and severity of the graft versus host disease (GVHD), (5) lower risk of transmission of latent infections such as cytomegalovirus and Epstein Barr Virus, (6) absence of risk to the donor, and (7) higher incidence of rare haplotypes than those found in the records of BM donors [4]. Thus, this source of SCs has been successfully replacing BM and apheresis in transplants, such that in many countries the transplants using UCB has outnumbered those with other sources of SCs.

The first transplantation using UCB was performed by Gluckman and colleagues [5], in 1988. The successful use of these cells in transplants brought about the need for storing UCB. Therefore, the first public UCB bank, for allogeneic transplantation, was established in 1993 by Rubinstein at The New York Blood Center [6]. This procedure encouraged the establishment of other human umbilical cord banks in various parts of the world, and the number of transplants using cord blood cells has increased remarkably since 1997 [1]; until March 2006, according to NetCord, 109,771 UCB units had already been stored (www.netcord.org).

Since then, the studies have progressed as to the procedures of collection, processing, characterization, quantification, cultivation, cryopreservation, thawing, and transportation of UCB around the world [7].

Some types of SCs were identified in UCB, such as HSCs, MSCs, and EPCs. The characterization of the SCs from the UCB units facilitates the understanding of factors affecting the quality and improvement of transplant outcomes [8]. For this reason, standards for processing, quantifying, manipulating, cultivation, and freezing must be established and followed to ensure the minimum characteristics of the unit to be used.

Hematopoietic Stem Cells

General Characteristics of Hematopoietic Stem Cells

Hematopoietic tissues contain a small population of primitive and multipotent HSCs. These cells are defined by their ability of self-renewal and proliferation, as well as to differentiate into all of the blood cell lineages, generating committed progenitors of the different myeloid and lymphoid compartments [9, 10, 11]. The complexity of this system is enormous, since as many as 10^{10} erythrocytes and 10^8–10^9 white blood cells are produced each hour each day during the lifetime of the individual [12].

A single SC has been proposed to be capable of more than 50 cell divisions or doublings and has the capacity to generate up to 10^{15} cells, or sufficient cells for up to 60 years [13]. The proliferation and differentiation of cells is controlled by a group of proteins called hematopoietic growth factors and interleukins [13, 14]. If it could replicate this cell amplification in vitro with hematopoietic growth factors, it might be possible to generate large numbers of cells that could be used for a variety of clinical applications [13].

Besides hematopoietic growth factors, the self-renewal, proliferation, differentiation, homing, and mobilization of hematopoietic progenitors are regulated by a complex mechanism involving the BM microenvironment. The adhesion molecules expressed in the hematopoietic progenitors play an important role in these processes. The expression of these molecules has been of particular interest in the studies with UCB.

Phenotypic Characteristics of Hematopoietic Stem Cells

Surface Molecules Expressed in Stem and Progenitor Cells from Umbilical Cord Blood

The most primitive human hematopoietic progenitor cells have demonstrated expression of CD34, CD45^{low}, Thy-1 (CDw90), c-kit receptor (CD117), and CD133, being negative for CD38 and lineage markers (Lin$^-$) [11, 12, 15, 16, 17, 18].

Besides these, several other molecules, including adhesion molecules, have been described as present in the cellular surface of HSCs and will be described below.

CD34

The CD34$^+$ protein is a surface glycoprotein of 90–120 kDa expressed on developmentally early hematopoietic stem and progenitor cells in UCB and in BM [10, 19] as well as endothelial cells [20, 21, 22]. It has been suggested that this molecule works by regulating the adhesion of the hematopoietic cell to the stroma of the hematopoietic microenvironment [20, 23].

Although the CD34 antigen is the classic marking molecule of HSCs, there is evidence that the progenitors of a yet uncommitted population of SCs do not express this marker. Depending on the stage of differentiation, a CD34 negative SC may generate not only hematopoietic progenitors but also more specific mesenchymal precursors, such as osteoclasts, chondrocytes, myocytes, adipocytes, and others. Recent studies have demonstrated the remarkable plasticity of the population of primitive SCs, comprising cells designed to form the hematopoietic stroma, as well as hematopoietic and mesenchymal progenitors [24].

It has been suggested that CD34 may be a marker of activated SCs, since $CD34^-$ (negative) cells in culture originate $CD34^+$ cells [25]. Other studies demonstrate that $CD34^+$ cells may be reservoirs of $CD34^-$ cells, showing that the expression of CD34 may be reversible in the HSCs [26].

In several reference centers, the quantification of the CD34 marker has been used to choose a unit of UCB. However, the knowledge and standardization of UCB $CD34^+$ cells phenotype is critical since the volume of UCB is limited [27].

Frequency of Hematopoietic Stem Cells from Umbilical Cord Blood

Parameters commonly used to evaluate an UCB unit and predict transplant outcomes have been total nucleated cells (TNCs) and $CD34^+$ cells counts [28].

Approximately 1–3% of TNCs of the BM, including HSCs and endothelial cells, are $CD34^+$ cells [29, 30, 31]. In UCB, the number of $CD34^+$ cells is around 1–2% among mononuclear cells (MNCs) [33, 34, 35, 36] and it has previously been shown that UCB contains a ten times more $CD34^+$ cells than peripheral blood, in which the percentage of $CD34^+$ cells among the TNCs is smaller, ranging from 0.01% to 0.1% [29].

However, studies have shown great variation in the number of HSCs of UCB. The number of $CD34^+$ cells among the leukocyte marker, the $CD45^+$ molecule, has already been described as being $0.28 \pm 0.15\%$ [37] or $0.4 \pm 0.03\%$ of total $CD45^+$ cells, in UCB samples in term newborn [38]. Among cord blood MNCs, the frequency of $CD34^+$ cells was found to be $1.4 \pm 0.9\%$ [36] or $0.36 \pm 0.33\%$ [39] with a large variation among samples (range 0.4–4.9% and 0.02–1.43%, respectively). The absolute number of $CD45^+$ cells in UCB of a term newborn has been shown to be about $12 \pm 1.3 \times 10^6$/mL, while the concentration of $CD34^+$ cells is around $5.6 \pm 3.9 \times 10^4$/mL [38]. Several studies have estimated that the number of $CD34^+$ cells ranges from 15 to 100 cells/mL of UCB [37, 40, 41]. However, some studies showed a greater variation of these cells, from 22 to 600 $CD34^+$ cells/mL of UCB [42]. These differences may be a result of the heterogeneity proper of UCB cells as well as of differences between the techniques used by the various group [43].

These findings show the importance of using standardized methods in the quantification of $CD34^+$ cells of UCB.

Clinical Relevance of the Quantification of $CD34^+$ Cells

Besides HLA compatibility, the parameter commonly used in choosing an UCB unit for a probable successful transplant has been the count of TNCs and $CD34^+$ cells [28]. The quantity of TNCs present in the sources of HSCs is of paramount importance for myeloid, lymphoid, and platelet recovery in transplants of HSCs, as well as in post-transplant survival [44].

Nevertheless, as yet there is no consensus about the minimum number necessary for a successful transplant. It has been suggested though that the minimum number of nucleated cells in UCB to be used in transplants in order to reduce the time of hematopoietic recovery should be 1.5×10^7 [45] or 2.0×10^7/kg [4] of recipient body weight. The number of CD34$^+$ cells is also an important issue in HSCs tranplants, since it has been suggested to have an correlation between the number of these cells with TNCs [46]. Studies designed to determine the role of the quantity of CD34$^+$ cells show that a precise dose is yet unknown and that this factor may suffer variations depending on the source of HSCs, donor type, relative or non-relative, number of incompatible HLA alleles, and the type of recipient disease [47]. Recent works suggest that a minimum of 2.0×10^5 CD34$^+$ cells/kg of patient should be used [4], since high doses of CD34$^+$ cells result in increased myeloid and platelet recovery [48], and other data evidence that a more slow graft "catch" is due to a low number of primitive CD34 cells [49]. The "catch" refers to the ability of infused cells, as they reach the BM, to generate mature cells, detected in the blood flow [50].

Quantification of CD34$^+$ Cells from Umbilical Cord Blood

In many transplant centers throughout the world, the total number of positive CD34 cells is used as a parameter when selecting umbilical cord units suitable for transplantation since the adequate quantity of these cells is an important factor for hematopoietic reconstitution [51].

As it is a matter of searching for rare events, given the low frequency of CD34$^+$ cells, standardized, well-established techniques should be used [52]. The use of validated protocols, with a proven coefficient of low inter-laboratory variation, is of paramount importance as regards the control of quality in these UCB banks. In using a protocol which has less than 10% of inter-laboratory variation for this single-platform technique [49], it is certainly adding quality to the samples stored and which may come to be used by any recipient in need.

The two most widely employed methods of quantification of human UCB CD34$^+$ cells are the ISHAGE (International Society of Hematotherapy and Graft Engineering) protocol and the ProCOUNT™ (BD) method (Becton Dickinson) [29].

As a method for standardized analysis of CD34$^+$ cells and use by worldwide banks, Sutherland et al. proposed the ISHAGE guidelines in 1996, currently called ISCT protocol (International Society for Cellular Therapy). This protocol is based on the combination of cell characteristics measured by flow cytometry [29]. This technique uses a sequential gating strategy allowing the selection of populations of interest [51], using four parameters: size, complexity, CD34, and CD45, evaluated by flow cytometry and able to detect one CD34$^+$ cell among 10,000 cells.

However, this protocol has been suffering modifications in order to further improve the techniques of analysis and achieve more accurate quantification. In this way, Gratama and colleagues [53] introduced a marker of cell viability 7AAD (7-Amino Actinomycin D) for determination of the number of viable and inviable CD34$^+$ cells [54]. In 2001, Brocklebank and Sparrow [42] described a protocol combining the attributes of the ISHAGE method, use of 7AAD, and use TRUCOUNT tubes, which contain a lyophilized pellet of a known number of fluorescent beads. A reliable rapid method is thus obtained, which employs a single platform and makes it possible to quantify absolute CD34$^+$ cells and assess cell viability using a single technique and the same equipment, thus increasing its sensitivity.

It is known that 7AAD identifies dead or apoptotic cells. Many studies in the literature show that 7AAD is very important for the quantification of $CD34^+$ cells in the ISHAGE protocol, since this dye identifies dead $CD34^+$ cells and weakly labels $CD34^+$ cells in apoptosis [55], and are therefore, not contributing to engraftment. It has been showed that the use of 7AAD can decrease by 50% the presence of $CD34^+$ cells/mL of blood, suggesting that these were unviable cells [49]. However, the use of 7AAD shows controversial results too when protocols using or not using it are compared [56]. However, where the samples are processed within 36 h post-partum, it reduces the possibility of there being dead or apoptotic cells, since the viability of UCB cells is around 95% [57, 58, 59]. Nevertheless, notwithstanding these conflicting results and the detection of unviable cells remaining problematic, there are situations in which the use of 7AAD may be justified and its use remains consensual. It is particularly important in cases where $CD34^+$ cells are clinically used, such as in UCB banks, the measurement of cell viability through 7AAD is important, since the number of these cells is used to choose an UCB sample. Also, in cases where the samples are cryopreserved, as in UCB banks, after thawing of samples, or after cell cultivation, whose aim is to transplant frozen or expanded cells, cell viability may be much affected [36, 55, 59, 60]. It is thus suggested that 7AAD should be routinely used for quantification of $CD34^+$ cells in the ISHAGE protocol [49].

CD33

The CD33 molecule is expressed in myeloid progenitors (CFU-GEMM, CFU-GM, CFU-G, BFU-E), monocytes/macrophages and in granulocyte precursors. Expression decreases with maturation and differentiation. It is expressed at a low level on mature granulocytes. Expression outside of the hematopoietic system is unknown. The expression of CD33 is a feature of multipotential HSCs, but not of "true stem cells" (www.ncbi.nlm.nih.gov/prow). It has been shown that less than 30% of $CD34^+$ cells express the CD33 marker [10].

CD38

The CD38 molecule is variously expressed by most hematopoietic cells, particularly during early differentiation and cell activation (www.ncbi.nlm.nih.gov/prow). It is expressed, too, in subgroups of $CD34^+$ cells, primitive or activated T and B cells, plasmocytes and thymocytes [61], monocytes, NK cells, and myeloid progenitors [32], as well as in brain, muscle, and kidney cells and other tissues (www.ncbi.nlm.nih.gov/prow). Regarding function, it may play a role in cell activation, proliferation, or cell survival [32]. It downregulates and upregulates cell activation and proliferation, depending on the cell microenvironment. It is also involved in the adhesion between human lymphocytes and endothelial cells (www.ncbi.nlm.nih.gov/prow).

The most primitive human hematopoietic progenitor cells, $CD34^+$, express little or no express CD38 [11, 12, 15, 16]. In this way, expression of the CD38 molecule identifies a $CD34^+$ cell that is already committed, while the $CD34^+CD38^-$ phenotype identifies a subset of more primitive HSCs [28], with greater ability to generate clones and to allow the expansion of $CD34^+$ cells in culture [62], besides being responsible for the "catch" of the graft in the long run [63]. The presence of the CD38 antigen appears to reflect cell activation and differentiation, since cells with the $CD34^+CD38^-$ phenotype are capable of dividing and proliferating in vitro, for long periods, without undergoing differentiation [64].

About 1% of BM cells express CD34, and generally less than 1% of these cells are CD38-negative. Hence, the frequency of this population is about 1 in 10,000, or even lower. Phenotypic analysis of several cell surface markers reveals that even this rare population is highly heterogeneous. However, it has been observed that the number of $CD34^+CD38^-$ cells is significantly higher in cord blood than in BM (16 $\pm$ 8.8% and 4.7 $\pm$ 3% of total $CD34^+$ cells, respectively) [65].

On the other hand, controversial results have been published regarding the frequency of $CD38^-$ cells among cord blood $CD34^+$ cells. It has been showed that among $CD34^+$ cells 2.6 $\pm$ 2.1% (range 0.55–5.57) [36], 3.9 $\pm$ 0.9% [38], 11.94 $\pm$ 2.09% [17], 13.9% [39], 16 $\pm$ 8.8% [65], 34.9 $\pm$ 3.4%, [66] or 67.9 $\pm$ 7.2% [67] are CD38 negative. These findings show the great difficulty in quantifying these events, considered as rare.

It has been demonstrated that phenotype $CD34^+CD38^-$ characterizes a cell as a candidate of being a "true hematopoietic stem cell". The fact that the frequency of $CD34^+CD38^-$ cells is greater in the UCB [65, 67, 68, 69], than in the other two available sources (BM and peripheral blood), might explains the successful clinical of its use in transplants [70] even when low number of cells are used, and candidates these antigens as the predictive parameter for clinical use of UCB samples [8, 70], since these cells are responsible for long-term graft survival [63].

The great variability and controversial results reported for $CD34^+CD38^-$ cells in freshly collected cord blood can be explained by the natural heterogeneity of the $CD34^+$ population or by factors that can change the number of the $CD34^+$ cells, for instance differences in the gestational age [48, 71]. Alternatively, different volumes of cord blood collected might be responsible for this variation, since it was hypothesized there are more $CD34^+CD38^-$ cells in the last fraction of the cord and placenta blood than in the first ones [28, 70]. In these studies, the authors found in the first fraction 1.61 $\pm$ 1.12% $CD34^+CD38^-$ cells in comparation with the last fraction, where they found 18.98 $\pm$ 13.96% of these cells [28]. This suggests that the higher the volume collected, the higher the probability of obtaining more residual, immature cells from the placenta.

Although the success of UCB cells transplantation is largely related to the number of total nucleated and $CD34^+$ cells, UCB $CD34^+CD38^-$ cells possess high potential of proliferation and expansion of $CD34^+$ cells [62], suggesting possible advantages concerning the homing and engrafment of more undifferentiated cells [68]. The proliferative capacity is also negatively correlated with gestational age [48], corroborating the hypothesis that $CD34^+CD38^-$ cells are more primitive

HSCs with higher clonogenic capacity. On the other hand, it has been suggested that the superiority of using UCB in hematopoietic cells transplantation is more related to the ability to generate progenitors than to the frequency of $CD34^+CD38^-$ cells proper [72].

CD45

Expressed, typically at high levels, on all hematopoietic cells, the CD45 molecule is known as the leukocyte marker. This expression occurs at a higher density on lymphocytes, approximately 10% of the surface area is CD45. While still abundant, the expression is lower on other leukocytes (www.ncbi.nlm.nih.gov/prow).

Thy-1

CD90, or Thy-1, is expressed by HSCs, neurons and highly expressed in connective tissue and various fibroblast and stromal cell lines (http://mpr.nci.nih.gov/prow). It has been suggested that Thy-1 is involved in the inhibition of cell proliferation [30]. The Thy-1 molecule is expressed on 10–40% of $CD34^+$ cells in BM (http://mpr.nci.nih.gov/prow). Thy-1 co-expression profiles on the cell subsets defined by internal/external CD34 phenotyping are different when comparing BM with cord blood. Although the $extCD34^+$/Thy-1 immunophenotype reportedly highlights a primitive cord blood hematopoietic stem and progenitor cells population, many groups have found that a significant proportion of primitive cord blood MNCs do not express Thy-1 [17].

CD117

Others names for the molecule CD117 are c-kit (c-kit receptor) or SCFR [stem cell factor (SCF) receptor] [32] (www.ncbi.nlm.nih.gov/prow). This marker is expressed in hematopoietic stem and progenitor cells [32, 61] (www.ncbi.nlm.nih.gov/prow), mastocytes, melanocytes, spermatogonia, oocytes in cells of the embryonic brain, and some NK cells [32] (www.ncbi.nlm.nih.gov/prow).

The CD117 molecule is the receptor of the SCs growth factor and it induces his tyrosine kinase activity [32] (www.ncbi.nlm.nih.gov/prow). A member of the immunoglobulin superfamily adhesion molecules, this marker is involved in the interactions of $CD34^+$ cells with stromal and other cells in the BM, MPB, and UCB. This marker has a relevant role in the viability, differentiation, and proliferation of HSCs [73, 74].

The expression of c-kit receptor has been reported for characterizing the primitive HSCs [75], since this molecule can be detected in most $CD34^+$ cells [16]. This marker was detected on the majority of $CD34^+$ HSCs, particularly in human UCB, where it was found $80.7 \pm 8.2\%$ of the $CD34^+$ cells, positive for CD117, while on the $CD34^+$ cells from BM and peripherical blood the c-kit was found in $72.3 \pm 13.1\%$ and $64.2 \pm 17\%$, or lower, of these cells, respectively [16, 76].

The literature findings, however, are still conflicting as to whether these more primitive, HSCs express this molecule in higher [11, 12, 16, 36, 75, 77], or lower levels [78], or do not express it at all [79]. The expression of this marker can vary as well according to the subset of HSCs, since its expression among $CD34^+CD38^+$ and $CD34^+CD38^-$ cells can be $80 \pm 10\%$ and $56 \pm 24\%$ of these cells, respectively, in the UCB [36]. In evaluating the expression of surface and intracytoplasmic antigens among cells containing intracytoplasmic CD34 (int CD34) yet non-expressed on the surface, $86.36 \pm 7.83\%$ of $CD34^+$ cells were found be positive for CD117 [17].

Studies showed that cells with $CD34^+CD117^{low}$ phenotype have been used to describe quiescent progenitor cells, based on the fact that the low c-kit expression on the cell surface might "protect" the cells, preventing it to receive stimuli and differentiate itself, thus characterizing it as a more primitive cell [80]. Other studies showed that cells with $CD117^{high}$ phenotype may be ones related to the formation of cell colonies [17].

It has been demonstrated that myeloid progenitors are enumerated in $CD34^+$ c-kit^{high} cells and erythroid progenitors are more enriched in $CD34^+$c-kit^{low} cells [81]. In contrast, it has been found that erythroid progenitors are highly enriched in MPB $CD34^+$c-kit^{high} cells, and that CFU-GM is enriched in MPB $CD34^+$ c-kit^- cells. Primitive progenitors with self-renewal potential may present in the MPB $CD34^+$c-$kit^{-/low}$ cell populatoin [76]. It was reported that the human UCB-derived $CD34^+$c-kit^{low} cell population contains the majority of cell cycle dormant progenitors and blast cell colony forming cells. The expression of c-kit may therefore be useful in identifying human UCB progenitors with long-term engraftment capability [82].

CD133

The CD133, or AC133, molecule is a 120 kDa transmembrane glycoprotein, belonging to the family of mucoproteins [18]. This marker is expressed on primitive cell populations, such as CD34 hematopoietic stem and progenitor cells, neural, and endothelial SCs, developing epithelium (neuroepithelium, kidney, and gut) in 5 weeks human embryos, retina and retinoblastoma cell lines, and endothelial cell precursors (hemangioblasts). The population of CD133 positive cells contain CD90 (Thy-1) positive, most of the CD117 (c-kit) positive, most of the HLA-DR positive population of progenitors (http://mpr.nci.nih.gov/prow).

The CD133 antigen has been used to characterize more immature HSCs, since in cord blood, the expression of internal CD34 ($intCD34^+$) could be detected on co-expressing $CD133^+$ cells before expression of external CD34 antigen ($extCD34^+$) [17]. It is important to observe that $intCD34^+$ cell subsets are consistently and significantly enriched for cells with more primitive phenotypes. It has also been reported that $CD133^+$ cells demonstrated a higher proliferation potential and contain long-term culture-initiating cells (LTC-IC) at a higher frequency than $CD34^+$ cells [17, 83]. CD133 antibody has been used for positive selection of hematopoietic stem and progenitor cells for transplantation studies as an alternative to the widely used CD34 (http://mpr.nci.nih.gov/prow).

$CD34^+CD133^+$ cells indicate primitive SCs that are important in reparation of lesions to an organ, as well migration of SCs to the site of the lesion. Molecule CD133, expressed in EPCs, contribute to vasculogenesis [84, 85, 86, 87]. As CD133 populations are know to have the ability to develop into endothelial lineage, it is hypothesized that following cardiac insertion, damaged capillary beds are reseeded by CD133 positive cells that have migrated to the site of injury [17].

FLT3

The Flt3 receptor, or CD135, is a growth factor receptor for early hematopoietic progenitors (http://mpr.nci.nih.gov/prow). FLT3 is expressed on primitive human and murine hematopoietic progenitors cells [11]. It enhances hematopoietic cell proliferation and facilitates HSC mobilization in vivo [88]. The class III receptor tyrosine kinase, FLT3 represents an important molecule involved in early steps of hematopoiesis. In cord blood, the majority of $CD34^+CD117^+$ (c-kit$^+$), $CD34^+CD90^+$ (Thy-1$^+$), and $CD34^+CD109^+$ cells coexpress FLT3 [89].

CD164

The molecule CD164 is a 80- to 90-kDa transmembrane glycoprotein sialomucins expressed by human $CD34^+$ hematopoietic progenitor cells and it have been implicated in cell-to-cell interactions and activations. The CD164 antigen, expressed on early hematopoietic populations, is reported to have a possible function facilitating $CD34^+$ cells to adhere to BM stroma [90]. CD164 has been also demonstrated to be highly expressed on strongly positive $CD133^+$ $CD38^{low/-}$ cells than on those more mature weakly positive $CD133^+CD38^+$ cells [17]. $CD164^+$ cells represents about 20% of cord blood MNCs and about 60% of cord blood cells coexpressing $CD34^+CD164^+$ cells also expressed AC133 [90].

This receptor may play a key role in hematopoiesis by facilitating the adhesion of $CD34^+$ cells to BM stroma and by negatively regulating $CD34^+$ hematopoietic progenitor cell growth. It has been reported that the majority of $CD34^+$ human cord blood cells that were $CD38^{low/-}$ or that coexpressed AC133, CD90 (Thy-1), CD117 (c-kit), or CD135 (FLT-3) are $CD164^+$ [91].

CXCR4

CXCR4 or CD184, is the receptor for the the stromal-derived factor (SDF-1) [88, 92, 93, 94]. CXCR4 is a common marker of hematopoietic, endothelial, neural, muscle, and liver SCs. SDF-1, the CXCR-4 ligand, is secreted in various organs to which circulating SCs are chemoattracted and "home/reside." Circulating SCs may compete for common tissue-specific niches with the result that SCs committed to other tissues may be detected in various organs. Furthermore, CXCR4 has recently been reported to be present on primordial germ cells, neural SCs, and retinal pigment epithelial SCs as well as liver oval SCs. More importantly, CXCR4 is functional on all of these cells and CXCR4-positive tissue-committed SCs respond by chemotaxis to an SDF-1 gradient [95].

In a study comparing the CXCR-4 expression among different sources of HSCs like peripherical blood, BM, and fetal blood, the frequency of this marker in $CD34^+$ cells from cord blood is the highest [96]. About 90% of $CD34^+$-cord blood cells are positive for this marker [96, 97]. Because the CXCR-4 receptor is expressed in umbilical cord hematopoietic stem/progenitor cells, it plays a crucial role in the homing of these cord cells to the BM microenvironment [95].

The Importance of CXCR4 in Homing

Homing is the first and a rapid process in which circulating hematopoietic cells actively cross the blood/BM endothelium barrier and lodge at least transiently in the BM compartment by activation of adhesion interactions prior to their proliferation. SCs also home to other organs, especially in response to stress signals, transmitted in response to alarm situation [98].

The ligand for CXCR4, SDF-1, is secreted by BM fibroblast and plays an important role in the homing/retention of HSCs in the BM microenvironment. SDF-1, however, is also secreted in several other organs and, for example, is detectable in heart and skeletal muscles, liver, neural tissue, and kidney. The secretion of SDF-1 increases during muscle ischemia, toxic liver damage, or total body irradiation. Thus, it has been hypothesized that SDF-1 plays an important role in heart regeneration by attracting CXCR4-positive muscle SCs. On the other hand, SDF-1 secreted during tissue damage may play an important role in directing tissue-committed SCs necessary for organ/tissue regeneration [95].

When there is tissue damage, $CD34^+CXCR4^+$ cells migrate to the site of the lesion, attracted by the secretion of the SDF-1, the ligand of receptor CXCR4. Niches of SDF-1 are found in injured organs and are released during tissue damage. It is well-known that the organization of cells niches has a key role in the normal regulation of SC differentiation and regeneration [99]. Thus, $CXCR4^+$ cells are important in the regeneration of injured organs, indicating the regenerative ability of SCs [94, 97]. The BM and the skeletal muscle also contain a population of CXCR4 cells which express specific genes for muscle progenitor cells and which can be mobilized to the peripheral blood. SDF-1 is an important factor that influences the mobilization of BM cells [100]. After myocardial infarction, for example, the CXCR4 cells are mobilized from BM into the peripheral blood and chemoattracted to the infarcted myocardium [101]. Other studies have shown that SDF-1 can regulate the lengthening of the axons [102]. This growth factor also performs leukocyte chemotaxis to the site of the brain injury, the hippocampal neurons being the target for the CXCR4 cell receptor. The SDF-1/CXCR4 system may therefore contribute to neuronal plasticity induced by ischemia [103]. The neurons express a variety of cytokine receptors that regulate neuronal signaling and survival [104]. The CXCR-4 molecule is expressed in the adult rat brain cells, in glial cells (astrocytes and microglia, but not in oligodendrocytes) as well as in neurons [92].

These findings show the importance of CXCR4 in homing and, since the cord blood cells are rich in these molecules, this is an advantage of using the UCB cells.

Other Markers and Adhesion Molecules Expressed in Hematopoietic Stem and Progenitor Cells from Umbilical Cord Blood

Adhesion molecules play a role in the migration of hematopoietic progenitor cells and regulation of hematopoiesis [105]. There is evidence that cord blood, BM, and peripheral blood-derived HSCs are highly heterogeneous for a number of antigens useful for HSCs enumeration by flow cytometry [106]. Cell adhesion molecules are highly expressed in both human UCB and BM $CD34^{+}CD38^{+}$ cells. Since the expression of such molecules has been related to the repopulating capacity of hematopoietic progenitor cells, there is a possible advantage in homing and engraftment of more undifferentiated human UCB as opposed to BM hematopoietic progenitor cells [65]. The blood release of hematopoietic progenitor cells is probably due to a perturbation of the adhesive interactions between these cells and the expression on $CD34^{+}$ hematopoietic progenitor cells found in the three hemopoietic compartments evaluated it can lead to new knowledge about the mobilization kinetics in which the adhesion molecules are involved [16].

The adhesion molecules allow interaction with various regulatory elements present in the microenvironment, which include stromal cells, molecules of the extracellular matrix, and soluble regulatory factors such as cytokines or growth and cell differentiation factors [107]. The hematopoietic stem and progenitor cells, most of which expressing the CD34 antigen, have multiple adhesion receptors. These receptors allow binding of stem or progenitor cells to the components of the extracellular matrix within the medullary sinusoids, thus facilitating its homing in the BM and promoting a close cell–cell contact necessary for cell survival and cell proliferation regulation. There are several adhesion receptors and their ligands, present in stem and progenitor cells and in components of the hematopoietic microenvironment [61]. Some of the subgroups of receptors are: integrins (such as CD11c and CD49e), molecules of the superfamily of immunoglobulins (such as CD31 and CD117), lectins or selectins (such as CD62L), sialomucins (such as CD34), CD38, among others.

CD11c

The CD11c molecule is an integrin of the leukocyte surface found in em macrófagos, NK cells, subpopulation of T and B cells (www.ncbi.nlm.nih.gov/prow), monocytes and polymorphonuclear neutrophils [32]. This adhesion molecule has a role in the linkage to receptors on the estimulated endothelium (www.ncbi.nlm.nih.gov/prow).

It has been shown that the expression of CD11c is rare in $CD34^{+}$ cells of both human UCB [36, 108] and BM [109].

CD31

Also known as PECAM-1 (platelet endothelial cell adhesion molecule-1) the molecule is present in myeloid cells, leukocyte and their precursors, endothelial cells, CD34$^+$ cells, monocytes, neutrophils [32, 61], platelets, NK cells, T cells subgroups, but not on circulating B cells (www.ncbi.nlm.nih.gov/prow). CD31 binding activates leukocyte integrins [32]. This molecule is involved with the adhesion between cells such as endothelial and leukocytes (www.ncbi.nlm.nih.gov/prow), as well as with the interaction between hematopoietic cells and extracelullar matrix components in BM [110].

Several reports have shown high expression of CD31 on BM [105, 109] and UCB [36, 113] CD34$^+$ cells.

CD49e

The CD49e molecule corresponds to the alpha chain of the VLA-5 integrin, (www.ncbi.nlm.nih.gov/prow) [32, 61], and it is expressed on cellular surface of thymocytes, T cells, monocytes, activated platelets, and primitive B cells [32] and in CD34$^+$ cells [61]. VLA-5 is strongly involved in the binding of BM progenitor cells to extracellular matrix components [111].

It is interesting that different reports have conflicting results regarding this molecule. It was already shown that all CD34$^+$ cells in normal BM express CD49e, while cord blood and mobilized CD34$^+$ cells have a lower expression of this molecule [109]. Other studies showed opposite results [65] or that cord blood CD34$^+$ cells have a remarkably similar [112, 113] expression of VLA-5 on BM CD34$^+$ cells. By studying the subpopulation of CD34$^+$ cells, it has already been shown a large number of CD34$^+$CD38$^+$ and CD34$^+$CD38$^-$ cells positive for CD49e, before and after culture of UCB-derived CD34$^+$ cells with some combinations of hematopoietic growth factors [36].

CD61

The CD61 molecule is the beta 3 integrin chain, also called GPIIb/IIIa (www.ncbi.nlm.nih.gov/prow). It is present in platelets, megakaryocytes, monocytes, macrophages, and endothelial cells whose function is to facilitate platelet aggregation [32].

CD61 has been observed in small levels on human UCB CD34$^+$ cells, with less [27, 36] or around than 20% [28] of these cells positive for CD61.

CD62L

The CD62L molecule is also called L-selectina, LAM-1 (leukocyte adhesion molecule-1) and LECAM-1 [32, 61, 114, 115] (www.ncbi.nlm.nih.gov/prow) and it is present in T and B cells, monocytes, neutrophils, thymocytes, eosinophils, basophils, erythroid and myeloid progenitor, and NK cells ([32], www.ncbi.nlm.nih.gov/prow). The molecule is also present in a few lymphocytes of the spleen and BM and in myeloid cells of the BM, as well as in certain hematopoietic malignant cells (www.ncbi.nlm.nih.gov/prow).

L-selectin takes part in the homing of lymphocytes and facilitates cell binding to the endothelium at inflammatory sites [32]. This molecule is involved in the homing of $CD34^+$ cells after peripheral blood MNC transplantation [108] and it is suggested that it can increase the clonogenic capacity of $CD34^+$ cells [116].

The majority of the $CD34^+$ cells also have CD62L on the surface membrane. Cord blood and mobilized blood $CD34^+$ have been shown to present a higher expression of CD62L than BM $CD34^+$ cells [109]. However, the results are controversial, since in other studies the expression of this molecule seems to be similar [112] ou smaller [65] in the SCs from UCB than in SCs from the BM. It has been showed that CD62L is more expressed, also, in cord blood than in BM $CD34^+CD38^-$ subset, suggesting a possible advantage in homing and engraftment [65, 68]. The great heterogeneity of positive cells in fresh samples as well as small differences after culture, in CD62L molecules could be explained by the natural heterogeneity of $CD34^+$ cells or, perhaps, by the differences in gestational age, since it was showed that CD62L on $CD34^+$ stem and progenitor cells in UCB change during gestation [117].

HLA-DR

The HLA molecule Class II is expressed in monocytes, macrophages, and lymphocytes, and its function is the presentation of exogen antigens to Th lymphocytes (CD4). HLA-DR is expressed in the majority of human UCB [27, 28] and peripheral blood $CD34^+$ cells [27, 76]. Some studies showed that the coexpression of CD34 with HLA-DR was not significantly different in human UCB and BM (respectively, $86.3 \pm 2.7\%$ and $92.7 \pm 5.1\%$) [67], while other showed that among MNCs, $CD11^+HLA\text{-}DR^+$ cell frequencies did not differ significantly among the three hematopoietic compartments [69].

A great variation was also shown in the expression of HLA-DR molecule, in fresh or cultivated cells. This finding may be ascribed to the heterogeneity of $CD34^+$ cells or to differences in gestational age [117]. Fetal liver cells, for instance, have been shown to present lower proportions of $CD34^+HLA\text{-}DR^+$ than human UCB, showing that the composition of fetal leukocytes changes during development and with gestational age [118]. The frequency of HLA-DR-positive cells is a little higher among $CD34^+CD38^+$ than $CD34^+CD38^-$ cells. These findings support the hypothesis that these molecules are more expressed in more differentiated cells [36].

Conflicting Results in the Expression of Surface Molecules in Hematopoietic Stem Cells

The controversial results presented in the literature about the co-expression of markers in $CD34^+$ cells of UCB probably reflect the phenotypic and functional heterogeneity of the $CD34^+$ cell population. However, it is known that the handling of HSCs, as well as their freezing, for example, changes the distribution of such surface molecules as CD34 [119]. The mobilization induced by cytokines can also alter the profile of markers, especially adhesion molecules, in $CD34^+$ cells of the BM [120]. Finally, it is known that the adhesion molecules and their receptors present interaction between one another and even functional overlay [121].

Culture of Hematopoietic Stem Cells from Umbilical Cord Blood

Clearly, the UCB is an excellent source of SCs and its clinical utilization has increased in recent years, even for disorders other than those usually treated with BM transplantation. One problem, however, is that the number of HSCs in UCB samples often is limited [3]. Identification of conditions that support the self-renewal and expansion of human HSCs remains a major goal of experimental and clinical hematology [122]. The expansion of human SCs ex vivo will likely have important applications in transplantation, SC marking, and gene therapy [15, 123, 124].

Because the volume of UCB is a limiting factor for the number of SCs [1, 13], the number of hematopoietic progenitors and SCs in cord blood is enough to support the BM engraftment in children, but many times it is not enough to successfully engraft an adult [125]. Of the 5,220 UCB units transplanted from the Netcord Network until March 2007, 2,940 were transplanted in children and 2,477 in adults (www.netcord.org).

The possibility of increasing the dose of cells to be used in the transplantation of human HSCs is very important since the efficacy of cord blood transplantation is limited by the low cell dose available [9, 122, 126, 127, 128, 129, 130]. Low cell doses at transplant are correlated with delayed engraftment, prolonged neutropenia and thrombocytopenia and elevated risk of graft failure. To potentially improve the efficacy of UCB transplantation, approaches have been taken to increase the cell dose available. One approach is the transplantation of multiple cord units, another is the use of ex vivo expansion [131].

Transplantation of multiple UCB units could be a strategy to overcome cell dose limitations [132]. Nevertheless, to find a HLA match in two UCB units could be difficult. Ex vivo expansion of HSCs is suggested as the best way of overcoming problems caused by limited hematopoietic cell number for cord blood transplantation [133, 134]. As a result, the expansion of human SCs will have important clinical applications, because their ex vivo expansion might be required to successfully engraft an adult [125].

Therefore, two important aspects of the biology of ex vivo expanded cells relate to cultured cells: either maintaining their self-renewal capacity and multilineage differentiation potential, or improving their short-term engraftment ability when transplanted into myeloblated recipients. Several growth factor combinations have been tested to identify suitable culture conditions to induce expansion of primitive SCs. So far, only a few studies have shown that primitive non-obese diabetic severe combined immunodeficient (NOD/SCID) mouse repopulation SCs from cord blood can be expanded (a few or several-fold) after in vitro culture [125].

Currently, the UCB cells ex vivo expansion processes include: (1) liquid expansion: $CD34^+$ or $CD133^+$ cells are selected and cultured in medium containing factors targeting the proliferation and self-renewal of primitive hematopoietic progenitors; (2) co-culture expansion: unmanipulated cord blood cells are cultured with stromal components of the hematopoietic microenvironment, specifically MSCs, in medium containing growth factors; and (3) continuous perfusion: cord blood hematopoietic progenitors cells are cultured with growth factors in 'bioreactors' rather than in static cultures. Ultimately, the goal of ex vivo expansion is to increase the available dose of the cord blood cells responsible for successful engraftment, thereby reducing the time to engraftment and reducing the risk of graft failure [131].

Countless are the factors regulating hematopoiesis. Hematopoietic growth factors are soluble factors influencing the growth or differentiation of hematopoietic progenitor cells. These factors can act directly or indirectly on the cells, binding to cell receptors [14]. The interaction of these factors and their receptors on cell membranes is an important mechanism of regulation of survival, proliferation and differentiation of hematopoietic cells [78].

The hematopoietic growth factors are the so-called: colony-stimulating factors (CSFs), such as granulocyte-macrophage colony-stimulating factor (GM-CSF), granulocyte-CSF (G-CSF), and macrophage-CSF (M-CSF); steel factor or SCF or kit ligand (KL); erythropoietin (EPO); thrombopoietin (TPO); tumor necrosis factor (TNF); FLT-3 ligand or FL; interleukins (IL); and others [11, 14]. The proliferation and differentiation of HSCs is controlled not only by soluble growth factors, but also by adhesion to stromal cells and matrix molecules [115].

Several culture systems were developed to try to expand HSCs [9, 36, 126, 127, 135]. According to literature, several different combinations of growth factors have been used. Some studies showed the differential ability of combination of some growth factors like FLT-3, TPO, KL, GM-CSF, IL-3, and IL-6, to support different stages of hematopoiesis in long term and suspension cultures of progenitor cells from human UCB [9, 18, 136].

Several studies showed the effects of thrombopoietin alone in culture, where it can stimulate the early proliferation, survival [128], or differentiation of progenitor cell in cord blood [129] or BM [130]. TPO is a primary regulator of megakaryocyte and platelet production and might also play an important role in early hematopoiesis [15]. It is an important cytokine in the early proliferation of human primitive as well as committed hemopoietic progenitors, and in the ex vivo manipulation of human hematopoietic progenitors [128]. TPO has also been observed to suppress apoptosis of $CD34^+CD38^-$ cells in culture, showing a potential role in maintaining quiescent primitive human progenitor cells viable [137]. In studies using a combination of growth factors with and without TPO, a significant expansion of $CD34^+$ cells from UCB and neonatal blood to early and committed progenitors was shown, in the presence of this factor [138].

SCF or KL, also called mast cell growth factor, stimulates the survival and growth of primitive SCs in synergy with several factors [11, 74].

FLT3 ligand or FL co-stimulates the multipotent SCs, especially with TPO and KL. It stimulates the generation of dendritic cells and induces regression of tumors in vivo [11]. It is able to induce proliferation of $CD34^{+}CD38^{-}$ cells that are non-responsive to other early acting cytokines and to improve the maintenance of progenitors in vitro [127].

It has already been shown that, although TPO alone can stimulate limited clonal growth, it synergizes with SCF, FL, or IL-3 to potently enhance clonogenic growth [15]. Several published studies have shown the increase of this cell population, even with TPO alone. However, in many studies using UCB, the expansion of non-adherent cells was greater with TPO, FL, and SCF than with TPO and FL, and greater in this combination than with TPO alone [9, 123], especially in the sense of achieving expansion of $CD34^{+}CD38^{-}$ cells in vitro [139] based on the proliferative potential of these cells present in the UCB [36, 72].

Some cell surface molecules can change their expression after cultivation with growth factors. For example, the number of CD62L-positive $CD34^{+}CD38^{-}$ and $CD34^{+}CD38^{+}$ cells and the CD62L expression on these cells increase during short-term culture with TPO, FL and SCF [36]. It has already been showed that a short exposure to cytokines increases L-selectin expression in the more differentiated hematopoietic progenitors, $CD34^{+}CD38^{+}$ cells which could improve their homing in a transplant setting. After transplantation of HSCs, adhesion molecules play a major role in the multistep process of engraftment in which L-selectin is suggested to be of relevance [36, 65]. The expression of c-kit (CD117) on $CD34^{+}CD38^{+}$ and $CD34^{+}CD38^{-}$ cells decreases, in some studies, after culture with TPO, FL, and SCF. Culture of $CD34^{+}$ cells with TPO, FL, and SCF thus significantly increases the number of candidate SCs with the $CD34^{+}CD38^{-}$ (c-kit) phenotype. On the other hand, the downregulation of c-kit may be due to the presence of SCF in the growth factor combination, since this factor is essential to expand $CD34^{+}CD38^{-}$ cells. In the same growth factor combination, the number of cells positive for HLA-DR and the intensity of fluorescence increased in both $CD34^{+}CD38^{+}$ cells and $CD34^{+}CD38^{-}$ cells [36].

A number of cultivation strategies have been tested for cell expansion. A stroma-free culture with FL, SCF, and TPO allows the maintenance and expansion for several weeks of a cord blood $CD34^{+}$ cell population capable of multilineage and long-lasting hematopoietic repopulation in NOD/SCID mice. Moreover, a long-lasting severe post-transplant thrombocytopenia is often observed even in pediatric patients [125].

Selected $CD34^{+}$ cells, after a 4-week expansion with FL, SCF, and TPO, appear to be more efficient in megakarocyte engraftment than the same number of unmanipulated cells [125]. In a comparative study carried out with two groups of irradiated NOD-SCID mice transplanted with expanded and non-expanded cells from the same UCB, the BM was analyzed for the presence of human cells. Both groups of mice showed successful engraftment and the cell population obtained after 12 days expansion consisted mainly of myeloid and megakaryocytic progenitors [140].

In many studies cells are cultured with fetal calf serum (FCS) or pooled human serum (HS) [9]. However, for clinical use, cell expansion in the absence of serum is a clear advantage. In trials performed with mice receiving human SCs expanded in serum-free medium with a combination of three (FL, TPO, SCF) or four

(FL, TPO, SCF, IL6) growth factors were compared with the results obtained using FCS or HS. The engraftment of human cells in mice was higher for serum-replete than for serum-free expanded cells. Nevertheless, serum-free cultured cells were also able to engraft both marrow and spleen in all animals. In addition, engrafted human cells still maintained clonogenic ability. With SCF, FL, TPO $\pm$ IL6 it is possible to expand hematopoietic progenitor cells in a serum-free medium [136]. It is believed that serum-free medium allows a better control of the role that individual cytokines and their combination have on cell growth and differentiation [36]. However, compared with serum-replete cultures, the absolute number of clonogenic cells and in vivo repopulating cells is lower when serum-free medium is used. Although the degree of expansion remains significant, a clinical trial still needs to be carried out to address the question of whether this expansion might be useful in reducing post-transplant aplasia [136].

Another important factor influencing the efficiency and practicality of UCB cell cultivation is the choice of length of cell cultivation. Some studies use long-term cultures, while others, short-term cultures. While long-term cultures allow the expansion of a greater number of cells, in short-term culture the expansion is lower. On the other hand, in the face of the need for transplantation in a patient with cells from UCB, the expansion of $CD34^+CD38^-$ cells within a short period of time could be better suit the necessity of having available cells rapidly [36].

Finally, another strategy that has been studied, particularly for adult patients where the amount of UCB cells would not be enough for the transplant, is the autologous transplant concomitantly with the use of UCB cells, whether expanded or not. Therefore, it is fundamental that short-time culture systems are perfected so that more patients can benefit from the transplantation of these cells.

Physiological, Hematological, and Immunophenotypical Correlations of Umbilical Cord Blood

Many factors can influence the concentration of progenitor and SCs in UCB. The quantity of TNCs is correlated with the percentage value of $CD34^+$ cells/mL of blood as there is correlation between collected volume and number of $CD34^+$ cells both per microliter of UCB and in the percentage of these cells among $CD45^+$ ones [46, 141].

It is known that higher volume of blood is collected with the placenta still in the uterus [148, 143, 144]. Nevertheless, this procedure is not performed in public UCB banks collections. It was observed, also, that high volume samples are correlated with high doses of TNCs, $CD34^+$ cells and GM-CFU [7].

In addition, factors like newborn and placental weight [144, 145], longer umbilical cord, cesarean section, and advanced gestational age can influence the volume of collected blood and the number of TNCs [145]. The volume collected could be larger, also, according the effect of "upper" and "lower" positions of the term neonates, vaginally delivered, increasing the progenitor cell ($CD34^+$) content of the UCB [146]. Other findings can also explain the variability of $CD34^+$ frequency among UCB samples. Longer duration stress (a prolonged first stage of labor) of the infant during delivery, for instance, demonstrated increased numbers of nucleated cells, granulocytes, $CD34^+$ cells, and hematopoietic progenitor cells in UCB from children with lower venous pH [147].

Also were found positive correlations of advanced gestational age with volume [148] and number of CD34 cells [46]. The quantity of $CD34^+$ cells/mL of UCB is inversely proportional to gestational age [10, 43, 48]. Yet, if on the one hand the UCB of prematures presents a higher quantity of $CD34^+$ cells/mL, the collected volume is lower than that obtained from term fetuses, because the more advanced the gestational age, the higher the placental weight and the higher the volume of blood that can be collected [145].

Although some form of linear correlation between TNC and $CD34^+$ cells in cord blood has been reported, within groups of samples with similar TNCs counts a high degree of variation (at times exceeding tenfold) in $CD34^+$ cells is observed [36, 43]. Different explanations have been given to the variability found on the frequency of $CD34^+$ cells in UCB. There is evidence that, although the CD34 population is a reliable indicator of the progenitor potential of human UCB it is nevertheless heterogeneous in nature. On the other hand, these heterogeneous results can reflect differences in the sensitivity of the methods employed by the different groups. Besides gestational age, $CD34^+$ HSCs have also been shown to vary with mode of delivery and positioning of the delivered neonate after delivery, inasmuch as these factors can affect the volume of collected blood [43, 146].

The frequency of $CD34^+$ cells was shown to decline linearly with gestation age, being significantly higher in the early gestational age than in term gestation fetuses [10, 48, 71, 117, 149, 150, 151], decreasing rapidly in the peripheral blood of neonates soon after birth [152]. In fetal liver, also, there seems to be a strong and highly significant inverse correlation between $CD34^+$ cells (as a proportion of total leukocytes) and gestational age [118]. The proliferative capacity also shows an inverse correlation with gestational age [48].

Some studies report that the number of $CD34^+$ cells/mL of blood is significantly higher in samples coming from cesarean deliveries, due to the higher volume collected [153]. On the other hand, in other studies, the association of cesarean delivery with the number of TNCs, $CD34^+$ cells [46, 148, 154] and $CD34^+CD38^-$ cells [47] was not observed. It has also been shown a correlation between the number of erythroblasts with $CD34^+$ cells and $CD34^+CD38^-$ [46].

With regard to the percentage of $CD34^+CD38^-$ cells, as previously mentioned there is great data disagreement, which may be accounted for by the difficulty in analyzing such rare events. Moreover, the factors affecting the number of $CD34^+$ cells might also influence the number of $CD34^+CD38^-$ cells in the UCB. The variation in relation to gestational age has already been reported as a factor that is inversely proportional to the number of $CD34^+CD38^-$ cells in cord blood [48, 71]. Though the relation between ethnic origin and quantity of these cells was little investigated so far, it has been found that $CD34^+CD38^-$ subsets were significantly lower in African American and Asian persons compared to Caucasian and Hispanic persons [46].

It was also shown that cells presenting CD34$^+$CD117$^-$ phenotype, or low expression on the surface, appear to vary with the volume obtained, as well as with the presence of TNCs, CD34$^+$, and CD34$^+$CD38$^-$ cells. In addition, it was already found positive correlations concerning the relative presence of CD34$^+$CD117$^-$ cells among the CD34$^+$ cells population with the parameters volume, total leukocytes, number of CD34$^+$ cells/mL of UCB, and percentage of CD34$^+$CD38$^-$ cells. On the other hand, the same parameters presented negative correlations with CD34$^+$CD117$^+$, as is shown in Fig. 3.1 [155].

Therefore, several factors may influence TNCs and CD34$^+$ cell counts and, hence, the success of a transplant. Procedures such as clamping the umbilical cord as closely as possible to the infant's body, in order to obtain a longer cord, and

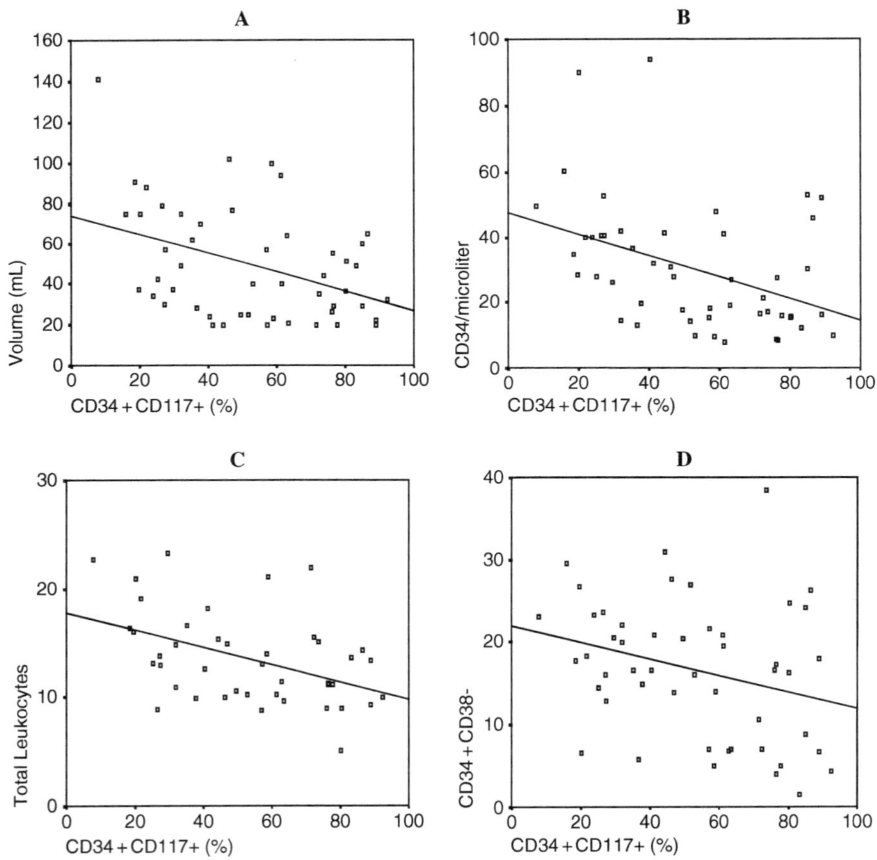

Fig. 3.1 Significance by Pearson's correlation between the relative number of CD34$^+$CD117$^+$ cells with volume and immunophenotypical parameters. A significant negative correlation between the relative number of CD34$^+$CD117$^+$ cells and (**A**) the volume of UCB ($r = -0.41, p < 0.01$); (**B**) the CD34$^+$ cells ($r = -0.41, p < 0.01$); (**C**) the leukocytes, ($r = -0.45, p < 0.01$); and (**D**) the CD34$^+$CD38$^-$ cells ($r = -0.45, p < 0.01$) [155]

collecting cord blood as promptly as possible after birth, surely provide higher collected volume [145]. In addition, it is suggest that a shorter time interval between collection and handling of the sample (cell counting) can increase the concentration of $CD34^+$ cells [141]. Measures like these may be highly valuable in the acquisition and storage of samples with higher quality standards, thus avoiding that such a rich material with so much proliferative potential will not be used to the fullest.

As the volume of collected UCB directly affects the quantity of $CD34^+$ cells/mL of blood and possibly the quantity of TNCs, some measures must be taken at the moment of collection in order to increase the collected volume. These measures include the advice that this procedure must be performed by individuals trained to this end, because the longer it takes from the removal of the placenta and cord, the smaller the yield obtained and, hence, the lower the number of $CD34^+$ and TNCs.

Clinical Importance of the Quantification of Hematopoietic Stem Cells in the Umbilical Cord Blood

Since the UCB constitutes a very rich source of hematopoietic cells that can thus be used to reconstitute the blood system [156], an accurate quantification of SCs in the UCB is crucial.

At present, an increasing number of cases are been studied in order to compare the use of UCB with other sources of HSCs, particularly the BM, as regards the "catch" potential, GVHD induction, immune reconstitution, effect of graft against the tumor, patient survival, in relation to the dose used, and the number of incompatible HLA alleles. As main advantage of UCB, we can point the rapid availability of the unit, which once located can be promptly used, thus reducing approximately the time in searching for a marrow donor from 4 months to around 13.5 days in searching for a unit of donated UCB [44, 157, 158].

Doses above 3.0×10^7 TNCs/kg appear to compensate the negative effect of one incompatible HLA allele [159]. The risk of developing acute and chronic GVHD in recipients of UCB with up to two incompatible HLA alleles is similar to that of receiving a BM from an identical HLA donor [157], and the disease-free survival time turned out to be similar [160]. However, though the UCB constitutes a good alternative to be used in allogeneic transplantation, the number of immature cells is limited by blood volume that is possible to collect, which can bring about a delay in engraftment "catch", particularly in adult patients.

However, the UCB can be used as an alternative in adult patients when an identical BM donor is not available [161], since in a study of 68 adult patients receiving transplant of UCB, a mean 1.6×10^7 TNCs and 1.2×10^5 $CD34^+$ cells/kg of the recipient's body weight were enough to ensure engraftment [162]. Another alternative would be the utilization of more than one UCB unit to increase engraftment "catch". This technique can provide for fast hematopoietic recovery and total chimerism of one of the units at day 100 post-transplantation, i.e., at least 90% of donor cells present in the recipient, confirming "engraftment catch" [44].

Moreover, it is suggested that UCB cells, when transplanted, possess a reduced potential for homing toward the BM, as compared to more mature cells. However, this difference is compensated by the fact that the UCB cells are more easily maintained in their immature state, guaranteeing the levels of progenitor cells for longer, as compared to BM transplantation [98]. A more rapid engraftment and better graft survival are obtained when the cord blood provides at least 2.0×10^7 TNCs and 2.0×10^5 $CD34^+$ cells/kg of the recipient's body weight [4].

It is known that the number of TNCs and the number of HLA mismatches interact in the engraftment and in the frequency of GVHD, and a higher number of TNCs might be thought to partially suppress the negative impact of HLA mismatches. However, this hypothesis has not yet been totally confirmed. A higher number of TNCs and a lower number of HLA mismatches were correlated with a higher likelihood of engraftment. On the other hand, higher HLA mismatch is related to higher incidence of GVHD grades III–IV and a lower incidence of relapse of acute leukemias, evidencing the graft effect against leukemia. Thus, the choice of a good unit of UCB to be used must be based on the number of TNCs and on the number of compatible HLA alleles [163].

As a result, the increasing use of UCB cells makes it necessary to expand the public (allogeneic) bank network for storage of these cells, since the more units stored, the greater the ethnic diversity that can be achieved, eventually permitting the identification of units which also contemplate racial minorities with all their haplotypes [40].

On this account, it is crucial that further research must be done to increase our knowledge of the biology, quantification, and factors that may affect UCB collections, for each day new results have shown us that we are faced with a material, which has great proliferative capacity and from which, according to recent studies, cells with embryonic characteristics have already been obtained [164]. With this, research has shown that the UCB may be in the future a source of SCs to treat not only hematological disorders but also several other diseases, since investigations into the plasticity of SCs have demonstrated the importance of these cells in restoring various other organs. Thus, a better understanding of these cells may generate outstanding findings, highly useful for preserving life, given that hitherto many questions remain unanswered. For example, if we have to choose between a unit with more nucleated cells (6×10^7) with one HLA incompatible allele, and another with less cells (4×10^7) but no HLA mismatch, which is the best for the patient? [163]. Although some studies show that the best option is to use the first sample [159, 163], since the risk of developing acute and chronic GVHD in UCB recipients with up to two HLA incompatible alleles is similar to that of a recipient of BM from an identical HLA donor [157], further studies must be performed. Doubts like this may be minimized as the biological properties of these cells are investigated and integrated into the issue that these UCB cells do include cells that are immature and highly capable of dividing before differentiating themselves, which may be crucial in evaluating transplant outcomes.

Cord Blood of Preterm Neonates

Human UCB has been recognized as a source of HSCs for transplantation. While hematopoietic properties of neonatal cord blood from full-term pregnancies have been well characterized, little is known about cord blood from early gestational ages [165]. Most studies involving UCB refer to term neonates, which are more than 37 weeks of gestational age [155, 166, 167, 168, 169] and few refer to preterm newborns with 25–37 weeks of gestation.

Hematopoietic cells appear in the embryo at the 3rd to 4th week of gestation [48]. In the fetus, these SCs originate in the yolk sac and are believed to be transferred to all other hematopoietic organs via the circulation [166], migrating from the yolk sac to the liver and spleen during the 5th to 12th week. Ultimately HSCs reach the BM throughout fetal circulation at the second to third trimester of gestation [48].

Umbilical cord blood from the early gestational human fetus is recognized as a rich source of HSCs [170]. By 34 weeks of gestation, preterm infant cord blood had a similar concentration of circulating SCs when compared with that of term infants. This gestational age-dependent decrease in HSCs of all lineages supports the hypothesis of a blood-borne transfer of hematopoiesis that appears largely complete by 34 weeks of gestation. Infants born after less than 32 weeks of gestation have high levels of circulating HSCs that may reflect the active transfer of hematopoiesis from liver to BM [166].

The absolute numbers and proportion of $CD34^+$ cells in MNCs is inversely correlated with gestational age [10, 48, 165]. The frequency of $CD34^+$ cells declines with advancing gestational age [48, 150, 151], thus both the percentage and the absolute number of $CD34^+$ cells detectable in human UCB are significantly higher in very preterm fetuses with more than 25 weeks of gestation compared with more mature preterm (about 29–35 weeks) [48]. On the other hand, in these preterm newborns, show a higher number of $CD34^+$ cells when compared to term newborns [10, 48, 169].

Other molecules change their expression in cord blood cells during ontogenesis with the initiation of the development of the human hematopoietic system. In premature newborns, the immunophenotypic profile of cord blood $CD34^+$ cells show a significantly higher expression of CD33, and a lower expression of CD38, CD117, and HLA-DR [10, 48, 150, 151, 165].

CD33 is expressed on a majority of cord blood $CD34^+$ cells of preterm neonates but only on a minor population of them in full-term neonates. In neonates with gestational age among 24 and 29 weeks, about 80% of the $CD34^+$ cells are positive for CD33 antigen. In preterm neonates with 30–36 weeks of gestational age, the frequency of $CD33^+$ cells in $CD34^+$ cells is about 50%, whereas the frequency of these cells is less than 30% in full-term newborn, with gestational age 37–41 weeks. In addition, CD33 is dominantly expressed on $CD38^-CD34^+$cells or $CD117^{low}CD34^+$ cells in cord blood of preterm neonates [10]. Thus, the gestational age is inversely correlated with the number of $CD34^+CD33^+$, and positively correlated with the number of $CD34^+CD38^+$ cells, which are increased in term infants [48].

The numbers of $CD34^+CD45^+$ cells is also significantly higher in the preterm neonates, whereas the number of $CD34^-CD38^+$ and $CD34^-CD45^+$ cells is higher in term infants. Furthermore, a significant correlation between advancing gestational age and $CD34^-CD38^+$ or $CD34^-CD45^+$ cells is found [48].

The proliferative capacity is also higher at lower gestational ages [48]. $CD33^+$ $CD34^+$ cells of preterm cord blood had high proliferative and reproducible potentials compared with $CD33^-CD34^+$ cells [10]. In addition, on a cell-to-cell basis, the proliferative potential of the primitive progenitors from immature infants (23–31 weeks) is greater than in adult BM or cord blood of term newborns [169], because the proliferative activity progressively decreased with advancing gestational age [48].

The number of CFU in preterm cord blood is correlated with the content of $CD34^+$ progenitors and twice that of cord blood from term newborn. Since preterm cord blood is richer in hematopoietic progenitors compared with term cord blood, the precursors from preterm cord blood can be extensively expanded ex vivo and this may have implications for the development of transplantation and gene transfer strategies targeting circulating fetal SCs [165].

These data suggest that the development and lineage commitment of fetal cord blood hematopoietic progenitor cells are very active during the last two trimesters of pregnancy. The most significant changes of hematopoietic cells maturation seem to occur within 25 weeks of gestation [48]. The presence of hematopoietic progenitor cells at various stages of development seems to support the migratory theory of ontogenesis of the human hematopoietic system. The relatively high number of the most primitive progenitor cells ($CD34^+$ non-coexpressing cells) at the very low gestational ages may relate to the migration process that starts in the fetal liver and only in a later stage colonizes the marrow. In addition, the presence of colonies at 19–25 weeks of gestation in fetal blood supports the hypothesis that the transfer from one anatomic location of hematopoiesis to another is via fetal circulation [48].

It has also been shown that human fetal cord blood progenitors are amenable to genetic modification by lentiviral vectors and may serve as a target for gene therapy of hematopoietic disorders by pre-natal autologous transplantation [170].

Endothelial Progenitor Cells

Introduction

Stem cells have the capacity to renew or to give rise to specialized cell types. Human UCB has been explored as an alternative source of different types of SCs [171]. Human fetal cord blood contains subsets of MNCs with the potential to form both hematological and endothelial cells [172]. EPCs and HSCs are believed to derive from common precursor cells, the hemangioblasts [173, 174]. The transmembrane glycoprotein CD34, as well as being expressed on HSCs, is also expressed on endothelial cells [175]. Moreover, EPCs and HSCs share other cell-surface antigens, including KDR and Tie-2 [173]. However, EPCs comprise less than 1% of HSCs [176].

Vasculogenesis and angiogenesis are two different processes defining the formation of new blood vessels [177]. Embryonic vascular system undergoes a series of complex, highly regulated series of events involving differentiation, migration, and association of primitive endothelial cells. This process is termed vasculogenesis. Further remodeling of the primitive vascular system forms the mature cardiovascular system. This process is known as angiogenesis (sprouting of new capillary vessels from pre-existing vasculature) (http://www.researchd.com/miscabs/tieab.htm).

Vascular and hemopoietic cells originate from the common precursor not only during embryogenesis but also in single cell transplants, thus, showing that a common precursor contributes to both the hemopoietic and endothelial lineages and demonstrating the presence of an adult hemangioblast [174]. Vascular progenitor cells which can produce all the elements of mature blood vessels, including smooth muscle, have been identified in animals [172].

In angiogenesis, where new capillaries proliferate, this process is in response to environmental stress, such as tissue ischemia [178]. EPCs have properties similar to those of embryonic angioblasts, in that they have the capacity to circulate, proliferate, and differentiate into mature endothelial cells [176].

Thus, EPCs represent a new source of cells for possible therapeutic use in an important field of health and new clinical approaches may emerge as a consequence of the current research.

General Characteristics of Endothelial Progenitor Cells

In 1997, the presence of EPC was shown in adult peripheral blood. After this discovery, many experimental studies revealed that EPCs have a potent ability for neovascularization and that the transplantation of EPC improves ischemic tissue [179, 180, 181]. EPCs exist in BM [173, 179, 181], in small percentages are found in peripheral blood [173, 179] and, recently, it was shown that human UCB [173, 179, 181] contains a large number of these cells [182].

Endothelial progenitor cells are known to propagate the neovascularization process by promoting vasculogenesis and angiogenesis [176, 183]. Human blood contains BM-derived EPCs that, besides contributing to post-natal neovascularization [184], have the capacity to colonize vascular grafts and hold promise for therapeutic neovascularization [176] and secrete angiogenic growth factors [185]. There is still some controversy in relation to the origin of EPCs [178, 184] as well as their function and phenotype. It is also not clear, if EPCs in adults originate from the BM or migrate from other sites earlier in development [178].

While mature endothelial cells have limited capacity of proliferation, endothelial cells on the site of new blood vessels may differentiate from EPCs released from the BM where the EPC originated from their precursor cells [177]. It has been reported that EPCs isolated from cord blood have a greater proliferative potential and a higher cell cycle rate than EPCs from other sources, suggesting that cord blood-derived EPCs may more effectively contribute to therapeutic vasculogenesis [179].

Phenotypic Characteristics of Endothelial Progenitor Cells

Surface Molecules Expressed in Endothelial Progenitor Cells from Umbilical Cord Blood

In 1997, a method was described to isolate EPCs from human peripheral blood [176, 186]. Nevertheless, the isolation, identification, and characterization of EPCs have been difficult due to the absence of specific endothelial markers or functional assays that differentiate EPCs from HSCs [176]. The peripheral blood of adult species contains EPCs derived from $CD34^+$ MNCs [173]. The role of human $CD34^+$ cells in human neovascularization has been investigated [184]. Several studies have suggested that in human post-natal life, analogous to the existence of the embryonic hemangioblast, the $CD34^+$ HSC population contains cells that can give rise to EPCs and endothelial cells [184].

Endothelial progenitor cells were first described as $CD34^+CD133^+$ cells in the BM [173, 178] and it was suggested that circulating EPCs are likely present in a $CD34^+CD133^+$ fraction of circulating MNCs in human peripheral blood [173]. The AC133 marker is expressed on a large subset of EPCs and HSCs, but not on the mature endothelium [176] (more information about CD133 can be obtained in the section on HSCs in this chapter). Despite many investigations, no consensus exists on the morphology or other characteristics of the cultured EPC, except that they probably express CD34 [178]. However, CD34-null mice display no vascular abnormalities, demonstrating that CD34 antigen expression is not required for normal vascular development. A $CD34^-$ cell population, that includes endothelial cell precursors, can be isolated from cord blood [175], showing evidence for the existence of $CD34^-$ endothelial cell precursors in cord blood and suggesting the use of *ex vivo*-expanded cord blood $CD34^-$ cells as a unique tool for the investigation of post-natal lineage diversification [175].

In human UCB cells, the endothelial precursors make up only approximately 1 in 10^7 MNCs but are highly enriched in the $CD133^+$ cell population. By ruling out cell fusion, the existence of an adult hemangioblast has been clearly demonstrated, but the differentiation of marrow SCs toward the endothelial lineage is an extremely rare event [174]. Interactions between $CD34^+$ cells and $CD34^-$ cells can contribute to stimulation of capillary growth.

It has been shown that coculturing of $CD34^+$ cells with $CD34^-$ cells significantly enhances EPC differentiation *in vitro* [184], and it has been suggested that $CD34^-$ and $CD14^+$ cells yield the "early EPC" [184]. *In vitro*, the EPCs differentiate into endothelial cells (ECs). Prior studies have suggested that circulating human $AC133^+$ cells have the capacity to differentiate into endothelial cells as progenitor cells. However, recent studies have demonstrated that circulating $CD34^-CD14^+$ cells also have EPC-like properties *in vitro* and *in vivo*.

It has been shown that $AC133^-CD14^+$ cells from human UCB have the potential to differentiate into endothelial cells with expression of endothelial-specific surface markers and even form cord- and tubular-like structures *in vitro* as progenitor cells [183]. These findings corroborate the hypothesis of the origin of the EPCs, since CD14 is expressed strongly on the surface of monocytes and macrophages (http://mpr.nci.nih.gov/prow).

As yet it is not completely clear how EPCs differentiate into endothelial cells and what are their characteristics. Nevertheless, EPC and endothelial cells may express similar endothelial-specific markers, including vascular endothelial growth-factor receptor-2 (VEGFR-2, KDR, Flk-1), Tie-1, Tie-2, CD34, VE-cadherin, and E-selectin. In addition to that, HSCs and progenitor cells express markers similar to endothelial cells, such as VEGRF-1, CD34, Tie-1, and PECAM (platelet-endothelial cell adhesion molecule) [177, 181]. Because EPCs and HSCs share several cell-surface antigens including KDR, Tie-2/Tek, and CD34, these premature cells should derive from common mesodermal precursor cells (i.e., hemangioblasts). Cell surface molecules such as CD34, KDR, Tie-2/Tek, and VE-cadherin are expressed by endothelial cells at the early stage of vasculogenesis. CD34 is also expressed by mature endothelial cells in adults [181].

Human vascular endothelial growth factor (VEGF), angiopoietin (ANG) and tyrosine kinase with immunoglobulin and epidermal growth factor (EGF) homology domains (TIE)-2 consist of a grouping of proteins that are involved in vascular homeostasis, vascular integrity, and angiogenesis [188].

Tie-1, Tie-2

The family of receptor tyrosine kinases Tie-1 and Tie-2 or Tek has been identified in the blood islands of the yolk sac and in endothelial cells. It is also expressed by human hematopoietic progenitor cells. A large fraction of $CD34^+$ cells from UCB and BM express Tie protein, however, peripheral blood MNCs are Tie-negative [189]. The Tek/Tie2 receptor tyrosine kinase plays a pivotal role in vascular and hematopoietic development [190]. In humans, the Tie receptor and presumably its ligand may function at an early stage of hematopoietic cell differentiation [189]. The other Tie family member, the Tie-1R, seems to be important in endothelial vascular integrity [188]. Tie-1 is a type 1 membrane receptor protein specifically expressed in developing vascular endothelial cells. Mice lacking Tie-1 or Tie-2 are lethal. Ties may represent the earliest endothelial cell lineage marker and may regulate the endothelial cell proliferation, differentiation, and proper patterning during vasculogenesis. Ties appear to be acting downstream of the VEGFRs (http://www.researchd.com/miscabs/tieab.htm).

The VEGF protein can modulate the Tie-1R via its complex with the Tie-2R. This complex provides a mechanism whereby this initiator of vessel growth and remodeling can directly modulate receptors involved in vessel stabilization [188].

Vascular Endothelial Growth-Factor Receptor

The formation of new blood vessels, angiogenesis, is critical for both embryonic development and a variety of normal post-natal physiological processes. Various pathological processes, most notably tumor growth and chronic inflammation, are also known to be dependent on the new vessel formation [191]. Vascular endothelial growth-factor receptor (VEGFR) is a ligand of VEGF and this molecule is expressed on EPC [177, 181]. The VEGF family of proteins consists of nine different proteins. It is active in angiogenesis and endothelial cell growth and can affect blood vessel permeability [188]. Members of the VEGF family regulate various aspects of blood vascular and lymphatic growth and function. VEGF acts through the tyrosine kinase receptors VEGFR-2 (KDR, Flk-1) and VEGFR-1 (Flt-1), which conveys signals that are essential for embryonic angiogenesis and hematopoiesis. Amongst the variety of factors that contribute to the regulation of this complex process, VEGF or VEGF-A is arguably the most well-characterized [191].

The ANG family is a group of proteins that are associated with VEGF that modulates and refines its activity. There are five ANG proteins (ANG-1, 2, 3, 4, and 5). ANG-1 is expressed by periendothelial cells. It also regulates angiogenesis, vascular permeability, and effects the expression of VEGFR-2 through the tyrosine kinase with immunoglobulin and EGF homology domains (Tie)-2 receptor. ANG-2 is expressed in areas undergoing vascular remodeling and is involved in neovascularization. ANG-3 seems to be expressed in the lung and cultured human umbilical vein endothelial cells and it appears to be member of the ANG family because it binds to the Tie-2R [188].

PAR-1

Human EPCs express functional proteinase-activated receptor-1 (PAR-1). PAR-1 activation induced EPC proliferation. This marker is important in blood vessel development and it is expressed and expanded from human $CD34^+$ cord blood cells. PAR-1 activation also increased CXCR4 expression on EPC and induced SDF-1 secretion, leading to autocrine stimulation. PAR-1 activation promotes cell proliferation and CXCR4-dependent migration and differentiation, leading to a proangiogenic effect [192].

KDR

Kinase insert domain receptor is a type III receptor tyrosine kinase, also known as FLK1, CD309, VEGFR, VEGFR2. Perlecan secreted by VEGF165-stimulated endothelial cells may be involved in the regulation of cellular behavior during angiogenesis. VEGFR-2 plays a crucial role in VEGF-mediated regulation of cell activity. Endothelial cell tissue transglutaminase might be involved in modulation of the cellular response to VEGF by forming an intracellular complex with VEGFR-2, and mediating its translocation into the nucleus upon VEGF stimulation (http://mpr.nci.nih.gov/prow).

Other Molecules Expressed in Endothelial Progenitor Cells

Other markers can be found on EPCs. The surface molecule PECAM (CD31) is found on monocytes and on endothelial cells. EPCs express CD11b and CD11c, as well as a low percentage of the stem/progenitor cell marker, c-kit [185]. CXCR-4, the natural receptor of the chemokine SDF-1, is widely expressed on human endothelial cells [176, 193] mainly on endothelial cells from coronary arteries, iliac arteries, and umbilical veins [193]. The CXCR4 ligand, SDF-1, can evoke a wide variety of responses from human endothelial cells and it has been shown that deletion of the chemokine receptor, CXCR4, causes disordered angiogenesis in mouse models [193].

More details about these markers can be found in the section on HSCs in this chapter.

Frequency of Endothelial Progenitor Cells from Umbilical Cord Blood

In human UCB, a rich source of hematopoietic progenitors, the majority (about 90%) of EPCs originates from the $CD34^-$ MNC population [186]. Only a minor but significant subset of cultured EPCs (about 10%) originates from the HSC-containing $CD34^+$ cell fraction. Further studies should elucidate whether this subpopulation of cells contains "true progenitors cells" with a higher capacity for proliferation and differentiation into endothelial cells [186].

As yet, there is no consensus regarding the quantity of EPCs found in the UCB or peripehral blood. Some studies have found approximately 11% of EPCs from peripheral blood coexpressed CD34 and KDR. Other studies have identified EPCs from cord blood, fetal liver, and MPB, while only about 1–2% of these cells were found in MPB and cord blood coexpressed CD34, CD133, and KDR [176].

Other molecules expressed EPCs appear in variable quantities. It was found that about 96% of the EPCs express CD14, the monocyte/macrophage surface marker. About 50% of these cells express the CD11b molecule, and about 91% of the EPCs express CD11c marker. EPCs also express about 94% of PECAM antigen, however a much lower percentage of these cells, about 1–2%, express the stem/progenitor cell marker c-kit (CD117) [185].

Culture of Endothelial Progenitor Cells from Umbilical Cord Blood

Endothelial progenitor cells can be isolated from UCB and expanded exponentially ex vivo. In contrast, human umbilical vein endothelial cells or human aortic endothelial cells derived from vessel walls are widely considered to be differentiated, mature endothelial cells [194].

The vast majority of attached endothelial-like cells derived from culturing umbilical cord MNCs originate, as previously reported, from CD34-negative cells. The endothelial-like cells obtained by short-term culture of peripheral blood MNCs are primarily derived from the monocyte/macrophage lineage and secrete angiogenic growth factors. Nevertheless, it has also been possible identify and quantify a minor proportion of EPC that has its origin in the HSC-containing $CD34^+$ cell population [186].

These findings also highlight the need to distinguish between three different types of adherent endothelial-like cells that can be isolated by culturing circulating

MNCs in the presence of endothelial growth factors: (1) Monocyte/macrophage-derived cells can attain an endothelial-like phenotype in culture and do not have a significant proliferative capacity. Such cells express monocyte/macrophage markers such as CD14 and are mostly negative for stem/progenitor cell surface markers such as CD34, CD117, and AC133. (2) True EPCs exhibit an endothelial phenotype in culture and demonstrate significant proliferation. They do not express CD14 and are likely to express stem/progenitor cell markers as well as endothelial markers while they are in circulation. However, they probably lose the stem and progenitor markers in culture (3). Circulating mature endothelial cells have either differentiated from less mature EPCs or may represent cells that have "sloughed off" from the vasculature. In culture, these can be difficult to distinguish from EPCs, because the latter may gradually cease to express stem/progenitor cell markers in culture [186].

Culture of $CD34^+$ cells from cord blood MNCs can develop EPCs [181]. On the other hand, $CD34^-$ cells from MNCs might support EPC differentiation of $CD34^+$ cells from MNCs [181], due to an interaction between $CD34^+$ and $CD34^-$ cells. Coculturing of $CD34^+$ and $CD34^-$ cells led to a significant increase in differentiation of $CD34^+$ cells to EPC as compared with cultures in which $CD34^+$ cells were cultured alone or cultures in which $CD34^+$ and $CD34^-$ cells were separated. These findings suggest that cell–cell contact between $CD34^+$ and $CD34^-$ cells are necessary for endothelial differentiation of $CD34^+$ cells [184].

Endothelial progenitor cells are estimated to make up about 2% of CD34 cells in cord blood. Since the number of EPCs in each cord blood unit is so low, it has been difficult to characterize the EPCs prior to culture by flow cytometry [176].

Some culture systems have been used to verify the potential application of cord blood-derived EPCs. The growth factors most commonly used to induce the differentiation of cord blood cells into EPCs are human VEGF-1, human fibroblast growth factor-2 (FGF-2), human EGF, insulin-like growth factor-1, and ascorbic acid [176, 180]. Other studies have used these factors in combination with SCF, FL (FLT-3 ligand) and TPO. It has been suggested that TPO plays a major role in differentiation from EPCs to endothelial cells [176].

Some studies have shown that the numbers of EPC that outgrew from culture of cord blood-MNCs is higher than from BM. A possible reason of the rapid outgrowth of EPCs from UCB might be due to the fact that cord blood progenitors have proliferative advantages, such as longer telomeres and higher cell-cycle rate, compared with adult BM progenitors [181]. It has recently been described that the cord blood-derivated EPCs have a clonogenic population with high levels of telomerase activity and high proliferative potential-endothelial colony-forming cells [178]. Currently, it is unknown whether EPCs in the UCB derived from fetal BM [181].

Clinical Importance of the Endothelial Progenitor Cells from Umbilical Cord Blood

The development of blood vessels in response to tissue ischemia constitutes a natural host defense intended to maintain tissue perfusion required for physiologic organ function. Under certain circumstances, however, including advanced age, diabetes, and hypercholesterolemia, such native angiogenesis is impaired [180].

Endothelial progenitor cells from the BM play an important role in vascular response to injury and ischemia. The mediators involved in the mobilization, recruitment, proliferation, and differentiation of EPCs are not fully understood [179]. Because EPCs exist in BM and cord blood and small percentages are found in peripheral blood, clinical trials of the transplantation of MNCs from BM or peripheral blood were performed for the treatment of ischemic diseases [179].

The EPCs are responsible for post-natal vasculogenesis in physiological and pathological neovascularization and have been used for attenuating ischemic diseases. However, EPCs from UCB were not well understood and the homing mechanisms of EPCs remain unclear [195]. The UCB-SCs differentiate into epithelial cells under *in vitro* conditions and thereby, might serve as a starting material for isolation and expansion of cells for transplantation in patients with large skin defects [171]. These findings suggest that endothelial cells progenitors may be useful for augmenting collateral vessel growth to therapeutic angiogenesis [188].

The tissue engineering is a scientific field that aims at *in vitro* fabrication of living autologous grafts with the capacity of growth, repair, and regeneration. The tissue engineered vascular grafts using human UCB derived EPCs is a non-invasive cell source for pediatric applications [196].

Human umbilical cord derived EPCs indicated exceptional growth characteristics used for tissue engineering of vascular grafts. These cells demonstrated a constant endothelial phenotype and related functional features. EPCs seem to be a promising autologous cell source with regard to cardiovascular tissue engineering, particularly for the repair of congenital defects [196]. Although little is known about generating EPC from human UCB [197], these cells appear to represent an excellent alternative source of cells in therapeutic vasculogenesis [181, 187].

Homologous or autologous transplantation of cord blood-derived EPCs may augment post-natal neovascularization in ischemic tissues. The fact that transplanted EPCs are incorporated into sites of neovascularization in adult tissues, it has been suggested a potential use of EPCs as cell vectors for gene delivery to angiogenic sites *in vivo* [181]. Because EPCs have been identified in adult human peripheral blood, many studies have shown that transplantation of EPCs improves circulation to ischemic tissues. In some studies, it has been demonstrated that therapeutic neovascularization using expanded EPCs derived from human UCB reversed diabetic neuropathy [179].

Type 1 diabetes is associated with reduced vascular repair, as indicated by impaired wound healing and reduced collateral formation in ischemia. Recently, EPCs have been identified as important regulators of these processes, and it has been shown that EPCs could be dysfunctional in diabetes [198]. Recent human studies also revealed that proliferation, adhesion, and incorporation of EPCs into vasculature were impaired in type 1 and type 2 diabetic patients, showing the beneficial effect of transplantation of cord blood-derived EPCs on diabetic neuropathy [179]. Thus, the ex vivo cell therapy, consisting of culture-expanded EPC transplantation, may be a novel therapy for diabetic neuropathy [179].

The cord blood-derived EPCs could have a potentially powerful therapeutic advantage in other ischemic diseases, especially myocardial infarction and stroke [178]. From the viewpoint of vasculogenesis, the ischemic diseases may be caused by an insufficient supply of EPCs. A number of experimental and clinical studies have revealed that ischemic heart diseases and arteriosclerosis obliterans can effectively be treated by EPC transplantation, causing post-natal neovascularization. [179, 182].

The use of UCB as an alternative source of SCs seems promising particularly in cases where the use of adult SCs for myocardial tissue repair might be limited in elderly and sick people because their cells are depleted and exhausted [85]. The $CD133^+$ cells from UCB are shown to be able to migrate, colonize, and survive in the infarcted myocardium. These cells play an important role for myocardial tissue repair in models of extensive myocardial infarction [85]. Studies have also shown that the therapeutic use of EPCs may contribute to atherosclerosis [184], and for vascular repair and targeted tumor therapy [197].

In conclusion, it has been suggested that UCB is a precious source for isolating EPCs, and transplantation of EPCs significantly augmented post-natal neovascularization [181].

Mesenchymal Stem Cells

Introduction

Stem cells have been the object of great interest for some time because of their biological features and unlimited range of use [199]. The umbilical cord contains an inexhaustible, non-controversial source of SCs for therapy [200]. In addition to HSC, human UCB contains a population of MSCs, which comprise a rare population of undifferentiated and multipotent SCs that differ from HSCs [201, 202]. MSCs are capable of supporting hematopoiesis and differentiating into three (osteogenic, adipogenic, and chondrogenic) or more (myogenic, cardiomyogenic, among others) lineages. Due to this ability, confirmed by the results of either *in vitro* experiments or *in vivo* studies, MSCs appear to be an attractive tool in the context of tissue engineering and cell-based therapy [203, 204].

Mesenchymal stem cells rapidly self-replicate, proliferate, and differentiate into mesenchymal tissues [205]. Self-renewal is a process during which a SC can divide symmetrically and give rise to two daughter SCs or divide asymmetrically and give rise to one SC and one more mature cell. In the first scenario, the number of SCs is increased, an important feature for SCs regeneration. In the second scenario, SC number is maintained as it happens in steady-state conditions [206].

Currently, BM represents the main source of MSCs for both experimental and clinical studies [203]. MSCs are an important cell population in the BM microenvironment and are considered to be engaged mainly in the support of hematopoiesis [207], since these cells differentiate into BM stroma [205]. However, UCB also contains MSCs, which can be isolated and cultured [204] and UCB-derived MSCs were highly similar to BM-derived MSCs [208]. Multipotent mesenchymal cells derived from human UCB represent promising candidates for the development of future strategies in cellular therapy [209]. Therefore, umbilical cord/placenta stroma could be regarded as an alternative source of MSCs for experimental and clinical needs [203].

Mesenchymal stem cells distribute to a wide variety of tissues following systemic or intraperitoneal injection. Numerous reports involving different animal models indicate that MSCs contribute to tissue repair and may be used in the regeneration of bone, cartilage, skeletal, muscle, and myocardium [210], since these cells have the capacity to give rise to fat, bone, and cartilage as well as to neuronal progenitors and muscle cells [210, 211]. These cells are ease to gene modification [213, 214], and immunosuppressive ability, thus holding promise for tissue engineering, gene therapy, and immunotherapy [214].

Due to their plasticity and high proliferation capacity *in vitro* [208, 212, 213], human MSCs have generated a great deal of interest because of their potential use in regenerative medicine and tissue engineering [215, 212] and there are some dramatic examples, derived from both pre-clinical and clinical studies, that illustrate their therapeutic value [215].

General Characteristics of Mesenchymal Stem Cells

Mesenchymal stem cells were first reported to reside [215, 216, 217] within the stromal compartment of BM in 1966 [215]. Previously known as stroma cells, MSCs are also recognized as colony-forming unit fibroblasts (CFU-F) [202]. These cells represent a very small fraction, 0.001–0.01% of the total population of nucleated cells in BM. However, they can be isolated and expanded with high efficiency, and induced to differentiate to multiple lineages under defined culture conditions [202, 218]. Morphologically, MSCs in their undifferentiated state are spindle shaped and resemble fibroblasts [203, 218, 219]. The fate of BM- and UCB-derived MSCs is not confined to the mesoderm layer, as they can traverse embryonic germ layer boundaries [208]. It has also been found that MPB- and UCB-MSCs express Oct4, a transcriptional binding factor present in undifferentiated cells with high proliferative capacity [87]. Some studies have suggested that the plasticity of MSCs is somewhat similar to that of embryonic stem cells (ESCs) [220, 221]. This plasticity of MSCs and the molecular mechanisms underlying it should be more extensively studied in the future [208].

Although UCB and BM are reported to be the main sources of MSCs, some studies have shown that human MSCs can be isolated from many kinds of adult or fetal human tissues [222], and they had no difference in their origin [223]. MSCs isolated from umbilical cord veins are functionally similar to BM-MSCs, but differentially expressed genes may reflect differences related to their sites of origin: BM-MSCs would be more committed to osteogenesis, whereas umbilical cord-MSCs would be more committed to angiogenesis [222].

Mesenchymal stem cells from UCB or from BM had the same biological characteristics and the function of secreting hematopoietic growth factors [224]. In a study comparing different sources of MSCs, such as adult BM, fetal BM, and human UCB it was shown that the shapes of three kinds of cells were same. There was no difference in number, size, and the expansion speed in these three kinds of MSCs [223]. MSC-like cells are also present within the umbilical vein endothelial/subendothelial layer and may be expanded in culture successfully [203].

Mesenchymal stem cells give rise to the marrow stromal environment that supports hematopoiesis [203, 222, 225], plays an important role in the process of homing [225] and enhances HSCs engraftment [225, 226]. The microenvironment also plays a fundamental role in the transdifferentiation of SCs [227]. MSCs present a wide range of differentiation potentials and a complex relationship with HSCs and endothelial cells [222]. MSCs are capable of homing to the BM and survive in the long term, for more than 1 year. Due to their particular function in the marrow microenvironment, it has been speculated that MSCs could improve allogeneic HSCs transplantation by replacing the damaged marrow stroma after myeloablative chemotherapy. Although several studies in animal models have clearly shown that MSCs help hematopoietic recovery [226].

Mesenchymal Stem Cells from Umbilical Cord Blood

Despite the fact that currently BM represents the main available source of MSCs [203], the use of BM-derived cells is not always acceptable due to some disadvantages in the clinical use of BM [203, 228]. Among these disadvantages are the highly invasive donation procedure and the decline in MSCs number and proliferative/differentiation potential with increasing age [203, 228], besides the high degree of viral infection [203]. More recently, UCB was introduced as an alternative source of hematopoietic and MSCs as its collection is less invasive [216]. As UCB is well accepted as a source of HSCs, transplantation of cord blood cells has been part of clinical practice for more than 10 years [228]. Since it has been discovered that UCB is a good source of MSCs, its use in many clinical applications has been proposed, mainly due to the good pluripotentiality and self-renewal capacity of MSCs [223, 227].

As the number of BM-MSCs significantly decreases with age, the search for adequate alternative sources of these cells for autologous and allogenic use becomes necessary. In this connection, most attention should be paid to tissues containing cells with higher proliferative potency, capability of differentiation, and lower risk of viral contamination [203], such as UCB. So, the cryopreserved human UCB fractions [219] stored in public umbilical cord banks represent a promising alternative source of MSCs for clinical use.

Umbilical cord blood has a number of advantages in cell procurement, such as vast abundance, lack of donor attrition, and low risk of transmission of herpes family viruses. Moreover, SCs in this neonatal blood are less mature than other adult cells so that they do not produce strong immune rejection in unrelated donor transplantation [208]. It is now known that the UCB graft can tolerate 1 or 2 mismatch in HLA types between a donor and recipient, which expands significantly the available donor pool [208]. This strongly implies that they may have potential application in allograft transplantation. Since placenta and UCB are homogeneous, the MSCs derived from human placenta can be transplanted combined with HSCs from UCB to reduce the potential GVHD in recipients [229]. More importantly, a large quantity of UCB units can be cryopreserved and maintained in public banks so that the unrelated donor UCB can be instantly available from the stored pool. Therefore, UCB-derived MSCs, provided that they can be routinely isolated and expanded in culture, would be the most practical tool for SC-based therapy and transplantation [208]. Furthermore, umbilical cord SCs have other properties that make them of interest as a source of cells for therapeutic use. They are isolated in large number, grow robustly and can be frozen/thawed, can be clonally expanded, and can easily be engineered to express exogenous proteins [200].

While UCB is widely accepted as a rich source of HSCs [203, 204, 219, 228] with practical and ethical advantages [219], there is still controversy in the literature as to whether UCB can serve as a source of MSCs [203, 204, 208, 219, 228, 230, 231, 232]. Though several studies have shown that full-term UCB is a rich source of MSCs [208, 223, 219, 228, 232, 233, 234], some investigators have suggested that these cells are found in early fetal blood [231], in first and mid-trimester fetal blood [208] and in preterm UCB [203], but not in full term UCB [203, 205, 231].

Where MSCs migrate at the end of gestation is not clear. Questions have arisen regarding the destination of these cells after they leave the circulation and whether excess MSCs are deposited in placenta/umbilical cord stroma, including that of blood vessels [203]. On the one hand some results indicate that UCB-MSCs had a significantly stronger osteogenic potential but less capacity in adipogenic differentiation than BM-MSCs. On the other hand, controversy exists as to whether cord blood can serve as a source of MSCs, which can differentiate into cells of different connective tissue lineages such as bone, cartilage, and fat, and little success has been reported in the literature about the isolation of such cells from cord blood [228].

Despite increasing experimental and clinical interest in recent years because of the powerful proliferation and pluripotent differentiating ability of MSCs [231], our understanding of these cells biology remains rudimentary. In fact, the basic question of how to define the MSCs remains a point of discussion and controversy. In addition, there are no quantitative assays to assess the presence of MSCs in any given population. Therefore, MSCs are currently defined by a combination of physical, morphologic, phenotypic, and functional properties, many of which are clearly non-physiologic [213].

However, despite doubts expressed in the literature [203, 204, 208, 219, 228, 230, 231, 232], it has been strongly suggested that UCB is a source of MSCs [208, 219, 223, 228, 232, 233, 234], and this biological material appears to be a rich and inexhaustible source of primitive MSCs [200] opening a new field for therapeutic research.

Other Sources of Mesenchymal Stem Cells

Besides adult BM and UCB there are other sources of MSCs. These cells are present in several fetal organs and circulate in the blood of preterm fetuses simultaneously with hematopoietic precursors [203]. MSCs have been found in human first-trimester fetal blood [218, 234], UCB from preterm fetuses [203], fetal BM [218, 223, 234], fetal lung [235], and fetal liver [218, 234, 236, 237]. These cells have also been described in periosteum, trabecular bone, adipose tissue, synovium, skeletal muscle, deciduous teeth [215], as well as in blood vessel walls in adult human saphena vein [238], and umbilical cord vein [222], and in low frequencies in adult peripheral blood [218].

Differentiation of Mesenchymal Stem Cells

If MSCs are isolated from human UCB and cultured [239] under appropriate conditions, they may differentiate into cell types of all three germ layers [228]. Recent reports demonstrate that UCB-derived MSCs can differentiate into other germ layer cells such as hepatic cells of endodermal origin and neuroglial cells of neuroectodermal origin [208].

Nevertheless, most studies on the plasticity of MSCs are performed with MSCs from BM. *In vitro* differentiation assays have shown that MSCs have the capacity to differentiate into mesodermal lineages [202, 208] toward adipogenic, osteogenic [208, 239, 225], and chondrogenic lineages [208, 225], skeletal myogenic lineages [208] including bone [202, 215, 218, 227], fat [202, 215, 227], muscle [202, 215, 218, 227], cartilage [202, 215, 218, 227], tendon [202, 218], marrow stroma [202, 218, 227], and nerve [218]. Hence, under appropriate conditions, these cells, can give rise to different types of cells *in vitro* such as osteoprogenitor cells [131, 240] or osteoblasts [201, 203, 208, 225, 241], and osteocytes [226, 242], adipocytes [131, 201, 202, 208, 225, 226, 242], chondrocytes [131, 208, 226, 242] and chondoroblasts [225], endothelial [243], neuronal cells [201, 225, 227, 232, 242], neuroglial- [204, 228] and hepatocyte-like cells [228], smooth muscle [243], skeletal myoblasts [208, 242], cardiac myocytes [225, 226, 242], astrocytes [226], and fibroblasts [225]. Given this capacity for differentiation, MSCs can contribute to the regeneration of many tissues, such as bone [215, 223, 228, 230, 232, 234, 241], cartilage [215, 223, 228, 230, 232, 234], adipose [230], muscle [215, 223, 230, 232, 234], stroma [223, 230, 234], neural [230], fat [215, 223, 228, 232, 234], tendon [223, 230, 234], and ligament [223, 234].

In a study with MSCs isolated from the umbilical cord veins, which are also morphologically and immunophenotypically similar to MSCs obtained from the BM, these cells were capable of differentiating *in vitro* into adipocytes, osteoblasts, and chondrocytes [222]. UCB-derived MSCs showed the capacity to differentiate into hepatocytes by induction of FGF-4 and hepatocyte growth factor.

These findings suggest that UCB-derived MSCs could be a new source of cell types for transplantation therapy, and it should not be regarded as medical waste because it can serve as an alternative source of MSCs to BM [228, 243].

Phenotypic Characteristics of Mesenchymal Stem Cells

Mesenchymal stem cells can be identified by flow cytometry through the use of monoclonal antibodies [210]. Phenotypically, these non-hematopoietic cells are characterized by their negativity of the hematopoietic cell markers, CD34 and CD45, and for expressing the MHC class I, but do not express MHC class II [217, 226]. Several monoclonal antibodies have been raised against MSCs, providing a panel of markers for their characterization [217]. Flow cytometric analysis shows that MSCs can be identified by the presence and absence of many other markers, as shown in Table 3.1.

Numerous proteins are secreted by MSCs, such as IL-1([241], IL-6 [244], IL-7, IL-8 [241], IL-11 [241, 244], IL-12, IL-14 [241], IL-15, LIF [241, 244], SCF, FLT-3 ligand, GM-CSF, G-CSF [241], and M-CSF [241, 244]. MSCs also express receptors for some cytokines and growth factors such as: IL-1 R (CD121a), IL-3 R (CD123), IL-4 R (CDw124), IL-6 R (CD126), IL-7 R (CD127) [241, 245], LIFR, SCFR, G-CSFR [241], VCAM-1 (CD106) [226, 241, 245], ALCAM-1 (CD166) [217, 219, 223, 225, 232, 239, 241, 245, 246, 247, 248], LFA-3 (CD58), TGF(1R, TGF(2R, IFN(R (CDw119), TNF1R (CD120a), TNF2R (CD120b), bFGFR, PDGFR (CD140A), EGFR [241, 245] and CXCR-4 [245, 252, 250, 251, 252, 253, 254, 255, 256].

CXCR4

Many studies showed that MSCs express CXCR-4 [252, 250, 251, 252, 253, 254, 255, 256]. This molecule was also shown to be strongly expressed in UCB-progenitor cells [95, 96, 97] and plays a crucial role in the homing of these cord cells to the BM microenvironment [95] after cord cell transplant.

The plasticity, differentiation, and migratory functions of MSCs in a given tissue are dependent on the specific signals present in the local micro-environment of the damaged tissue. Recent studies have identified that specific molecular signals, such as SDF-1/CXCR4, are required for the interaction of MSCs and damaged host tissues [256].

Modulation of homing capacity may be instrumental for harnessing the therapeutic potential of MSCs [255]. The engraftment of MSCs is in part explained by their expression of CXCR4, the receptors for SDF-1 [250] and studies *in vitro* suggest that the SDF-1-CXCR4 is involved in recruitment of expanded MSCs to damaged tissues [251]. However, substantial improvements in engraftment will be required in order to derive clinical benefit from transplantation, since chemokines are the most important factors controlling cellular migration. SDF-1 has been shown to be critical in promoting the migration of cells to the BM, via its specific receptor CXCR4 [254].

More details about this marker can be found in the section on HSCs in this chapter.

Table 3.1 Cell markers in mesenchymal stem cells

Presence of markers	References	Absence of markers	References
CD13	[200, 208, 239, 241, 246, 247]	CD3	[231, 246]
CD29 (ß1-integrin)	[200, 208, 217, 223, 232, 238, 239, 241, 246, 247, 248]	CD11a	[223]
CD44 (H-CAM)	[200, 208, 213, 217, 223, 231, 232, 238, 239, 241, 246, 247, 248, 263]	CD14	[87, 200, 208, 223, 232, 238, 244, 247]
CD49e	[208, 213, 249]	CD19	[246]
CD54	[208, 246]	CD28	[223]
CD59	[223]	CD31	[200, 208, 238, 247]
CD62	[213]	CD33	[200, 223, 238, 246]
CD71 (transferrin receptor)	[231, 241, 245]	CD34	[87, 200, 208, 213, 217, 223, 226, 231, 232, 238, 239, 244, 246, 247, 248, 263]
CD73 (ecto-5-′ nucleotidase, SH-3 and SH-4)	[87, 208, 210, 217, 225, 226, 219, 239, 241, 248]	CD38	[246, 247, 263]
CD90 (Thy-1)	[200, 208, 217, 223, 225, 226, 231, 232, 238, 239, 241, 246, 247, 248, 263]	CD40	[213, 232]
CD95	[232, 239]	CD45	[87, 200, 208, 217, 223, 225, 226, 231, 232, 238, 239, 244, 246, 247, 248, 263]
CD105 (SH-2, endoglin)	[87, 208, 210, 217, 219, 223, 225, 226, 231, 232, 239, 241, 246, 247]	CD80	[213, 232]
CD117 (c-kit)	[248, 261, 262]	CD86	[213, 232]
CD106 (VCAM-1, vascular cell adhesion molecule-1)	[226, 241, 245]	CD106	[208, 238, 247]
CD166 (SB-10, ALCAM)	[217, 219, 223, 225, 232, 239, 241, 245, 246, 247, 248]	CD133	[238, 247, 263]
STRO-1	[202, 217, 241, 248]	CD152	[232]
HLA-ABC (MHC-class I)	[208, 213, 226, 232, 238, 239, 241, 247]	HLA-DR (MHC Class II)	[87, 200, 208, 213, 217, 226, 232, 239, 239, 246, 247, 263]

CD29

The CD29 or fibronectin receptor, molecule belongs to the family of integrin. Integrin family members are membrane receptors involved in cell adhesion and recognition in a variety of processes including embryogenesis, hemostasis, tissue repair, immune response, and metastatic diffusion of tumor cells. The protein encoded by this gene is a beta subunit (http://mpr.nci.nih.gov/prow). Flow cytometric analysis shows that MSCs express CD29. [217, 232, 233, 239, 246, 247].

CD44

The CD44 expression has also been demonstrated on human MSCs [223, 232, 239, 241, 246, 247]. CD44 is involved in leukocyte attachment to and rolling on endothelial cells, homing to peripheral lymphoid organs and to sites of inflammation, and leukocyte aggregation. Signaling through CD44 induces cytokine release and T cell activation. The ability of CD44 to bind its ligands and growth factors changes with pattern of glycosylation (http://mpr.nci.nih.gov/prow).

CD90

The human Ig superfamily glycoprotein Thy-1 (CD90) is characterized as an adhesion molecule [257, 258]. The CD90 molecule is highly expressed in MNCs, connective tissue, various fibroblast cell lines, as well as being expressed by HSCs and neurons in several species studied. In humans, this molecule is expressed only on small percentage of fetal thymocytes and in 10–40% of $CD34^+$ cells in BM, and less than 1% of $CD3^+CD4^+$ lymphocytes in peripheral circulation (www.ncbi.nlm.nih.gov/prow). Thy-1 is identified as an activation-associated cell adhesion molecule on human dermal microvascular endothelial cells and it plays an important role in the regulation of leukocyte [257]

More details about this marker can be found in the section on HSCs in this chapter.

STRO-1

The Stro-1 molecule is present on CFU-F cells in adult human BM and potentially defines a progenitor subpopulation (E6). Stro-1^+ cells can be isolated from long-term cultures of human marrow cells by magnetic immunobeads linked to the antibody Stro-1 [259, 260].

Human marrow-derived Stro-1^+ cells have been tested for their ability to differentiate into multiple mesenchymal phenotypes [260] and studies are showing that the functions of MSCs depend on their Stro-1 phenotype [259]. Subset of marrow cells that express the Stro-1 antigen is capable of differentiating into multiple mesenchymal lineages including hematopoiesis-supportive stromal cells with a vascular smooth muscle-like phenotype, adipocytes, osteoblasts, and chondrocytes [260].

Phenotypic Heterogeneity of Mesenchymal Stem Cells

Studies have shown the heterogeneity of MSCs and the difficulty in determining some MSCs markers, since their expression is the cause of controversy. For example, while some reports indicate the presence of CD117 on MSCs [248, 261, 263], others show the absence of this marker [232, 263]. This heterogenity can also be found in the expression of CD90 (Thy1.1), SH2 (CD105 or endoglin), SH3 or SH4 (CD73), and STRO-1 have also been often observed. Characteristics of MSCs can differ between laboratories and these discrepancies arise due to the differences in isolation methods, tissues and species of origin, and culture conditions [213] as well as due to the heterogeneous nature of the samples.

Culture of Mesenchymal Stem Cells

Although BM-MSCs occur at very low frequencies of 2–5/1 × 10^6 MNCs in BM harvest, the rapid proliferation of these cells *in vitro* allows expansion of this population by a factor of 10^3 within 14–21 days of culture [227].

Mesenchymal stem cells can be isolated by selecting the CD45 negative cells (i.e., non-hematopoietic) [225]. UCB- and BM-derived MNCs are able to generate an adherent layer [208, 230, 231] [208, 264] and show a high proliferation capacity [208, 216, 264]. Adherent cells are negative for the hematopoietic markers CD34 and CD45 and HLA-DR antigen [217, 230] and these adherent cell populations exhibit fibroblast-like morphology [202, 219] and express mesenchymal markers [203]. Human placental MSCs may be a suitable feeder layer for expansion of hematopoietic progenitors from UCB *in vitro* [264]. Some results suggest that fetal have higher proliferative capacity and are less lineage committed than adult [265].

Various preparative protocols have been proposed for the acquisition and cultivation of MSCs [266]. MSCs can be extensively expanded *in vitro* and, when cultured under specific permissive conditions [218]. A MNCs fraction obtained from the full-term UCB harvest yielded an adherent layer of heterogenous cells in the primary culture, but upon the first passage of culture, highly proliferative fibroblast-like cells arose, and became predominant over cells of other types [208]. The growth of MSCs *in vitro* has been well-documented, and is of variable ease depending on the source of cells, with human MSCs being one of the less difficult types to grow [241].

For the selective isolation of BM-MSCs, total cells are washed, counted, resuspended in culture medium, and plated. Non-adherent cells are removed 24–72 h later by changing the medium. After 1 week, a heterogeneous culture develops, which is generally referred to as BM stroma. Maintenance of the culture with a twice-weekly medium change and removal of non-adherent cells results, after 2 or 3 weeks, in a relatively homogeneous culture of morphologically and immunophenotypically similar MSCs. The batch of FCS employed to cultivate these cells may introduce phenotypic variations, which show that unknown factors influence the selection and expansion of these cells. Ideal culture conditions would maintain MSCs with (a) phenotypic and functional characteristics similar to those exhibited in their original niche, (b) indefinite proliferation, and (c) a capacity to differentiate into multiple lineages. It has been shown that FGF-2 was shown to increase the lifespan of human MSCs [245].

Panepucci and colleagues cultivated MSCs obtained from umbilical vein. When these cells were cultured with dexamethasone and ascorbic acid they underwent osteogenic differentiation, as demonstrated by alkaline phosphatase expression and positive calcium staining by the von Kossa reaction. On the other hand, in culture with insulin, dexamethasone, and indomethacin, they originate adipocytes, which are identified by numerous vacuoles that stain positively with Sudan III. When cultured as a pellet in the bottom of the tube, they originate a mass of cells with chondrocyte or condroblast features such as rounded shape with a large vacuolated and basophilic cytoplasm on hematoxylin and eosin stains. The cells are disposed in nests intermingled by an extracellular matrix rich in type II and IV collagen [222].

However, many laboratories have been unable to culture MSCs from UCB. Therefore, one approach to overcome the engraftment delay after transplantation of UCB is to support these grafts by addition of significant numbers of MSCs from other sources that might improve the microenvironment [225].

Clinical Importance of the Mesenchymal Stem Cells

Stem cell transplantation is a promising treatment for many conditions. Although SCs can be isolated from many tissues, blood is the ideal source of these cells due to the ease of collection [231] and, in recent years, UCB has been used as an alternative source of MSCs to BM [204]

A potential clinical application of MSCs is their use for enhancing HSC engraftment [226]. UCB-MSCs not only have the ability to expand the primitive HSCs but also sustain their proliferation, which can amplify mainly myeloid and megakaryocytoid progenitor subsets. These findings may have clinical significance in reducing infection and hemorrhage [224].

The use of MSCs from UCB or BM in transplants has been shown to have many advantages in clinical therapy. First, MSCs are capable of homing to the BM and survive in the long term (for more than 1 year). Second, due to their particular function in the marrow microenvironment, it has been speculated that MSCs could improve allogeneic HSC transplantation by replacing the damaged marrow stroma after myeloablative chemotherapy [226].

Since it has been shown that adult BM CD45-negative cells were also able to enhance the engraftment of UCB $CD34^+$ cells [225], new therapeutic procedures can be used. Preliminary reports on cotransplantation of autologous ex vivo-expanded MSCs and HSCs from HLA-identical siblings may enhance HSC engraftment and also indicate a significant reduction in acute and chronic GVHD [210]. This strongly implies that they may have potential application in allograft transplantation. Since placenta and UCB are homogeneous, the derived from human placenta can be transplanted combined with HSCs from UCB to reduce the potential GVHD in recipients [229].

Mesenchymal stem cells represent the promise of tissue regeneration not only in hematologic diseases but also in a variety of other diseases. However, while most studies refer to the clinical use of MSCs obtained from bone morrow, recent studies have shown that MSCs from UCB can be of significant therapeutic application [208, 219, 223, 228, 232, 233, 234].

Mesenchymal stem cells have been shown to have potential clinical use in a variety of cardiovascular, neural, and orthopedic applications. These cells can be indicated in cases of myocardial infarction, muscular dystrophy, lung fibrosis, spine fusion, segmental bone defects, craniotomy defect, tendon defect, tendom defect, and meniscus, osteogenesis imperfecta, large bone defect, metachromatic leukodystrophy, Hurler syndrome, and severe idiopathic aplastic anemia [215].

It is known that spontaneous repair is limited after central nervous system (CNS) injury or degeneration because neurogenesis and axonal regrowth rarely occur in the adult brain. Fetal brain tissue has already been shown to have significant effects in patients with Parkinson's disease. Clinical use of the fetal brain tissue is, however, limited by ethical and technical problems as it requires high numbers of grafted fetal cells and immunosuppression [267]. SCs are a valuable resource for treating disease, but limited access to SCs from tissues such as brain restricts their utility [268]. However, when thinking carefully about MSCs as candidates for cellular therapy in neurological diseases, their effects on resident neural cell fate have to be considered [267]. Neurotransplantation has been used to explore the development of the CNS and for repair of diseased tissue in many diseases, and MSCs have shown several advantages as cells for neurotransplantation [269]. MSCs can migrate throughout forebrain and cerebellum, without disruption to the host brain architecture. Some MSCs within the striatum and the molecular layer of the hippocampus expressed glial fibrillary acidic protein and, therefore, differentiated into mature astrocytes. A large number of MSCs also were found within the external granular layer of the cerebellum. In addition, neurofilament positive donor cells were found within the reticular formation of the brain stem, suggesting that MSCs also may have differentiated into neurons. These results suggest that MSCs are potentially useful as vectors for treating a variety of CNS disorders [268].

The transplantation of autologous MSCs can enhance angiogenesis and cardiac function in ischemic hearts [270]. BM cells are reported to contribute to the process of regeneration following myocardial infarction [271]. Although many cell types related to BM contribute to organ repair in infarction models [227], it has been suggested that the origin of the vast majority of BM-derived cardiomyocytes is MSCs [271]. BM-MSCs have the greatest potential for repairing myocardia, since these cells have a strong capability of penetrating the myocardium from the coronary artery and significantly regenerate the myocardium [227, 272]. The time window was the key problem for transplantation of BM-SCs in patients with myocardial infarction and remained unclear. It has been suggested that the best time for transplantation was 7–14 days after acute myocardium infarction [227]. The use of skeletal myoblasts has invariably succeeded in reconstituting the structure of heart muscle, that is, the myocardium and coronary vessels [227]. MSCs isolated from adult BM provide an excellent model for development of SC therapeutics, and their potential use in the cardiovascular system is currently under investigation in laboratory and clinical settings [273]. Hence, cellular cardiomyoplasty is also a promising approach to improve post-infarcted cardiac function [274].

Full-term UCB may act as an appropriate source of osteoprogenitor cells will impact significantly on the development of autologous tissue- engineered bone constructs [240]. Osteocytes are the most abundant cells in bone and there is increasing evidence that they control bone remodeling via direct cell-to-cell contacts and by soluble factors. Osteocytes have an active stimulatory role in controlling bone formation [275].

Buerger's disease is a vaso-occlusive disease for which there is no curative medication or surgery. The necrotic skin lesions were healed within 4 weeks. Because an animal model of Buerger's disease is absent and also in order to understand human results. Therefore, it is suggested that human UCB-derived MSCs transplantation may be a new and useful therapeutic armament for Buerger's disease and other similar ischemic diseases [276].

Mesenchymal stem cells are believed to modulate the immune system and may have applications in both the induction of tolerance in transplantation in both the induction of tolerance in transplantation and in the treatment of autoimmune diseases [207]. Reinjecting mesenchymal cells associated with hematopoietic cells ensured effective treatment of the autoimmune disease, confirming the key therapeutic role for MSCs. Thus, mesenchymal cells hold promise for the treatment of autoimmune disease. Their therapeutic effects are mediated by immunosuppressive properties, which have been abundantly documented in xeno-allogeneic graft experiments. In addition, these cells can be used to achieve targeted expression of anti-inflammatory molecules such as cytokines or TNF receptor within diseased tissues [243].

Mesenchymal stem cells can retain hepatogenic potential suitable for cell therapy and transplantation against intractable liver diseases since they are able to differentiate into hepatocyte-like cells [277]. Cartilage engineered from cord blood may prove useful for the treatment of select congenital anomalies [278], as articular cartilage is frequently damaged in different pathological situations such as osteoarthritis, rheumatoid arthritis, and trauma [273]. The function of adipocytes derived from human MSCs from fetal liver and adult BM was investigated for the first time in the study by Ryden and colleagues in 2003 [236]. MSCs differentiate readily into chondrocytes, adipocytes, osteocytes, and they can also support embryonic SCs in culture. Evidence suggests MSCs can also express phenotypic characteristics of endothelial, neural, smooth muscle, skeletal myoblasts, and cardiac myocyte cells [273].

In summary, these findings open the possibility of expanding clinical research with MSCs from UCB.

Immunoprivileged and Immunosuppressed Effects of Mesenchymal Stem Cells

Mesenchymal stem cells derived from postpartum human placenta, an important and novel source of multipotent SCs, suppress blood lymphocyte proliferation, thus they may be used to reduce GVHD in recipients [239]. The negative GVHD correlated markers might result from the fact that MSCs had no significant HLA barrier but had broad clinical use [223]. Undifferentiated MSCs do not express immunologically relevant cell surface markers [212]. These cells expressed class MHC-I, but they did not express MHC-II molecules [212, 229, 244].

Recent studies have shown that MSCs have profound immunomodulatory function [207, 225]. Thus, MSCs ought to be seen as immunoprivileged or immunomodulating cells which are potentially available for HLA-incompatible cell replacement therapies [212]. However, as yet little is known regarding these mechanisms [225].

The ability of MSCs to regulate immune response might also be harnessed to reduce GVHD, the idea underlying a multicenter clinical trial in which patients with advanced hematologic malignancies received donor MSCs at the time of hemopoietic stem-cell infusion as prophylaxis for GVHD. Some studies have shown that the incidence of acute and chronic GVHD is significantly lower among the patients infused with MSCs compared with controls [206].

The immunoregulatory feature of MSCs is important for clinical therapies [237]. MSCs are able to suppress proliferation of T lymphocytes [212, 225] playing a role in the functional activation of lymphocytes [225]. It has been shown that undifferentiated and differentiated MSCs do not stimulate alloreactive lymphocyte proliferative responses and modulate immune responses [210, 212, 237]. Thus, MSCs are not rejected by the immune system, even after allogeneic transplantation, because they are not recognized by T cells [244]. These findings indicate that MSCs can be transplantable between HLA-incompatible individuals [210] and strongly implies that they may have a potential application for allogenic [237] or xenogenic transplantation [212].

Since it is possible to obtain placenta and UCB from the same donor, placenta is an attractive source of MSCs for co-transplantation in conjunction with UCB-derived HSCs to reduce the potential GVHD in recipients.

Side Effects of Immunosuppression

Recently, there has been a great deal of interest in the immunosuppressive role of MSCs [226]. However, MSCs also suppress some T-cell functions in transplanted hosts [241], and could favor tumor growth, so a cautious approach is needed [241, 226]. Nevertheless, side effects of immunosuppressive agents and mobidity resulting from lifelong immunosuppression, especially high cancer incidence among recipients, remain substantial problems [207].

In allogeneic transplantations in which the graft versus tumor effect is expected, the presence of MSCs in the cell transplant might counteract the graft anti-tumor response. Furthermore, it has been clearly demonstrated that stromal cells in total BM transplantation were responsible for the immunosuppressive effect in patients suffering from lupus and was shown, in that case, to be beneficial in treating the disease. Regardless of the mechanisms underlying the tolerigenic properties of MSCs, their role in cancer development, as well as in autoimmune diseases, remains unclear [226].

Thus, caution is needed whenever MSCs are to be used clinically, particularly allogeneic cells, especially with those recipients who may be at risk of tumor growth (smokers, families with hereditable cancers, etc) [241]. Although the potential side effects of immunosuppression induced by MSCs have to be considered in further clinical studies [226] and clearly need much further investigation [241], the usefulness of MSCs for various therapeutic applications still remains of great interest [226].

Homing of Mesenchymal Stem Cells

Human MSCs are increasingly being considered in cell-based therapeutic strategies for regeneration of various organs/tissues. However, the signals required for their homing and recruitment to injured sites are not yet fully understood [251].

It is known that MSCs can also attract hematopoietic cells by expressing chemokine receptors and secreting SDF-1 [244]. Some studies have shown that the SDF-1-CXCR4 system may be involved in recruitment of expanded BM- and CB-derived MSCs to damaged tissues [251].

In an animal model study of myocardial infarction, where BM-MSCs were delivered by left ventricular cavity infusion, there was drastically lower lung uptake, better uptake in the heart, and specifically higher uptake in infarcted compared with sham-myocardial infarcted hearts. Histological examination at 1 week after infusion identified labeled cells either in the infarcted or border zone but not in remote viable myocardium or sham-myocardial infarction hearts and labeled cells were also identified in the lung, liver, spleen, and BM [272].

In another animal model study of myocardial infarction using autologous MSCs, 2 months after the cell transplantation, there was significant improvement of left ventricular function, showing that autologous MSCs transplantation may represent a promising therapeutic strategy for neovascularization in ischemic heart diseases, free of ethical concerns and immune rejection [270].

Several studies have shown that after infusion of MSCs labeled with green fluorescent protein into sublethally irradiated recipients in an animal model, the animals showed the homing of these cells in different tissues/organs after 7, 14, and 28 days following infusion. These cells were found mainly in gut, liver, lung, kidney, skin and spleen, and, to a lesser extent, but also in significant percentage, in brain, muscle, and heart [211]. These findings show the homing of the MSCs to different tissues, proving their clinical importance.

Gene Therapy with Mesenchymal Stem Cells from Umbilical Cord Blood

Human UCB may be used not only in cell transplantation but also in a wide range of gene-therapy treatments [232], since MSCs are vehicles for gene therapy in a variety of diseases [202, 213, 269].

Mesenchymal stem cells are easily transduced by a variety of vectors and therefore can be envisioned as vehicles for either short-term or long-term gene transfer. This could be to facilitate the therapeutic effect of MSCs, as in bone morphogenetic protein expression for bone repair, or MSCs could be used as "factories" for secreted protein deficiency disorders such as the hemophiliac [213].

Comparison with a library of $CD34^+$ cells revealed that MSCs had a larger number of expressed genes in the categories of cell adhesion molecule, extracellular, and development. MSCs express several transcripts for various growth factors and genes suggested to be enriched in SCs. Some studies have already reported the profile of gene expression in MSCs and identified the important contribution of extracellular protein products, adhesion molecules, cell motility, TGF-ß signaling, growth factor receptors, DNA repair, protein folding, and ubiquination as part of their transcriptome [279].

Mesenchymal stem cells have also been successfully used to express therapeutic genes such as EPO and anti-hemophilia factors, with effects that lasted more than 3 months [244]. Another intriguing strategy is the use of genetically engineered MSCs as delivery agents for chemotherapy. This is supported by the observation of specific homing of intravenously administered MSCs, engineered to produce interferon-β, to tumors with subsequent regression of tumor in a xenogeneic mouse model [213].

Other studies analyzed gene expression profiles of human MSCs isolated from different sources such as adipose tissue, UCB, and BM under the same growth conditions and compared them to terminally differentiated human fibroblasts. No phenotypic differences were observed by flow cytometry using a panel of 22 surface antigen markers, however many genes were differentially expressed in MSCs from different ontogenetic sources or from different culture conditions [263]. These findings should be taken into consideration when choosing the sources of MSCs for gene therapy.

Other Stem Cells

Accumulated evidence suggests that in addition to HSCs, MSCs and EPCs, UCB, or BM can also harbor other SCs, such as unrestricted somatic stem cells (USSCs), multipotential adult progenitor cells (MAPCs) [280, 281], pluripotent stem cells (PSC) [280], marrow isolated adult multilineage inducible (MIAMI) cells [281], as well as tissue committed stem cells (TCSC) [280]. With the exception of the USSCs, most of these cells have been described in research on BM, but not in umbilical cord cells. On the other hand, some studies have suggested that some of these cells can be subsets of MNCs.

Although it is not known if these cells can be found in other tissues besides BM, it is important to know some of their characteristics.

Unrestricted Somatic Stem Cells

Recently a new, intrinsically pluripotent, CD45-negative population from human cord blood, termed USSCs was described. USSCs are spindle-shaped and between 20 and 25 μm in size. The authors show that this rare population grows adherently and can be expanded to 10^{15} cells without losing pluripotency while maintaining a normal karyotype. *In vitro* USSCs showed homogeneous differentiation into osteoblasts, chondroblasts, adipocytes, and hematopoietic and neural cells including astrocytes and neurons that express neurofilament, sodium channel protein, and various neurotransmitter phenotypes [282]. Recent reports have shown the possibility of USSCs being able to differentiate under defined culture conditions into at least bone, cartilage, adipose, and muscle cells *in vitro* [283], and their use in repairing of lung, liver, skin, and skeletal muscle under conditions of tissue injury [284].

The phenotypic features show that USSCs are negative for CD14, CD33, CD34, CD45, CD49b, CD49c, CD49d, CD49f, CD50, CD62E, CD62L, CD62P, CD106, CD117, glycophorin A, and HLA-DR and expressed high levels of CD13, CD29, CD44, CD49e, CD90, CD105, vimentin, and cytokeratin 8 and 18, human Endo, low levels of CD10, and FLK1 (KDR), and showed variable but weak expression of HLA-ABC. Another interesting finding is that the average telomere length of USSCs obtained after several population doublings (or passages) is significantly longer than the telomere length of MSCs generated from an adult BM donor [282].

In vivo differentiation of USSCs along mesodermal and endodermal pathways was demonstrated in animal models and no tumor formation was observed in any of these animals. They found *in vitro* and *in vivo* differentiation of USSCs into neural cells, bone, cartilage, adipocytes, hematopoietic, hepatic, and myocardial cells and Purkinje fibers [282].

The authors reported several advantages regarding USSCs. While several groups were unable to generate MSCs or generated MSCs only in a limited number of cord blood specimens, the USSCs can be expanded to at least 10^{15} cells. Their study showed an adherent cell population that after ex vivo expansion allowed directed differentiation into bone, cartilage, hematopoietic cells, neural, liver, and heart tissue *in vivo* in various animal models [282]. USSCs also produce functionally significant amounts of hematopoiesis-supporting cytokines and seem to expand $CD34^{+}$ cells from cord blood better than MSCs from BM. This would suggest that USSCs are therefore a suitable candidate for stroma-driven ex vivo expansion of hematopoietic cord blood cells for short-term reconstitution [285].

One major difference compared to human MSCs is the distribution of USSC-derived cells in the heart. USSC-derived cells form both Purkinje fiber cells and cardiomyocytes. This would indicate that the USSCs are of an earlier cell type than multipotent MSCs, possibly representing also the precursor cell for MSCs. The ability of the USSCs to form more than one cell type suggests that these cells may be a valuable source of cells for the repair of the infarcted heart [282]. Other studies have found that USSCs isolated from UCB have great potential to differentiate into myogenic cells and induce angiogenesis. The effects of USSCs on myocardial regeneration and improvement of heart function after myocardial infarction were evaluated in a porcine model, and showed that USSCs implantation will be efficacious for cellular cardiomyoplasty [286].

Characterization of a cord blood-derived USSCs with capacity to differentiate into hematopoietic and non-hematopoietic tissues in the absence of cell fusion has highlighted the great potential of SC plasticity. A great variety of SC types have been defined and even the most pure marrow SCs are highly heterogeneous [284].

Multipotent Adult Progenitor Cells

Multipotent adult progenitor cells are a rare population within human BM-MSC cultures that can be expanded for more than 80 population doublings. They have been isolated from BM in several species of mammal. It has been shown that these cells differentiate not only into mesenchymal but also endothelium and endoderm lineage cells [221], suggesting that they have properties similar to ESCs, since they can differentiate in vitro to cells of the three germ layers.

These cells contribute to most somatic tissues when injected into tissue-specific cell types in response to cues provided by different organs. It is widely known that ESCs are pluripotent cells derived from the inner cell mass of the blastocyst that can be propagated indefinitely in an undifferentiated state. ESCs differentiate to all cell lineages in vivo and differentiate into many cell types in vitro. Although ESCs have been isolated from humans, their use in research as well as therapeutics is encumbered by ethical considerations. SCs also exist for most tissues, including hematopoietic, neural, gastrointestinal, epidermal, hepatic, and MSCs. However, when compared with ESCs, tissue-specific SCs have less self-renewal ability and, although they differentiate into multiple lineages, they are not pluripotent [221].

When injected into an early blastocyst, single MAPCs contribute to most, if not all, somatic cell types [221] including all of the cell types in the CNS [213]. On transplantation into a non-irradiated host, it was shown that MAPCs engraft and differentiate to the hematopoietic lineage, in addition to the epithelium of liver, lung, and gut. Engraftment in the hematopoietic system as well as the gastrointestinal tract was found to increase when MAPCs were transplanted in a minimally irradiated host [221].

Nevertheless, some important biological differences between human MAPCs generated from BM and USSCs were shown, such as the ease of generation of USSCs in cytokine-free cultures [282].

According to some studies, in contrast to classic MSCs, MAPCs are capable of in vitro differentiation into endothelial, epithelial, and mesenchymal cell types. However, although MAPCs may represent a more primitive, pluripotent progenitor of MSCs, the relationship between the two cell types remains speculative, and the in vivo correlation of either cell has not been definitively identified [213]. In spite of this, as MAPCs proliferate extensively without obvious senescence or loss of differentiation potential, they may be an ideal cell source for therapy of inherited or degenerative diseases [221].

Marrow Isolated Adult Multilineage Inducible Cells

Marrow isolated adult multilineage inducible cells are described as a population of non-transformed pluripotent human cells from BM after a unique expansion/

selection procedure. This procedure was designed to provide conditions resembling the in vivo microenvironment that is home for the most-primitive SCs. Marrow-adherent and -non-adherent cells when co-cultured on fibronectin, at low oxygen tension, for 14 days, colonies of cells express numerous markers found among ESCs as well as mesodermal-, endodermal-, and ectodermal-derived lineages. These cells have been differentiated to bone-forming osteoblasts, cartilage-forming chondrocytes, fat-forming adipocytes, and neural cells and to attachment-independent spherical clusters expressing genes associated with pancreatic islets. MIAMI cells proliferate extensively without evidence of senescence or loss of differentiation potential and thus may represent an ideal candidate for cellular therapies of inherited or degenerative diseases [287].

Tissue Committed Stem Cells

Another type of cell was identified in the BM in addition to other SCs already described. It is a rare population of heterogenous CD45-negative non-hematopoietic cells called TCSC [281]. These non-hematopoietic TCSC give rise to cells building particular tissues [206] and are enriched in population of $CXCR4^{+}$ $CD34^{+}$ $AC133^{+}$ lin^{-} $CD45^{-}$ in humans, in contrast to HSCs that are widely known be positive for CXCR4, CD34, AC133, and CD45 molecules [281].

Accumulated evidence suggests that in addition to HSCs, BM also harbors versatile subpopulations of TCSC and perhaps even more primitive pluripotent SCs [288].

The vast majority of research with different types of SCs has been performed with cells collected from BM. However, it is possible that different types of SCs can be found in human UCB in future studies, as more and more studies are being carried out on this source.

Final Remarks

Stem cells expressing CD34, CD133, and CXCR-4, and other markers, have been utilized in progenitor cell transplant regimes not only in BM transplant but also in many other therapeutic procedures. The success of the initial results of the use of SCs in the treatment of diseases other than those of hematologic origin has opened the possibility of new therapies based on the use of SCs from UCB, which has, among many other advantages, that of having greater donor availability. It is estimated that, as well as widening the clinical use of SCs for hematological and cardiac diseases, an extensive variety of diseases, such as auto-immune and neurodegenerative diseases, among others, will be treatable, in the near future, with cells obtained from human UCB.

However, many aspects need more in-depth understanding. The precise signaling pathways of SCs that determine their differentiated fate are not fully understood.

HSCs have been used in clinical approaches for more than three decades. Despite this, questions remain with regard the true plasticity of these cells. Clinical use of EPCs is interesting, however, their low quantity is an important inhibitory factor in their use and improved culture protocols need to be developed. Experiments with MSCs have highlighted a paradox: whereas they are easily manipulated in vitro to perform virtually on command, they have confirmed surprisingly resistant to in vivo manipulation. Moreover, although ease of expansion in culture is one of the primary advantages of MSCs, fundamental questions regarding the existence, phenotype, and function of MSCs from UCB in vivo remain to be answered [213].

Numerous papers in the literature show intriguing and interesting results. Some may lead us to ask whether "Umbilical cord blood" is "a perfect source of stem cells?" [199]. Others show that we have a long way to go before important questions can be answered: "Stem cell biology – a never ending quest for understanding" [206].

However, the wider use of BM in clinical studies has been impeded by a number of disadvantages, such as donor-invasive procurement, tight HLA restriction, and high risk of transmitting viral diseases. Hence, it has been suggested that UCB can be an alternative source of cells to BM [208]. As an inexhaustible source of cells, the cord blood seems to have more advantages than BM as it exhibits a lower frequency of GVHD after transplantation and lower risk of viral transmission, among other advantages.

Thus, it is of great importance that knowledge of the biology and plasticity of the SCs present in cord blood is expanded, with the aim of widening its clinical use, making it possible to develop new therapeutic procedures, including gene therapy. It is also necessary to expand the number of public umbilical blood banks in order to increase the supply of units of donated UCB, so that, in the future, the cells they possess can be made available for the treatment of a number of seriousor currently incurable diseases that affect so many patients

List of Abbreviations

UCB	Umbilical cord blood
HSCs	Hematopoietic stem cells
EPCs	Endothelial progenitor cells
MSCs	Mesenchymal stem cells
SCs	Stem cells
BM	Bone marrow
MNCs	Mononucleated cells
MPB	Mobilized peripheral blood
HLA	Human leukocyte antigen
GVHD	Graft-versus-host disease
MAPCs	Multipotential adult progenitor cells
PSC	Pluripotent stem cells
MIAMI	Marrow isolated adult multilineage inducible
TCSC	Tissue committed stem cells

References

1. McNiece I, Kubegov D, Kerzic P, et al. Increased expansion and differentiation of cord blood products using a two-step expansion culture. Exp Hematol 2000; 28: 1181–6.
2. Wagner JE, Barker JN, DeFork TE, et al. Transplantation of unrelated donor umbilical cord blood in 102 patients with malignant and nonmalignant diseases: influence of CD34 cell dose and HLA disparity on treatment-related mortality and survival. Blood 2002; 100: 1611–8.
3. Yamaguchi M, Hirayama F, Kanai M, et al. Serum-free coculture for ex-vivo expansion of human cord blood primitive progenitors and SCID mouse-reconstituting cells using human bone marrow primary stromal cells. Exp Hematol 2001; 29: 174–2.
4. Gluckman E, Koegler G, Rocha V. Human leukocyte antigen matching in cord blood transplantation. Semin Hematol 2005; 42: 85–9.
5. Gluckman E, Broxmeyer HA, Auerbach AD, et al. Hematopoietic reconstitution in a patient with Fanconi's anemia by means of umbilical-cord blood from an HLA-identical sibling. N Engl J Med 1989; 321: 1174–8.
6. Rubinstein P, Dobrila L, Rosenfield RE, et al. Processing and cryopreservation of placental/umbilical cord blood for unrelated bone marrow reconstitution. Proc Natl Acad Sci USA 1995; 92: 10119–22.
7. Bradley MB, Cairo MS. Cord blood immunology and stem cell transplantation. Hum Immunol 2005; 66: 431–46.
8. Aroviita P, Teramo K, Hiilesmaa V, et al. Cord blood progenitor cell concentration and infant sex. Transfusion 2005; 45: 613–21.
9. Piacibello W, Sanavio F, Garetto L, et al. Extensive amplification and self-renewal of human primitive hematopoietic stem cells from cord blood. Blood 1997; 89: 2644–53.
10. Jin CH, Takada H, Nomura A, et al. Immunophenotypic and functional characterization of $CD33^{+}CD34^{+}$ cells in human cord blood of preterm neonates. Exp Hematol 2000; 28:: 1174–80.
11. Quesenberry PJ, Colvin GA. Hematopoietic stem cells, progenitor cells, and cytokines. In: Williams W, Beutler E, Coller BS, Lichtman MA, Kipps TJ, Seligsohn U. editors. Hematology 6th ed. New York: McGraw-Hill; 2001. p. 153–74.
12. Williams DA. Stem cell model of hematopoiesis. In: Hoffman R, Benz EJ, Shattil SJ, Furie B, Cohen HJ, Silberstein LE, McGlave P. Hoffman R. editors. Hematology – Basic Principles and Practice 4th ed. New York: Elsevier Science Health Science; 2004. p. 2821.
13. McNiece I, Briddell R. *Ex vivo* expansion of hematopoietic progenitor cells and mature cells. Exp Hematol 2001; 29: 3–11.
14. Bagby Jr, Heinrich MC. Growth factors, cytokines, and control of hematopoiesis. In: Hoffman R, Benz EJ, Shattil SJ, Furie B, Cohen HJ, Silberstein LE, McGlave P. editors. Hematology – Basic Principles and Practice 3rd ed. New York: Churchill Livingstone; 2000. p. 154–202.
15. Ramsfjell V, Borge OJ, Cui L, et al. Thrombopoietin directly and potently stimulates multilineage growth and progenitor cell expansion from primitive ($CD34^{+}CD38^{-}$) human bone marrow progenitor cells. J Immunol 1997; 158: 5169–77.
16. D'Arena G, Musto P, Cascavilla N, et al. Carotenuto M. Thy-1 (CDw90) and c-kit receptor (CD117) expression on $CD34^{+}$ hematopoietic progenitor cells: a five dimensional flow cytometric study. Haematologica 1998; 83: 587–93.
17. McGuckin CP, Pearce D, Forraz N, et al. Multiparametric analysis of immature cell populations in umbilical cord blood and bone marrow. Eur J Haematol 2003; 71: 341–50.
18. Ruzicka K, Grskovic B, Pavlovic V, et al. Differentiation of human umbilical cord blood $CD133^{+}$ stem cells towards myelo-monocytic lineage. Clin Chim Acta. 2004; 343(1–2):: 85–92.
19. Mayani H, Landsdorf PM. Biology of umbilical cord blood-derived hematopoietic stem/progenitor cells. Stem Cells 1998; 16: 153–65.
20. Civin CI, Gore SD. Antigenic analysis of hematopoiesis: a review. J Hematother 1993; 2: 137–44.

21. Verfaillie CM. Anatomy and physiology of hematopoiesis. In: Hoffman R, Benz EJ, Shattil SJ, Furie B, Cohen HJ, Silberstein LE, McGlave P. editors. Hematology – Basic Principles and Practice 3rd ed. New York: Churchill Livingstone; 2000. p. 139–54.
22. Verfaillie CM. Hematopoietic stem cells for transplantation. Nat Immunol 2002; 3: 314–7.
23. Sutherland DR, Keating A. The CD34 antigen: structure, biology and potential clinical applications. J Hematother 1992; 1: 115–29.
24. Huss R. Perspectives on the morphology and biology of CD34-negative stem cells. J Hematother Stem Cell Res 2000; 9: 783–93.
25. Goodell MA. $CD34^+$ or $CD34^-$: Does it really matter? Blood 1999; 94(8): 2545–7.
26. Dao MA, Arevalo J, Nolta JA. Reversibility of CD34 expression on human hematopoietic stem cells that retain the capacity for secondary reconstitution. Blood 2003; 101(1): 112–8.
27. Belvedere O, Feruglio C, Malangone W, et al. Phenotypic characterization of immunomagnetically purified umbilical cord blood $CD34^+$ cells. Blood Cells Mol Dis 1999; 25: 141–6.
28. Malangone W, Belvedere O, Astori G, et al. Increased content of $CD34^+CD38^-$ hematopoietic stem cells in the last collected umbilical cord blood. Transplant Proc 2001; 33: 1766–8.
29. Sutherland DR, Anderson L, Keeney M, et al. The ISHAGE guidelines for $CD34^+$ cells determination by flow cytometry. J Hematother 1996; 5: 213–26.
30. Keeney M, Chin-Yee I, Weir K, et al. Single platform flow cytometric absolute $CD34^+$ cell counts based on the ISHAGE guidelines. Cytometry 1998; 34: 61–70.
31. Barnett D, Janossy G, Lubenko A, et al. Guideline for the flow cytometric enumeration of $CD34^+$ haematopoetic stem cells. Clin Lab Haematol 1999; 21: 301–8.
32. Kipps TJ. The cluster of differentiation antigens. In: Williams W, Beutler E, Coller BS, Lichtman MA, Kipps TJ, Seligsohn U. editors. Hematology 6th ed. New York: McGraw-Hill; 2001. p. 141–52.
33. Kinniburgh D, Russell NH. Comparative study of CD34 positive cells and subpopulations in human umbilical cord blood and bone marrow. Bone Marrow Transplant 1993; 12: 489–94.
34. Fritsch G, Stimpfl M, Buchinger P. Does cord blood contain enough progenitor cells for transplantation? J Hematother 1994; 3: 291–8.
35. Van Epps DE, Bender J, Lee W. Harvesting, characterization, and culture of $CD34^+$ cells from human bone marrow, peripheral blood and cord blood. Blood Cells 1994; 20: 411–23.
36. Pranke P, Hendrikx J, Debnath G, et al. Immunophenotype of hematopoietic stem cells from placental/umbilical cord blood after culture. Braz J Med Biol Res 2005; 38: 1775–89.
37. Pranke P, Hendrikx J, Alespeiti G, et al. Comparative quantification of umbilical cord blood $CD34^+$ and $CD34^+$ bright cells using the ProCount-BD and ISHAGE protocols. Braz J Med Biol Res 2006; 39(7): 901–6.
38. Campagnoli C, Fisk N, Overton T, et al. Circulating hematopoietic progenitor cells in first trimester fetal blood. Blood 2000; 95: 1967–72.
39. Hao QL, Shah AJ, Thiemann FT, et al. A functional comparison of $CD34^+CD38^-$ cells in cord blood and bone marrow. Blood 1995; 86: 3745–53.
40. Chin-Yee I, Anderson L, Keeney M, et al. Quality assurance of stem cell enumeration by flow cytometry. Cytometry 1997; 30: 296–303.
41. Barnett D, Granger V, Storie I, et al. Quality assessment of $CD34^+$ stem cell enumeration: experience of the United Kingdom National External Quality Assessment Scheme (UK NEQAS) using a unique stable whole blood preparation. Br J Haematol 1998; 102: 553–65.
42. Brocklebank AM, Sparrow RL. Enumeration of $CD34^+$ cells in cord blood: a variation on a single-platform flow cytometric method based on the ISHAGE gating strategy. Cytometry. 2001; 46: 254-2654-25ar sobre coletas e exames Lab.1.
43. Yap C, Loh MT, Heng KK, et al. Variability in $CD34^+$ cell counts in umbilical cord blood: implications for cord blood transplants. Gynecol Obstet Invest 2000; 50: 258–9.:

44. Barker JN, Weisdorf DJ, DeFor TE, et al. Rapid and complete donor chimerism in adult recipients of unrelated donor umbilical cord blood transplantation after reduced-intensity conditioning. Blood 2003; 102: 1915–19.
45. Gluckman E. Hematopoietic stem cell transplants using umbilical cord blood. N Engl J Med 2001; 344: 1860–1.
46. Cairo MS, Wagner EL, Fraser J, et al. Characterization of banked umbilical cord blood hematopoietic progenitor cells and lymphocyte subsets and correlation with ethnicity, birth weight, sex, and type of delivery: A Cord Blood Transplantation (COBLT) Study report. Transfusion 2005; 45(6): 856–66.
47. Heimfeld S. Bone marrow transplantation: how important is CD34 cell dose in HLA-identical stem cell Transplantation? Leukemia 2003; 17: 856–8.
48. Gasparoni A, Ciadella L, Avanzini MA, et al. Immunophenotypic changes of fetal cord blood hematopoietic progenitor cells during gestation. Pediatr Res. 2000; 47: 825–9.
49. Keeney M, Gratama JW, Sutherland R. Critical role of flow cytometry in evaluating peripheral blood hematopoietic stem cell grafts. Cytometry 2004; 58A: 72–5.
50. Frassoni F, Podesta M, Maccario R, et al. Cord blood transplantation provides better reconstitution of hematopoietic reservoir compared with bone marrow transplantation. Blood 2003; 102(3): 1138–41.
51. Gratama JW, Orfao A, Barnett D, et al. Flow cytometric enumeration of $CD34^+$ hematopoietic stem progenitors cells. European Working Group on Clinical Cell Analysis. Cytometry 1998; 34 (3): 128–42.
52. Sutherland DR, Keeney M, Gratama JW. Enumeration of $CD34^+$ hematopoietic stem and progenitor cells. Curr Protocol Cytom 2003; 6.4: 1–23.
53. Gratama JW, Keeney M, Sutherland DR. Enumeration of $CD34^+$ hematopoietic stem and progenitor cells. Curr Protocol Cytom 1999; 6.4: 1–22.
54. Keeney M, Sutherland DR. Stem cell enumeration by flow cytometry: current concepts and recent developments in $CD34^+$ cell enumeration. Cytotherapy 2000; 2: 395–402.
55. Philpott NJ, Turner AJC, Scopes J, et al. The use of 7-amino actinomycin D in identifying apoptosis: simplicity of use and broad spectrum of application compared with other techniques. Blood 1996; 87: 2244–51.
56. Cabezudo E, Querol S, Concelas JA, et al. Comparison of volumetric capillary cytometry with standard flow cytometry for routine enumeration of $CD34^+$ cells. Transfusion 1999; 39(8): 864–72.
57. Shen HP, Ding CM, Chi ZY, et al. Effects of different cooling rates on cryopreservation of hematopoietic stem cells from cord blood. Sheng Wu Gong Cheng Xue Bao 2003; 19(4): 489–92.
58. Xiao M, Dooley DC. Assessment of cell viability and apoptosis in human umbilical cord blood following storage. J Hematother Stem Cell Res 2003; 12(1): 115–22.
59. Bayer-Zwirello LA, Hoffman DE, Adams LA, et al. The effect of processing and cryopreservation on nucleated umbilical cord blood cells. J Perinat Med 2004; 32(5): 430–3.
60. Van Haute I, Lootens N, De Smet S, et al. Viable $CD34^+$ stem cell content of a cord blood graft: which measurement performed before transplantation is most representative? Transfusion 2004; 44(4): 547–54.
61. Abboud CN, Lichtman MA. Structure of the marrow and the hematopoietic microenvironment. In: Williams W, Beutler E, Coller BS, Lichtman MA, Kipps TJ, Seligsohn U. editors. Hematology 6th ed. New York: McGraw-Hill; 2001. p. 29–58.
62. Encabo A, Mateu E, Carbonell-Uberos F, et al. $CD34^+CD38^-$ is a good predictive marker of cloning ability and expansion potential of $CD34^+$ cord blood cells. Transfusion 2003; 43: 383–9.
63. Ishikawa F, Livingston AG, Minamiguchi H, et al. Human cord blood long-term engrafting cells are $CD34^+$ $CD38^-$. Leukemia 2003; 17: 960–4.

64. Tian H, Huang S, Gong F, et al. Karyotyping, immunophenotyping, and apoptosis analyses on human hematopoietic precursor cells derived from umbilical cord blood following long-term ex vivo expansion. Cancer Genet Cytogenet 2005; 157: 33–6.
65. Timeus F, Crescenzio N, Basso G, et al. Cell adhesion molecule expression in cord blood $CD34^+$ cells. Stem Cells 1998; 16: 120–6.
66. Almici C, Carlo-Stella C, Wagner JE, et al. Biologic and phenotypic analysis of early hematopoietic progenitor cells in umbilical cord blood. Leukemia 1997; 11: 2143–9.
67. De Bruyn C, Delforge A, Bron D, et al. Comparison of the coexpression of CD38, CD33 and HLA-DR antigens on $CD34^+$ purified cells from human cord blood and bone marrow. Stem Cells 1995; 13: 281–8.
68. Timeus F, Crescenzio N, Marranca D, et al. Cell adhesion molecules in cord blood hematopoietic progenitors. Bone Marrow Transplant 1998; 22(1): 61–2.
69. Cho SH, Chung IJ, Lee JJ, et al. Comparison of $CD34^+$ subsets and clonogenicity in human bone marrow, granulocyte colony-stimulating factor-mobilized peripheral blood, and cord blood. J Korean Med Sci 1999; 14: 520–5.
70. Belvedere O, Feruglio C, Malangone W, et al. Increased blood volume and $CD34^+CD38^-$ progenitor cell recovery using novel umbilical cord blood collection system. Stem Cells 2000; 18: 245–51.
71. Opie TM, Shields LE, Andrews RG. Cell-surface antigen expression in early and term gestation fetal hematopoietic progenitor cells. Stem Cells 1998; 16: 343–8.
72. Theunissen K, Verfaillie CM. A multifactorial analysis of umbilical cord blood, adult bone marrow and mobilized peripheral blood progenitors using the improved ML-IC assay. Exp Hematol. 2005; 33: 165–72.
73. Berardi AC, Wang A, Levine JD, et al. Functional isolation and characterization of human hematopoietic stem cells. Science 1995; 267: 104–8.
74. Broudy VC. Stem cell factor and hematopoiesis. Blood 1997; 90(4): 1345–64.
75. Papayannopoulou T, Brice M, Broudy VC, et al. Isolation of c-kit receptor-expressing cells from bone marrow, peripheral blood, and fetal liver: functional properties and composite antigenic profile. Blood 1991; 78: 1403–12.
76. Sakabe H, Ohmizono Y, Tanimukai S, et al. Functional differences between subpopulations of mobilized peripheral blood-derived $CD34^+$ cells expressing different levels of HLA-DR, CD33, CD38 and c-kit antigens. Stem Cells 1997; 15: 73–81.
77. Anderson DM, Lyman SD, Baird A, et al. Molecular cloning of mast cell growth factor, a hemopoietin that is active in both membrane bound and soluble forms. Cell 1990; 63: 235–42.
78. Xiao M, Oppenlander BK, Plunkett JM, et al. Expression of Flt3 and c-kit during growth and maturation of human $CD34^+CD38^-$ cells. Exp Hematol 1999; 27: 916–27.
79. Sakabe H, Yahata N, Kimura T, et al. Human cord blood-derived primitive progenitors are enriched in $CD34^+$c-kit^- cells: correlation between long-term culture-initiating cells and telomerase expression. Leukemia 1998; 12: 728–34.
80. Ikehara S. Pluripotent hemopoetic stem cells in mice and humans. Proc Soc Exp Biol Med 2000; 223: 149–155.
81. Gunji Y, Nakamura M, Osawa H, et al. Human primitive hematopoietic progenitor cells are more enriched in KITlow cells than KIThigh cells. Blood 1993; 82: 3283–9.
82. Laver JH, Abboud MR, Kawashima I, et al. Characterization of c-kit expression by primitive hematopoietic progenitors in umbilical cord blood. Exp Hematol 1995; 23: 1515–90.
83. Bonanno G, Perillo A, Rutella S, et al. Clinical isolation and functional characterization of cord blood $CD133^+$ hematopoietic progenitor cells. Transfusion 2004; 44(7): 1087–97.
84. He X, Gonzalez V, Tsang A, et al. Differential gene expression profiling of $CD34^+$ $CD133^+$ umbilical cord blood hematopoietic stem progenitor cells. Stem Cells 2005; 14: 188–98.
85. Leor J, Guetta E, Feinberg MS, et al. Human umbilical cord blood-derived $CD133^+$ cells enhance function and repair of the infarcted myocardium. Stem Cells 2006; 24(3): 772–80.
86. Massa M, Rosti V, Ramajoli I, et al. Circulating $CD34^+$, $CD133^+$, and vascular endothelial growth factor receptor 2-positive endothelial progenitor cells in myelofibrosis with myeloid metaplasia. J Clin Oncol 2005; 23: 5688–95

87. Tondreau T, Meuleman N, Delforge A, et al. Mesenchymal stem cells derived from CD133-positive cells in mobilized peripheral blood and cord blood: proliferation, Oct4 expression, and plasticity. Stem Cells 2005; 23(8): 1105–12.
88. Fukuda S, Broxmeyer HE, Pelus LM. Flt3 ligand and the Flt3 receptor regulate hematopoietic cell migration by modulating the SDF-1alpha (CXCL12)/CXCR4 axis. Blood 2005; 105(8): 3117–26.
89. Rappold I, Ziegler BL, Kohler I, et al. Functional and phenotypic characterization of cord blood and bone marrow subsets expressing FLT3 (CD135) receptor tyrosine kinase. Blood 1997; 90(1): 111–25.
90. McGuckin CP, Forraz N, Baradez MO, et al. Colocalization analysis of sialomucins CD34 and CD164. Stem Cells 2003; 21(2): 162–70.
91. Watt SM, Buhring HJ, Rappold I, et al. CD164, a novel sialomucin on CD34(+) and erythroid subsets, is located on human chromosome 6q21. Blood 1988; 92(3): 849–66.
92. Banisadr G, Fontanges P, Haour F, et al. Neuroanatomical distribution of CXCR4 in adult rat brain and its localization in cholinergic and dopaminergic neurons. Eur J Neurosci 2002; 16(9): 1661–71.
93. Khan MZ, Brandimarti R, Patel JP. Apoptotic and antiapoptotic effects of CXCR4: is it a matter of intrinsic efficacy? Implications for HIV neuropathogenesis. AIDS Res Hum Retroviruses. 2004; 10: 1063–71.
94. Lee YH, Lee YA, Noh KT, et al. Homing-associated cell adhesion molecules and cell cycle status on the nucleated cells in the bone marrow, mobilized peripheral blood and cord blood. J Korean Med Sci 2004; 19(4): 523–8.
95. Kucia M, Ratajczak J, Reca R, et al. Tissue-specific muscle, neural and liver stem/progenitor cells reside in the bone marrow, respond to an SDF-1 gradient and are mobilized into peripheral blood during stress and tissue injury. Blood Cells Mol Dis 2004; 32(1): 52–7.
96. Dabusti M, Lanza F, Campioni D, et al. CXCR-4 expression on bone marrow $CD34^+$ cells prior to mobilization can predict mobilization adequacy in patients with hematologic malignancies. J Hematother Stem Cell Res 2003; 12(4): 425–34.
97. Denning-Kendall P, Singhs S, Bradley B, et al. Cytokine expansion culture of cord blood $CD34^+$ cells induces marked and sustained changes in adhesion receptor and CXCR4 expressions. Stem Cells 2003; 21: 61–70.
98. Lapidot T, Dar A, Kollet O. How do stem cells find their way home? Blood 2005; 106 (6): 1901–10.
99. Sipkins DA, Wei X, Wu JW, et al. In vivo imaging of specialized bone marrow endothelial microdomains for tumour engraftment. Nature 2005; 435: 969–73.
100. Wojakowski W, Tendera M, Michalowska A, et al. Mobilization of CD34/$CXCR4^+$, CD34/$CD117^+$, c-met^+ stem cells, and mononuclear cells expressing early cardiac, muscle, and endothelial markers into peripheral blood in patients with acute myocardial infarction. Circulation 2004; 110(20): 3213–20.
101. Kucia M, Dawn B, Hunt G, et al. Cells expressing early cardiac markers reside in the bone marrow and are mobilized into the peripheral blood after myocardial infarction. Circ Res 2004; 95(12): 1191–9.
102. Pujol F, Kitabgi P, Boudin H. The chemokine SDF-1 differentially regulates axonal elongation and branching in hippocampal neurons. J Cell Sci 2005; 118: 1071–80.
103. Stumm RK, Rummel J, Junker V, et al. A dual role for the SDF-1/CXCR4 chemokine receptor system in adult brain: isoform-selective regulation of SDF-1 expression modulates CXCR4-dependent neuronal plasticity and cerebral leukocyte recruitment after focal ischemia. J Neurosci 2002; 22(14): 5865–78.
104. Khan MZ, Brandimarti R, Musser BJ, et al. The chemokine receptor CXCR4 regulates cell-cycle proteins in neurons. J Neurovirol 2003; 9(3): 300–14.
105. Dercksen MW, Gerritsen WR, Rodenhuis S, et al. Expression of adhesion molecules on $CD34^+$ cells: $CD34^+$ L-$selectin^+$ cells predict a rapid platelet recovery after peripheral blood stem cell transplantation. Blood 1995; 85: 3313–9.

106. Bertolini F, Battaglia M, Lanza A, et al. Hematopoietic stem cells from different sources: biological and technical aspects. Bone Marrow Transplant 1998; 21(Suppl 2): 5–7.
107. Nardi NB, Alfonso ZZ. The hematopoietic stroma. Braz J Med Biol Res 1999; 32: 601–9.
108. Pranke P, Failace RR, Allebrandt WF, et al. Hematologic and immunophenotypic characterization of human umbilical cord blood. Acta Haematol 2001; 105: 71–6.
109. Asosingh K, Renmans W, Van der Gucht K, et al. Circulating $CD34^+$ cells in cord blood and mobilized blood have a different profile of adhesion molecules than bone marrow $CD34^+$ cells. Eur J Haematol 1998; 60: 153–60.
110. Watt SM, Williamson J, Genevier H, et al. The heparin binding PECAM-1 adhesion molecule is expressed by $CD34^+$ hematopoietic precursor cells with early myeloid and B-lymphoid cell phenotypes. Blood 1993; 82: 2649–63.
111. Coulombel L, Auffray I, Gaugler MH, et al. Expression and function of integrins on hematopoietic progenitor cells. Acta Haematol 1997; 97: 13–21.
112. Roy V, Verfaillie C. Expression and function of cell adhesion molecules on fetal liver, cord blood and bone marrow hematopoietic progenitors: implications for anatomical localization and developmental stage specific regulation of hematopoiesis. Exp Hematol 1999; 27: 302–12.
113. Saeland S, Duvert V, Caux C, et al. Distribution of surface-membrane molecules on bone marrow and cord blood $CD34^+$ hematopoietic cells. Exp Hematol 1992; 20: 24–33.
114. Greenberg AW, Kerr WG, Hammer DA. Relationship between selectin-mediated rolling of hematopoietic stem and progenitor cells and progression in hematopoietic development. Blood 2000; 95: 478–86.
115. McEver RP. Cell adhesion. In: Hoffman R, Benz EJ, Shattil SJ, Furie B, Cohen HJ, Silberstein LE, McGlave P. editors. Hematology – Basic Principles and Practice 3rd ed. New York: Churchill Livingstone; 2000. p. 49–56.
116. Koenig JM, Baron S, Luo D, et al. L-selectin expression enhances clonogenesis of $CD34^+$ cord blood progenitors. Pediatr Res 1999; 45: 867–70.
117. Surbek DV, Steinmann C, Burk M, et al. Developmental changes in adhesion molecule expressions in umbilical cord blood CD34 hematopoietic progenitor and stem cells. Am J Obstet Gynecol 2000; 183: 1152–7.
118. Kilpatrick DC, Atkinson AP, Palmer JB, et al. Developmental variation in stem-cell markers from human fetal liver and umbilical cord blood leukocytes. Transf Med 1998; 8: 103–9.
119. Lanza F, Moretti S, Castagnari B, et al. Assessment of distribution of CD34 epitope classes in fresh and cryopreserved peripheral blood progenitor cells and acute myeloid leukemic blasts. Haematologica 1999; 84: 969–77.
120. Yano T, Katayama Y, Sunami K, et al. Granulocyte colony-stimulating factor and lineage-independent modulation of VLA-4 expression on circulating $CD34^+$ cells. Int J Hematol 2000; 71: 328–33.
121. Tada J, Omine M, Suda T, et al. A common signaling pathway via Syk and Lyn tyrosine kinases generated from capping of the sialomucins CD34 and CD43 in immature hematopoietic cells. Blood 1999; 93: 3723–35.
122. Conneally E, Cashman J, Petzer A, et al. Expansion in vitro of transplantable human cord blood stem cells demonstrated using a quantitative assay of their lympho-myeloid repopulating activity in nonobese diabetic-scid/scid mice. Proc Natl Acad Sci USA 1997; 94(18): 9836–41.
123. Piacibello W, Sanavio F, Severino A, et al. Engraftment in nonobese diabetic severe combined immunodeficient mice of human $CD34^+$ cord blood cells after *ex vivo* expansion: evidence for the amplification and self-renewal of repopulating stem cells. Blood 1999; 93: 3736–49.
124. Dorrell C, Gan OI, Pereira DS, et al. Expansion of human cord blood CD34(+)CD38(-) cells in ex vivo culture during retroviral transduction without a corresponding increase in SCID repopulating cell (SRC) frequency: dissociation of SRC phenotype and function. Blood 2000; 95(1): 102–10.

125. Bruno S, Gunetti M, Gammaitoni L, et al. Fast but durable megakaryocyte repopulation and platelet production in NOD/SCID mice transplanted with ex-vivo expanded human cord blood $CD34^+$ cells. Stem Cells 2004; 22(2): 135–43.
126. Koller MR, Bender JG, Papoutsakis ET, et al. Effects of synergistic cytokine combinations, low oxygen, and irradiated stroma on the expansion of human cord blood progenitors. Blood 1992; 80: 403–11.
127. Shah AJ, Smogorzewska EM, Hannum C, et al. Flt3 ligand induces proliferation of quiescent human bone marrow $CD34^+CD38^-$ cells and maintains progenitor cells in vitro. Blood 1996; 87: 3563–70.
128. Yoshida M, Tsuji K, Ebihara Y, et al. Thrombopoietin alone stimules the early proliferation and survival of human erythroid, myeloid and multipotential progenitors in serum-free culture. Br J Haematol 1997; 98: 254–64.
129. Schipper LF, Brand A, Reniers NCM, et al. Effects of thrombopoietin on the proliferation and differentiation of primitive and mature haemopoietic progenitor cells in cord blood. Br J Haematol 1998; 101: 425–35.
130. Matsunaga T, Kato T, Miyazaki H, et al. Thrombopoietin promotes the survival of murine hematopoietic long-term reconstituing cells: comparison with the effects of FLT3/FLK-2 ligand and interleukin-6. Blood 1998; 92: 452–61.
131. Robinson S, Niu T, de Lima M, et al. Ex vivo expansion of umbilical cord blood. Cytotherapy. 2005; 7(3): 243–50.
132. Nauta AJ, Kruisselbrink AB, Lurvink E, et al. Enhanced engraftment of umbilical cord blood-derived stem cells in NOD/SCID mice by cotransplantation of a second unrelated cord blood unit. Exp Hematol 2005; 33(10): 1249–1256.
133. Jang YK, Jung DH, Jung MH, et al. Mesenchymal stem cells feeder layer from human umbilical cord blood for ex vivo expanded growth and proliferation of hematopoietic progenitor cells. Ann Hematol 2006; 85(4): 212–25.
134. Araki H, Mahmud N, Milhem M, et al. Expansion of human umbilical cord blood SCID-repopulating cells using chromatin-modifying agents. Exp Hematol 2006; 34(2): 140–9.
135. Ye ZJ, Kluger Y, Lian Z, et al. Two types of precursor cells in a multipotential hematopoietic cell line. Proc Natl Acad Sci USA 2005; 102: 18461–6.
136. Berger M, Fagioli F, Piacibello W, et al. Role of different medium and growth factors on placental blood stem cell expansion: an in vitro and in vivo study. Bone Marrow Transplant 2002; 29(5): 443–8.
137. Borge OJ, Ramsfjell V, Cui L, et al. Ability of early acting cytokines to directly promote survival and suppress apoptosis of human primitive $CD34^+CD38^-$ bone marrow cells with multilineage potential at the single-cell level: key role of thrombopoietin. Blood 1997; 90: 2282–92.
138. Liu J, Li K, Yuen PM, et al. Ex vivo expansion of enriched $CD34^+$ cells from neonatal blood in the presence of thrombopoietin, a comparison with cord blood and bone marrow. Bone Marrow Transplant 1999; 24: 247–52.
139. Cohena Y, Nagler A. Hematopoietic stem-cell transplantation using umbilical cord blood. Leuk Lymphoma 2003; 44: 1287–99.
140. Astori G, Adami V, Mambrini G, et al. Evaluation of ex vivo expansion and engraftment in NOD-SCID mice of umbilical cord blood $CD34^+$ cells using the DIDECO "Pluricell System". Bone Marrow Transplant 2005; 35(11): 1101–6.
141. Nakagawa R, Watanabe T, Kawano Y, et al. Analysis of maternal and neonatal factors that influence the nucleated and $CD34^+$ cell yield for cord blood banking. Transfusion 2004; 44: 262–7.
142. Solves P, Mirabet V, Larrel L, et al. Comparison between two cord blood collection strategies. Acta Obstet Gynecol Scand 2003; 82: 439–42.
143. Pafumi C, Farina M, Bandiera S, et al. Differences in umbilical cord blood units collected during cesarean section, before or after the delivery of the placenta. Gynecol Obstet Invest 2002; 54(2): 73–7.

144. Solves P, Perales A, Moraga R, et al. Maternal, neonatal and collection factors influencing the haematopoietic content of cord blood units. Acta Haematol 2005; 113(4): 241–6.
145. Jones J, Stevens CE, Rubinstein P, et al. Obstetric predictors of placental/umbilical cord blood volume for transplantation. Am J Obstet Gynecol 2003; 188(2): 503–9.
146. Grisaru D, Deutsch V, Pick M, et al. Placing the newborn on the maternal abdomen after delivery increases the volume and CD34 cell content in the umbilical cord blood collected: an old maneuver with new applications. Am J Obstet Gynecol 1999; 180: 1240–3.
147. Lim FT, Scherjon SA, van Beckhoven JM, et al. Association of stress during delivery with increased numbers of nucleated cells and hematopoietic progenitor cells in umbilical cord blood. Am J Obstet Gynecol 2000; 183: 1144–52.
148. Askari S, Miller J, Chrysler G, et al. Impact of donor-and collection-related variables on product quality in ex utero cord blood banking. Transfusion 2005; 45: 189–94.
149. Meister B, Totsch M, Mayr A, et al. Identification of $CD34^+$ cord blood cells and their subpopulations in preterm and term neonates using three-color flow cytometry. Biol Neonate 1994; 66: 272–9.
150. Thilaganathan B, Nicolaides KH, Morgan G. Subpopulations of CD34-positive haemopoietic progenitors in fetal blood. Br J Haematol 1994; 87: 634–6.
151. Shields LE, Andrews RG. Gestational age changes in circulating $CD34^+$ hematopoietic stem/progenitor cells in fetal cord blood. Am J Obstet Gynecol 1998; 178: 931–7.
152. Li K, Yau FW, Fok TF, et al. Haematopoietic stem and progenitor cells in human term and preterm neonatal blood. Vox Sang 2001; 80: 162–9.
153. Yamada T, Okamoto Y, Kasamatsu H, et al. Factors affecting the volume of umbilical cord blood collections. Acta Obstet Gynecol Scand 2000; 79: 830–3.
154. Solves P, Moraga R, Saucedo E, et al. Comparison between two strategies for umbilical cord blood collection. Bone Marrow Transplant 2003; 31(4): 269–73.
155. Canabarro RL, Sporleder H, Gomes T, et al. Immunophenotypic evaluation and physiological and laboratory correlations of hematopoietic stem cells of umbilical cord blood. In: Canabarro R. Avaliação imunofenotípica e correlações fisiológicas e laboratoriais das células tronco hematopoéticas do sangue de cordão umbilical. Thesis. 111 pages. Universidade Federal do Rio Grande do Sul. Faculdade de Medicina. Programa de Pós-Graduação Medicina: Ciências Médicas. Porto Alegre, RS, Brazil, 2006.
156. Rogers I, Casper RF. Umbilical cord blood stem cells. Best Pract Res Clin Obstet Gynaecol 2004; 18: 893–908.
157. Grewal SS, Barker JN, Davies SM, et al. Unrelated donor hematopoietic cell transplantation: marrow or umbilical cord blood? Blood 2003; 101(11): 4233–44.
158. Barker JN, Wagner JE. Umbilical cord blood transplantation: current practice and future innovations. Crit Rev Oncol Hematol 2003; 48: 35–43.
159. Rubinstein P, Carrier C, Carpenter C, et al. Graft selection in unrelated placental/umbilical cord blood (PCB) transplantation: influence and weight of HLA match and cell dose on engrafment and survival (abstract). Blood 2000; 96: 588.
160. Rocha V, Cornish J, Sievers EL, et al. Comparison of outcomes of unrelated bone marrow and umbilical cord blood transplants in children with acute leukemia. Blood 2002; 97: 2962–71.
161. Laughlin MJ, Eapen M, Rubinstein P, et al. Outcomes after transplantation of cord blood or bone marrow from unrelated donors in adults with leukemia. N Engl J Med 2004; 351(22): 2265–75.
162. Laughlin MJ, Barker J, Bambach B, et al. Hematopoietic engraftment and survival in adult recipients of umbilical-cord blood from unrelated donors. N Engl J Med 2001; 344(24): 1815–22.
163. Gluckman E, Rocha V, Arcese W, et al. Eurocord Group. Factors associated with outcomes of unrelated cord blood transplant: guidelines for donor choice. Exp Hematol 2004; 32: 397–407.
164. McGuckin CP, Forraz N, Baradez MO, et al. Production of stem cells with embryonic characteristics from human umbilical cord blood. Cell Prolif 2005; 38: 245–55.

165. Wyrsch A, Dalle Carbonare V, Jansen W, et al. Umbilical cord blood from preterm human fetuses is rich in committed and primitive hematopoietic progenitors with high proliferative and self-renewal capacity. Exp Hematol 1999; 27(8): 1338–45.
166. Clapp DW, Baley JE, Gerson SL. Gestational age-dependent changes in circulating hematopoietic stem cells in newborn infants. J Lab Clin Med 1989; 113(4): 422–7.
167. Schibler KR, Liechty KW, White WL, et al. Production of granulocyte colony-stimulating factor in vitro by monocytes from preterm and term neonates. Blood 1993; 82(8): 2478–84.
168. Han P, Stacy D, Story C, et al. The role of haemopoietic growth factors in the pathogenesis of the early anaemia of premature infants. Br J Haematol 1995; 91(2): 327–9.
169. Haneline LS, Marshall KP, Clapp DW. The highest concentration of primitive hematopoietic progenitor cells in cord blood is found in extremely premature infants. Pediatr Res 1996; 39(5): 820–5.
170. Luther-Wyrsch A, Costello E, Thali M, et al. Stable transduction with lentiviral vectors and amplification of immature hematopoietic progenitors from cord blood of preterm human fetuses. Hum Gene Ther. 2001; 12(4): 377-89.
171. Kamolz LP, Kolbus A, Wick N, et al. Cultured human epithelium: human umbilical cord blood stem cells differentiate into keratinocytes under in vitro conditions. Burns. 2006; 32(1): 16–9.
172. Lu X, Dunn J, Dickinson AM, et al. Smooth muscle alpha-actin expression in endothelial cells derived from $CD34^+$ human cord blood cells. Stem Cells Dev 2004; 13(5): 521–7.
173. Aoki M, Yasutake M, Murohara T. Derivation of functional endothelial progenitor cells from human umbilical cord blood mononuclear cells isolated by a novel cell filtration device. Stem Cells 2004; 22(6): 994–1002.
174. Larrivee B, Niessen K, Pollet I, et al. Minimal contribution of marrow-derived endothelial precursors to tumor vasculature. J Immunol 2005; 175(5): 2890–9.
175. Murga M, Yao L, Tosato G. Derivation of endothelial cells from $CD34^-$ umbilical cord blood. Stem Cells 2004; 22(3): 385–95.
176. Shin JW, Lee DW, Kim MJ, et al. Isolation of endothelial progenitor cells from cord blood and induction of differentiation by ex vivo expansion. Yonsei Med J 2005; 46(2): 260–7.
177. Fan CL, Li Y, Gao PJ, et al. Differentiation of endothelial progenitor cells from human umbilical cord blood CD 34+ cells in vitro. Acta Pharmacol Sin 2003; 24(3): 212–8.
178. El-Badri NS. Endothelial progenitor cells from cord blood: a new therapeutic promise? Stem Cells Dev 2005; 14(3): 237–8.
179. Naruse K, Hamada Y, Nakashima E, et al. Therapeutic neovascularization using cord blood-derived endothelial progenitor cells for diabetic neuropathy. Diabetes 2005; 54(6): 1823–8.
180. Kalka C, Masuda H, Takahashi T, et al. Transplantation of ex vivo expanded endothelial progenitor cells for therapeutic neovascularization. Proc Natl Acda Sci USA 2000; 97(7): 3422–7.
181. Murohara T, Ikeda H, Duan J, et al. Transplanted cord blood-derived endothelial precursor cells augment postnatal neovascularization. J Clin Invest 2000; 105(11): 1527–36.
182. Zhang L, Yang R, Han ZC. Transplantation of umbilical cord blood-derived endothelial progenitor cells: a promising method of therapeutic revascularisation. Eur J Haematol 2006; 76(1): 1–8.
183. Kim SY, Park SY, Kim JM, et al. Differentiation of endothelial cells from human umbilical cord blood $AC133^-CD14^+$ cells. Ann Hematol 2005; 84(7): 417–22.
184. Rookmaaker MB, Verhaar MC, Loomans CJ, et al. $CD34^+$ cells home, proliferate, and participate in capillary formation, and in combination with $CD34^-$ cells enhance tube formation in a 3-dimensional matrix. Arterioscler Thromb Vasc Biol 2005; 25(9): 1843–50.
185. Rehman J, Li J, Orschell CM, March KL. Peripheral blood "endothelial progenitor cells" are derived from monocyte/macrophages and secrete angiogenic growth factors. Circulation 2003; 107(8): 1164–9.
186. Rookmaaker MB, Vergeer M, van Zonneveld AJ, et al. Endothelial progenitor cells: mainly derived from the monocyte/macrophage-containing $CD34^-$ mononuclear cell population and

only in part from the hematopoietic stem cell-containing CD34+ mononuclear cell population. Circulation 2003; 108(21): 150.
187. Asahara T, Murohara T, Sullivan A, et al. Isolation of putative progenitor endothelial cells for angiogenesis. Science 1997; 275(5302): 964–7.
188. Dormer A, Beck G. Evolutionary analysis of human vascular endothelial growth factor, angiopoietin, and tyrosine endothelial kinase involved in angiogenesis and immunity. In Silico Biol 2005; 5(3): 323–39.
189. Batard P, Sansilvestri P, Scheinecker C, et al. The Tie receptor tyrosine kinase is expressed by human hematopoietic progenitor cells and by a subset of megakaryocytic cells. Blood 1996; 87(6): 2212–20.
190. Jones N, Master Z, Jones J, et al Identification of Tek/Tie2 binding partners. Binding to a multifunctional docking site mediates cell survival and migration. J Biol Chem 1999; 274(43): 30896–905.
191. Salven P, Mustjoki S, Alitalo R, et al. VEGFR-3 and CD133 identify a population of CD34+ lymphatic/vascular endothelial precursor cells. Blood 2003; 101(1): 168–72.
192. Smadja DM, Bieche I, Uzan G, et al. PAR-1 activation on human late endothelial progenitor cells enhances angiogenesis in vitro with upregulation of the SDF-1/CXCR4 system. Arterioscler Thromb Vasc Biol 2005; 25(11): 2321–7.
193. Molino M, Woolkalis MJ, Prevost N, et al. CXCR4 on human endothelial cells can serve as both a mediator of biological responses and as a receptor for HIV-2. Biochim Biophys Acta 2000; 1500(2): 227–40.
194. Ingram DA, Mead LE, Moore DB, et al. Vessel wall-derived endothelial cells rapidly proliferate because they contain a complete hierarchy of endothelial progenitor cells. Blood 2005; 105(7): 2783–6.
195. Yang C, Zhang ZH, Li ZJ, et al. Enhancement of neovascularization with cord blood CD133+ cell-derived endothelial progenitor cell transplantation. Thromb Haemost 2004; 91(6): 1202–12.
196. Schmidt D, Breymann C, Weber A, et al. Umbilical cord blood derived endothelial progenitor cells for tissue engineering of vascular grafts. Ann Thorac Surg 2004; 78(6): 2094–8.
197. Eggermann J, Kliche S, Jarmy G, et al. Endothelial progenitor cell culture and differentiation in vitro: a methodological comparison using human umbilical cord blood. Cardiovasc Res 2003; 58(2): 478–86.
198. Loomans CJ, de Koning EJ, Staal FJ, et al. Endothelial progenitor cell dysfunction: a novel concept in the pathogenesis of vascular complications of type 1 diabetes. Diabetes 2004; 53(1): 195–9.
199. Stojko R, Witek A. Umbilical cord blood-a perfect source of stem cells? Ginekol Pol 2005; 76(6): 491–7.
200. Weiss ML, Medicetty S, Bledsoe AR, et al. Human umbilical cord matrix stem cells: preliminary characterization and effect of transplantation in a rodent model of Parkinson's Disease. Stem Cells 2006; 24(3): 781–92.
201. Hou L, Cao H, Wang D, et al. Induction of umbilical cord blood mesenchymal stem cells into neuron-like cells in vitro. Int J Hematol. 2003; 78(3): 256–61.
202. Caterson EJ, Nesti LJ, Albert T, et al. Application of mesenchymal stem cells in the regeneration of musculoskeletal tissues. Med Gen Med 2001: E1
203. Romanov YA, Svintsitskaya VA, Smirnov VN. Searching for alternative sources of postnatal human mesenchymal stem cells: candidate MSC-like cells from umbilical cord. Stem Cells 2003; 21(1): 105–10.
204. Ju XL, Huang ZW, Shi Q, et al. Biological characteristics and induced differentiation ability of in vitro expanded umbilical cord blood mesenchymal stem cells. Zhonghua Er Ke Za Zhi 2005; 43(7): 499–502.
205. Wexler SA, Donaldson C, Denning-Kendall P, et al. Adult bone marrow is a rich source of human mesenchymal 'stem' cells but umbilical cord and mobilized adult blood are not. Br J Haematol 2003; 121(2): 368–74.

206. Majka M, Kucia M, Ratajczak MZ. Stem cell biology – a never ending quest for understanding. Acta Biochim Pol 2005; 52(2): 353–8.
207. Zhao RC, Liao L, Han Q. Mechanisms of and perspectives on the mesenchymal stem cell in immunotherapy. J Lab Clin Med 2004; 143(5): 284–91.
208. Gang EJ, Hong SH, Jeong JA, et al. In vitro mesengenic potential of human umbilical cord blood-derived mesenchymal stem cells. Biochem Biophys Res Commun 2004; 321(1): 102–8.
209. Feldmann RE Jr, Bieback K, Maurer MH, et al. Stem cell proteomes: a profile of human mesenchymal stem cells derived from umbilical cord blood. Electrophoresis 2005; 26(14): 2749–58
210. Le Blanc K, Tammik C, Rosendahl K, et al. HLA expression and immunologic properties of differentiated and undifferentiated mesenchymal stem cells. Exp Hematol 2003; 31(10): 890–6.
211. Anjos-Afonso F, Siapati EK, Bonnet D. In vivo contribution of murine mesenchymal stem cells into multiple cell-types under minimal damage conditions. J Cell Sci 2004; 117(Pt 23): 5655–64.
212. Niemeyer P, Seckinger A, Simank HG, et al. Allogenic transplantation of human mesenchymal stem cells for tissue engineering purposes: an in vitro study. Orthopade 2004; 33(12): 1346–53.
213. Javazon EH, Beggs KJ, Flake AW. Mesenchymal stem cells: paradoxes of passaging. Exp Hematol 2004; 32(5): 414–25.
214. Sotiropoulou PA, Perez SA, Salagianni M, et al. Characterization of the optimal culture conditions for clinical scale production of human mesenchymal stem cells. Stem Cells 2006; 24(2): 462–71.
215. Barry FP, Murphy JM. Mesenchymal stem cells: clinical applications and biological characterization. Int J Biochem Cell Biol 2004; 36(4): 568–84.
216. Kern S, Eichler H, Stoeve J, et al. Comparative analysis of mesenchymal stem cells from bone marrow, umbilical cord blood or adipose tissue. Stem Cells 2006; 24 (5): 1294–301.
217. Etheridge SL, Spencer GJ, Heath DJ, et al. Expression profiling and functional analysis of wnt signaling mechanisms in mesenchymal stem cells. Stem Cells 2004; 22: 849–60.
218. Campagnoli C, Roberts IA, Kumar S, et al. Identification of mesenchymal stem/progenitor cells in human first-trimester fetal blood, liver, and bone marrow. Blood 2001; 98(8): 2396–402.
219. Lee MW, Choi J, Yang MS, et al. Mesenchymal stem cells from cryopreserved human umbilical cord blood. Biochem Biophys Res Commun 2004; 320(1): 273–8.
220. Reyes M, Verfaillie CM. Characterization of multipotent adult progenitor cells, a subpopulation of mesenchymal stem cells. Ann N Y Acad Sci 2001; 938: 231–3.
221. Jiang Y, Jahagirdar BN, Reinhardt RL, et al. Pluripotency of mesenchymal stem cells derived from adult marrow. Nature 2002; 418(6893): 41–9.
222. Panepucci RA, Siufi JL, Silva WA Jr, et al. Comparison of gene expression of umbilical cord vein and bone marrow-derived mesenchymal stem cells. Stem Cells 2004; 22(7): 1263–78.
223. Zhou DH, Huang SL, Wu YF, et al. The expansion and biological characteristics of human mesenchymal stem cells. Zhonghua Er Ke Za Zhi 2003; 41(8): 607–10.
224. Zhou DH, Huang SL, Zhang XC, et al. Effects of human umbilical cord blood mesenchymal stem cells on the expansion of $CD34^+$ cells from umbilical cord blood. Zhonghua Er Ke Za Zhi 2005; 43(7): 494–8.
225. Anker PS, Noort WA, Kruisselbrink AB, et al. Nonexpanded primary lung and bone marrow-derived mesenchymal cells promote the engraftment of umbilical cord blood-derived CD34(+) cells in NOD/SCID mice. Exp Hematol 2003; 31(10): 881–9.
226. Djouad F, Plence P, Bony C, et al. Immunosuppressive effect of mesenchymal stem cells favors tumor growth in allogeneic animals. Blood 2003; 102(10): 3837–44.
227. Chen SL, Fang WW, Ye F, et al. Effect on left ventricular function of intracoronary transplantation of autologous bone marrow mesenchymal stem cell in patients with acute myocardial infarction. Am J Cardiol 2004; 94(1): 92–5.

228. Lee OK, Kuo TK, Chen WM, et al. Isolation of multipotent mesenchymal stem cells from umbilical cord blood. Blood 2004; 103(5): 1669–75.
229. Li CD, Zhang WY, Li HL, et al. Mesenchymal stem cells derived from human placenta suppress allogeneic umbilical cord blood lymphocyte proliferation. Cell Res 2005; 15(7): 539–47.
230. Mareschi K, Biasin E, Piacibello W, et al. Isolation of human mesenchymal stem cells: bone marrow versus umbilical cord blood. Haematologica 2001; 86(10): 1099–100.
231. Yu M, Xiao Z, Shen L, et al. Mid-trimester fetal blood-derived adherent cells share characteristics similar to mesenchymal stem cells but full-term umbilical cord blood does not. Br J Haematol 2004; 124(5): 666–75.
232. Lu FZ, Fujino M, Kitazawa Y, et al. Characterization and gene transfer in mesenchymal stem cells derived from human umbilical-cord blood. J Lab Clin Med 2005; 146(5): 271–8.
233. Bieback K, Kern S, Kluter H, et al. Critical parameters for the isolation of mesenchymal stem cells from umbilical cord blood. Stem Cells 2004; 22(4): 625–34.
234. Kim JW, Kim SY, Park SY, et al. Mesenchymal progenitor cells in the human umbilical cord. Ann Hematol 2004; 83(12): 733–8.
235. Anker PS, Noort WA, Scherjon SA, et al. Mesenchymal stem cells in human second-trimester bone marrow, liver, lung, and spleen exhibit a similar immunophenotype but a heterogeneous multilineage differentiation potential. Haematologica 2003; 88(8): 845–52.
236. Ryden M, Dicker A, Gotherstrom C, et al. Functional characterization of human mesenchymal stem cell-derived adipocytes. Biochem Biophys Res Commun 2003; 311(2): 391–7.
237. Gotherstrom C, Ringden O, Tammik C, et al. Immunologic properties of human fetal mesenchymal stem cells. Am J Obstet Gynecol 2004; 190(1): 239–45.
238. Covas DT, Piccinato CE, Orellana MD, et al. Mesenchymal stem cells can be obtained from the human saphena vein. Exp Cell Res 2005; 309(2): 340–4.
239. Li CD, Zhang WY, Li HL, et al. Effect of human placenta derived mesenchymal stem cells on cord blood lymphocyte transformation. Zhonghua Yi Xue Za Zhi 2005; 85(24): 1704–7.
240. Hutson EL, Boyer S, Genever PG. Rapid isolation, expansion, and differentiation of osteoprogenitors from full-term umbilical cord blood. Tissue Eng 2005; 11(9–10): 1407–20.
241. Otto WR, Rao J. Tomorrow's skeleton staff: mesenchymal stem cells and the repair of bone and cartilage. Cell Prolif 2004; 37(1): 97–110.
242. Pittenger MF, Martin BJ. Mesenchymal stem cells and their potential as cardiac therapeutics. Circ Res 2004; 95(1): 9–20.
243. Kang XQ, Zang WJ, Bao LJ, et al. Fibroblast growth factor-4 and hepatocyte growth factor induce differentiation of human umbilical cord blood-derived mesenchymal stem cells into hepatocytes. World J Gastroenterol 2005; 11(47): 7461–5.
244. Jorgensen C, Djouad F, Fritz V, et al. Mesenchymal stem cells and rheumatoid arthritis. Joint Bone Spine 2003; 70(6): 483–5.
245. Beyer NN, da Silva ML. Mesenchymal stem cells: isolation, in vitro expansion and characterization. Handb Exp Pharmacol 2006; 174: 249–82.
246. Zhou Z, Jiang EL, Wang M, et al. Comparative study on various subpopulations in mesenchymal stem cells of adult bone marrow. Zhongguo Shi Yan Xue Ye Xue Za Zhi 2005; 13(1): 54–8.
247. Fan CG, Tang FW, Zhang QJ, et al. Characterization and neural differentiation of fetal lung mesenchymal stem cells. Cell Transplant 2005; 14(5): 311–21.
248. Gimeno MJ, Maneiro E, Rendal E, et al. Cell therapy: a therapeutic alternative to treat focal cartilage lesions. Transplant Proc 2005; 37(9): 4080–3.
249 Honczarenko M, Le Y, Swierkowski M, et al. Human bone marrow stromal cells express a distinct set of biologically functional chemokine receptors. Stem Cells 2006; 24(4): 1030–41.
250. Lee RH, Hsu SC, Munoz J, et al. A subset of human rapidly self-renewing marrow stromal cells preferentially engraft in mice. Blood 2006; 107(5): 2153–61.

251. Son BR, Marquez-Curtis LA, Kucia M, et al. Migration of bone marrow and cord blood mesenchymal stem cells in vitro is regulated by SDF-1-CXCR4 and HGF-c-met axes and involves matrix metalloproteinases. Stem Cells 2006; 24(5): 1254–64.
252. Bhakta S, Hong P, Koc O. The surface adhesion molecule CXCR4 stimulates mesenchymal stem cell migration to stromal cell-derived factor-1 in vitro but does not decrease apoptosis under serum deprivation. Cardiovasc Revasc Med 2006; 7(1): 19–24.
253. Ji JF, He BP, Dheen ST, et al. Interactions of chemokines and chemokine receptors mediate the migration of mesenchymal stem cells to the impaired site in the brain after hypoglossal nerve injury. Stem Cells 2004; 22(3): 415–27.
254. Wynn RF, Hart CA, Corradi-Perini C, et al. A small proportion of mesenchymal stem cells strongly expresses functionally active CXCR4 receptor capable of promoting migration to bone marrow. Blood 2004; 104(9): 2643–5.
255. Sordi V, Malosio ML, Marchesi F, et al. Bone marrow mesenchymal stem cells express a restricted set of functionally active chemokine receptors capable of promoting migration to pancreatic islets. Blood 2005; 106(2): 419–27.
256. Shyu WC, Lee YJ, Liu DD, et al. Homing genes, cell therapy and stroke. Front Biosci 2006; 11: 899–907.
257. Wetzel A, Chavakis T, Preissner KT, et al. Human Thy-1 (CD90) on activated endothelial cells is a counterreceptor for the leukocyte integrin Mac-1 (CD11b/CD18). J Immunol 2004; 172(6): 3850–9.
258. Wetzel A, Wetzig T, Haustein UF, et al. Increased neutrophil adherence in psoriasis: role of the human endothelial cell receptor Thy-1 (CD90). J Invest Dermatol 2006; 126(2): 441–52.
259. Bensidhoum M, Chapel A, Francois S, et al. Homing of in vitro expanded Stro-1- or Stro-1+ human mesenchymal stem cells into the NOD/SCID mouse and their role in supporting human CD34 cell engraftment. Blood 2004; 103(9): 3313–9.
260. Dennis JE, Carbillet JP, Caplan AI, et al. The STRO-1+ marrow cell population is multipotential. Cells Tissues Organs 2002; 170(2–3): 73–82.
261. Gojo S, Gojo N, Takeda Y, et al. In vivo cardiovasculogenesis by direct injection of isolated adult mesenchymal stem cells. Exp Cell Res 2003; 288(1): 51–9
262. Sun S, Guo Z, Xiao X, et al. Isolation of mouse marrow mesenchymal progenitors by a novel and reliable method. Stem Cells 2003; 21(5): 527–35.
263. Zhang L, Hong TP, Hu J, et al. Nestin-positive progenitor cells isolated from human fetal pancreas have phenotypic markers identical to mesenchymal stem cells. World J Gastroenterol 2005; 11(19): 2906–11.
264. Zhang Y, Li C, Jiang X, et al. Human placenta-derived mesenchymal progenitor cells support culture expansion of long-term culture-initiating cells from cord blood $CD34^+$ cells. Exp Hematol 2004; 32(7): 657–64.
265. Gotherstrom C, West A, Liden J, et al. Difference in gene expression between human fetal liver and adult bone marrow mesenchymal stem cells. Haematologica 2005; 90(8): 1017–26.
266. Wagner W, Wein F, Seckinger A, et al. Comparative characteristics of mesenchymal stem cells from human bone marrow, adipose tissue, and umbilical cord blood. Exp Hematol 2005; 33(11): 1402–16.
267. Wislet-Gendebien S, Bruyere F, Hans G, et al. Nestin-positive mesenchymal stem cells favour the astroglial lineage in neural progenitors and stem cells by releasing active BMP4. BMC Neurocsci 2004; 5: 33.
268. Kopen GC, Prockop DJ, Phinney DG. Marrow stromal cells migrate throughout forebrain and cerebellum, and they differentiate into astrocytes after injection into neonatal mouse brains. Proc Natl Acad Sci USA 1999; 96(19): 10711–6.
269. Azizi SA, Stokes D, Augelli BJ, et al. Engraftment and migration of human bone marrow stromal cells implanted in the brains of albino rats – similarities to astrocyte grafts. Proc Natl Acad Sci USA 1998; 95(7): 3908–13.
270. Tang YL, Zhao Q, Zhang YC, et al. Autologous mesenchymal stem cell transplantation induce VEGF and neovascularization in ischemic myocardium. Regul Pept 2004; 117(1): 3–10.

271. Kawada H, Fujita J, Kinjo K, et al. Nonhematopoietic mesenchymal stem cells can be mobilized and differentiate into cardiomyocytes after myocardial infarction. Blood 2004; 104(12): 3581–7.
272. Barbash IM, Chouraqui P, Baron J, et al. Systemic delivery of bone marrow-derived mesenchymal stem cells to the infarcted myocardium: feasibility, cell migration, and body distribution. Circulation 2003; 108(7): 863–8.
273. Noel D, Gazit D, Bouquet C, et al. Short-term BMP-2 expression is sufficient for in vivo osteochondral differentiation of mesenchymal stem cells. Stem Cells 2004; 22(1): 74–85.
274. Davani S, Marandin A, Mersin N, et al. Mesenchymal progenitor cells differentiate into an endothelial phenotype, enhance vascular density, and improve heart function in a rat cellular cardiomyoplasty model. Circulation 2003; 108(1): II253–8.
275. Heino TJ, Hentunen TA, Vaananen HK. Conditioned medium from osteocytes stimulates the proliferation of bone marrow mesenchymal stem cells and their differentiation into osteoblasts. Exp Cell Res. 2004; 294(2): 458–68.
276. Kim SW, Han H, Chae GT, et al. Successful stem cell therapy using umbilical cord blood-derived multi-potent stem cells for Buerger's disease and ischemic limb disease animal model. Stem Cells 2006; 24(6):1620–6.
277. Hong SH, Gang EJ, Jeong JA, et al. In vitro differentiation of human umbilical cord blood-derived mesenchymal stem cells into hepatocyte-like cells. Biochem Biophys Res Commun 2005; 330(4): 1153–61.
278. Fuchs JR, Hannouche D, Terada S, et al. Cartilage engineering from ovine umbilical cord blood mesenchymal progenitor cells. Stem Cells 2005; 23(7): 958–64.
279. Silva WA Jr, Covas DT, Panepucci RA, et al. The profile of gene expression of human marrow mesenchymal stem cells. Stem Cells 2003; 21(6): 661–9.
280. Ratajczak MZ, Kucia M, Majka M, et al. Heterogeneous populations of bone marrow stem cells-are we spotting on the same cells from the different angles? Folia Histochem Cytobiol 2004; 42(3): 139–46.
281. Kucia M, Reca R, Jala VR, et al. Bone marrow as a home of heterogenous populations of nonhematopoietic stem cells. Leukemia 2005; 19(7): 1118–27.
282. Kogler G, Sensken S, Airey JA, et al. A new human somatic stem cell from placental cord blood with intrinsic pluripotent differentiation potential. J Exp Med 2004; 200(2): 123–35.
283. Jager M, Wild A, Lensing-Hohn S, et al. Influence of different culture solutions on osteoblastic differentiation in cord blood and bone marrow derived progenitor cells. Biomed Tech 2003; 48(9): 241–4.
284. Quesenberry PJ, Dooner G, Colvin G, et al. Stem cell biology and the plasticity polemic. Exp Hematol 2005; 33(4): 389–94.
285. Kogler G, Radke TF, Lefort A, et al. Cytokine production and hematopoiesis supporting activity of cord blood-derived unrestricted somatic stem cells. Exp Hematol 2005; 33(5): 573–83.
286. Kim BO, Tian H, Prasongsukarn K, et al. Cell transplantation improves ventricular function after a myocardial infarction: a preclinical study of human unrestricted somatic stem cells in a porcine model. Circulation 2005; 112(9): I96–104.
287. D'Ippolito G, Diabira S, Howard GA, et al. Marrow-isolated adult multilineage inducible (MIAMI) cells, a unique population of postnatal young and old human cells with extensive expansion and differentiation potential. J Cell Sci 2004; 117(Pt 14): 2971–81.
288. Kucia M, Ratajczak J, Ratajczak MZ. Are bone marrow stem cells plastic or heterogenous – that is the question. Exp Hematol 2005; 33(6): 613–23.

Chapter 4
Ex Vivo Expansion of Cord Blood

Ian K. McNiece and Elizabeth J. Shpall

Umbilical cord blood (CB) provides an alternate source for patients undergoing high-dose chemotherapy for treatment of cancer or genetic diseases. In particular, CB has become a standard therapeutic option for selected patients with hematologic malignancies. Several studies have reported on the use of CB for transplantation in adult patients; however, the low cell doses have limited the use of CB in this setting due to subsequent delays in engraftment. Ex vivo expansion is an approach that is being explored as a means to provide larger cell numbers from CB products.

Cellular Content of CB

CB products contain similar cell populations to bone marrow (BM) and mobilized peripheral blood progenitor cell products (PBPC), including hematopoietic stem cells (HSC), primitive progenitor cells, mature progenitor cells, and mature functional cells. However, the total cell number and progenitor cells are much lower in CB as compared to BM and PBPC. For example, BM and PBPC contain approximately 10^8 CD34+ cells, whereas CB contains approximately 5×10^6 CD34+ cells. In contrast, the frequency of HSC, as determined by NOD/SCID engraftment, is enriched in the CD34+ cell population of CB compared to BM or PBPC. As few as 100,000 CB CD34+ cells can engraft NOD/SCID mice, while approximately one million BM CD34+ cells and five million PBPC CD34+ cells are required for the engraftment of human cells.

These numbers would suggest that CB contains similar levels of HSC to BM and PBPC but significantly lower levels of committed progenitor cells. The use of these cellular grafts in the clinical setting results in data that support this theory. Patients transplanted with CB grafts have delayed neutrophil and platelet engraftment compared to patients transplanted with BM or PBPC products; however, there does not appear to be any long-term engraftment problems in patients transplanted

I.K. McNiece (✉)
Interdisciplinary Stem Cell Institute, University of Miami, Miami, FL, USA

N. Bhattacharya, P. Stubblefield (eds.), *Frontiers of Cord Blood Science*,
DOI 10.1007/978-1-84800-167-1_4,

with CB grafts. This suggests that CB products contain sufficient long-term engrafting cells (HSC), but minimal short-term engrafting cells (mature progenitor cells).

Therefore, a simple goal of ex vivo expansion would be to generate more committed progenitor cells that have the potential to provide faster short-term engraftment. This can be achieved by an ex vivo culture in hematopoietic growth factors (HGFs); however, we must consider the potential negative impact of depleting HSC by driving their differentiation to mature progenitor cells. Therefore, the ideal protocol for evaluating ex vivo expanded CB cells involves the use of two products, one component which has been ex vivo expanded and the second that has not been manipulated.

Ex Vivo Expanded Cells Provide Rapid Engraftment

The potential enhancement of engraftment by ex vivo expanded cells has been demonstrated in clinical trials. Several studies [1, 2, 3, 4] have been reported using ex vivo expanded PBPC CD34+ cells in myeloablated patients. In these studies, the use of ex vivo expanded cells resulted in faster neutrophil engraftment, with patients having minimal days of neutropenia compared to patients receiving unexpanded PBPC products. Our own study conducted at the University of Colorado [4], resulted in neutrophil engraftment as early as 4 days post-transplant. Analysis of the patient data demonstrated minimal correlation of the time to engraftment to CD34+ cell dose, but demonstrated a highly significant correlation to the dose of total nucleated cells (TNC) per kg of body weight of the recipient [4]. Evaluation of cytospins prepared of the expanded cells demonstrated a high percentage of mature neutrophil cells. Based upon these data, we have focused our experimental protocols on driving differentiation of CB cells to produce a cellular product that contains a high proportion of mature neutrophil cells. In addition, these conditions drive the production of mature progenitor cells [4, 5]. These conditions also appear to deplete products of long-term engrafting cells as demonstrated by engraftment of fetal sheep [6]. Again indicating the need for developing clinical protocols that utilize two graft components, one expanded and the another unmanipulated.

Selection of CB Products for Ex Vivo Expansion

A number of systems have been explored for ex vivo expansion of CB products from liquid culture in bags to bioreactors. A number of groups have demonstrated that selection of CD34+ cells or CD133+ cells is necessary for optimal expansion. In 1997, we reported that culture of CB mono nuclear cells (MNC) in an HGF cocktail of stem cell factor (SCF) plus granulocyte colony stimulating factor (G-CSF) and thrombopoietin (Tpo) resulted in only a 1.4-fold expansion of total cells, 0.8-fold in mature progenitor cells (GM-CFC), and 0.3-fold in erythroid progenitors (BFU-E) [7]. In contrast, CD34+ selected CB cells resulted in 113-fold expansion of total cells, 73-fold expansion of GM-CFC, and 49-fold expansion of

BFU-E. Based upon these results, we have initiated expansion cultures in clinical trials with CD34-selected CB cells. Processing of clinical products has led us to two conclusions:

1. Although we can expand significantly the TNC and committed progenitor cells from CD34+ cells, we rarely reach pre-selection total cell numbers. For a typical CB product starting with a cell dose of 1×10^9 TNC and containing 0.5% CD34+ cells, we would obtain a maximum of 5×10^6 CD34+ cells post-selection. Therefore, after culture for 10–14 days, we would require a minimum of 200-fold expansion of TNC to obtain pre-processing levels.
2. The performance of clinical trials using CB grafts in the unrelated setting requires the use of frozen CB products. Selection of frozen CB products results in significant losses of CD34+ cells (50% or greater loss of CD34+ cells) and often results in low purities [8]. With a 50% recovery of CD34+ cells after selection, we now require at least a 400-fold cell expansion to obtain equivalent TNC as we started with. Again in our experience with clinical studies, the purity of the CD34-selected product impacted the levels of expansion achieved. The median purity of CD34+ cells was 47.5% (range: 14–81%) and the median expansion was 56-fold of TNC. Products with a purity greater than 50% resulted in a median of 139-fold, while products with a purity less than 50% resulted in only 32-fold expansion.

Therefore, in our experience to date, the use of CD34-selected products has rarely resulted in increased cell doses of ex vivo expanded cells compared to the starting unmanipulated product.

Availability of Clinical Grade Reagents

A number of approaches have been evaluated for ex vivo expansion of CB products including various culture media, HGF cocktails, and various culture vessels (flasks, bags, etc.). Most protocols utilize a 10- to 21-day culture in 5%CO_2 incubators, so the development of closed culture systems using clinical grade HGFs and media is essential to comply with regulatory body requirements. In our culture system, we have used three HGFs, namely, SCF, G-CSF, and Tpo as these HGFs have been manufactured to GMP (Good Manufacturing Practices) standards. It is most likely that addition of other HGFs could enhance the expansion potential of these cultures; however, the lack of GMP grade inhibits translation to clinical trials. Similarly, media must be manufactured to GMP standards and there are limited options available. In our initial clinical trials, we used a defined media that was manufactured by Amgen for clinical use; however, Amgen discontinued the production of this media and in subsequent expansion trials we have been using Sigma's Stemline II expansion media. This is a proprietary media with the formulation a trade secret to prevent duplication by other manufacturers. Sigma manufactures this defined media to GMP grade and we have recently initiated two expansion clinical trials using it.

Clinical Experience With Ex Vivo Expanded Cells

Despite hundreds of reports of pre-clinical studies evaluating ex vivo expansion of CB products, only a small number of clinical trials have been conducted to evaluate the clinical potential of ex vivo expanded CB cells. Kurtzberg et al. [9] ($n = 21$ patients) and Stiff et al. [10] ($n = 9$ patients) used the Aastrom system for the expansion of CB cells; however, no significant effects on engraftment kinetics were observed in these patients. We have reported the results of a clinical trial that we conducted at the University of Colorado [11], and again the conclusion was that the rate of engraftment was not significantly increased by the use of expanded cells. Several ongoing trials at MD Anderson have been reported at meetings by Dr. Shpall [12] and again the data suggest that the ex vivo expanded cells have had minimal impact on the rate of engraftment.

These studies suggest that the culture conditions currently being undertaken are not capable of expanding the appropriate cell population or that insufficient numbers are being generated to impact the time to recovery of neutrophils or platelets. Our conclusion from our own experience and data is that the requirement for selection of CD34+ cells or CD133+ cells from frozen CB products greatly minimizes the potential of generating a suitable expanded CB product to enhance the rate of engraftment. Therefore, in recent studies, we have evaluated methods for expanding CB products without an initial CD34- or CD133-selection.

Ex Vivo Expansion of CB-MNC on MSC

We have developed a co-culture system which is capable of expanding CB-MNC by culturing the CB-MNC on confluent mesenchymal stem cell (MSC) layers. The literature contains many reports of the ability of MSC to support the growth of hematopoietic cells. It has been demonstrated that MSC produce a number of HGFs and adhesion molecules that may stimulate growth of hematopoietic cells [13]. Our initial data reproducibly demonstrated a 10- to 20-fold expansion of TNC with 18-fold expansion of GM-CFC and 16- to 37-fold expansion of CD34+ cells.

In recent experiments, we have evaluated the potential of ex vivo expansion of frozen CB products using the co-culture on MSC. CB products were thawed and washed, and were resulting a median of 3.3×10^8 TNC (range: $1.4–3.6 \times 10^8$ TNC). For a 50-kg recipient, these CB products would provide only 0.73×10^7 TNC/kg with zero of five products reaching the minimal target dose of 1×10^7 TNC.

Each product was expanded by culturing the MNC fraction from each product on preformed layers of MSC. Ten T162-cm^2 flasks were used for each product such that each flask contained 10% of the CB MNC. After ex vivo culture for 14 days in the cocktail of SCF, G-CSF, and Tpo in Stemline II media, a median of 9-fold expansion of TNC was obtained with a range of 6.5- to 24-fold. The median TNC post-expansion was 21.6×10^8 TNC (range: $11–79 \times 10^8$ TNC) (Table 4.1). A median expansion of mature progenitor cells (GM-CFC) of 46-fold was also obtained in the co-culture. For a 50-kg recipient, the expanded CB product would be equivalent

Table 4.1 Ex vivo expansion of TNC from frozen CB products

	Exp #					
	1	2	3	4	5	Median
CB-MNC ($\times 10^8$ TNC)	3.6	2.2	1.4	3.3	3.3	3.3
Post-expansion ($\times 10^8$ TNC)	44.6	19	11	21.6	79.3	21.6
Fold expansion ($\times 10^8$ TNC)	12	9	7	6.5	24	9

Table 4.2 Cell doses based upon recipient weight of 50 kg and 100 kg

	Exp #					
	1	2	3	4	5	Median
Recipient weight 50 kg						
CB-MNC ($\times 10^7$ TNC/kg)	0.7	0.4	0.3	0.7	0.7	0.7
Post-expansion ($\times 10^7$ TNC/kg)	8.9	3.8	2.2	4.3	15.9	3.8
Recipient weight 100 kg						
CB-MNC ($\times 10^7$ TNC/kg)	0.4	0.2	0.1	0.3	0.3	0.3
Post-expansion ($\times 10^7$ TNC/kg)	4.5	1.9	1.1	2.2	7.9	2.2

to 4.3×10^7 TNC/kg (range: 2.2–16 $\times 10^7$ TNC/kg), with all five expanded products reaching the minimal target of 1×10^7 TNC/kg. In fact all expanded products contained more than 1×10^7 TNC/kg based upon a 100-kg recipient (Table 4.2).

We would propose two potential advantages to the use of co-culture for expansion based upon these results: first, the possible enhanced engraftment and, second, the ability to use better-matched CB products that may have a low cell dose. Wagner and colleagues have been transplanting two CB products to provide an increased cell dose; however, the majority of patients receive a two-antigen miss-matched CB unit [14]. Better-matched CB units are routinely identified but are not suitable due to low cell doses. The expansion of these CB units would enable at least on unit to be better matched to the recipient and potentially decrease the graft-versus-host disease that can result.

A clinical trial to evaluate the potential of ex vivo expanded cells generated using this co-culture approach is currently being conducted at MD Anderson Cancer Center.

Summary

Despite more than a decade of research, the clinical results for ex vivo expanded CB products have not provided a major impact on time to engraftment of the recipients. New approaches are currently being developed and it is hoped that these trials will demonstrate faster engraftment and provide a platform for optimization of the development of protocols for CB transplant. It is clear from the trials that have been undertaken to date, that we still have not clearly identified the cell population, required to provide rapid engraftment. We can only optimize culture of this cell population once we identify its phenotype. This highlights the need for continued clinical trials and the development of large animal models that may shed light on what cells and how many are required to provide an optimal hematopoietic cell graft.

Disclosure Statement

Under a licensing agreement between ViaCell Inc, and the Johns Hopkins University, Ian McNiece is entitled to a share of royalty received by the University on sales of products described in this article. The terms of this arrangement are being managed by the Johns Hopkisn University in accordance with its conflict of interest policies.

References

1. Reiffers J, Cailliot C, Dazey B, et al. (1999) Abrogation of post-myeloablative chemotherapy neutropenia by ex-vivo expanded autologous CD34-positive cells. Lancet 354:1092.
2. Paquette R, Dergham S, Karpf E, et al. (2001) Ex vivo expanded unselected peripheral blood: Progenitor cells reduce posttransplantation neutropenia, thrombocytopenia, and anemia in patients with breast cancer. Blood 96:2385–2390.
3. Prince MH, Simmons PJ, Whitty G, et al. (2004) Improved haematopoietic recovery following transplantation with ex vivo expanded mobilized blood cells. Br J Haematol 126:536–545.
4. McNiece I, Jones R, Bearman S, et al. (2000) Ex vivo expanded peripheral blood progenitor cells provide rapid neutrophil recovery in breast cancer patients following high dose chemotherapy. Blood 96:3001–3007.
5. McNiece I, Kubegov D, Kerzic P, Shpall EJ, Gross S (2000) Increased expansion and differentiation of cord blood products using a two step expansion culture. Exp Hematol 28(10): 1181–1186.
6. McNiece IK, Almeida-Porada G, Shpall EJ, Zanjani E (2002) Ex vivo expanded cord blood cells provide rapid engraftment in fetal sheep but lack long term engrafting potential. Exp Hematol 30(6):612–616.
7. Briddell R, Kern BP, Zilm KL, Stoney GB, McNiece I (1997) Purification of CD34+ cells is essential for optimal ex vivo expansion of umbilical cord blood cells. J Hematother 6: 145–150.
8. McNiece I, Harrington J, Turney J, Kellner J, Shpall EJ (2004) Ex vivo expansion of cord blood mononuclear cells on mesenchymal stem cells (MSC). Cytotherapy 6(4):311–317.
9. Jaroscak J, Martin PL, Waters-Pick B, et al. (1998) A phase I trial of augmentation of unrelated umbilical cord blood transplantation with ex-vivo expanded cells. Blood 92(10) Suppl. 1:646a.
10. Stiff P, Pecora A, Parthasarathy M, et al. (1998) Umbilical cord blood transplants in adults using a combination of unexpanded and ex vivo expanded cells: preliminary clinical observations. Blood 92(10) Suppl. 1:646a.
11. Shpall EJ, Quinones R, Giller R, et al. (2002) Transplantation of ex vivo expanded cord blood. Biol Blood Marrow Transplant 8(7):368–376.
12. Shpall EJ (2006) Workshop 3: Current Clinical Trials in HSC Transplantation. ISCT Annual Meeting, Berlin, Germany 2006.
13. Deans RJ, Moseley AB (2000) Mesenchymal stem cells: Biology and potential clinical uses. Exp Hematol 28:875–884.
14. Barker JN, Weisdorf DJ, DeFor TE, et al. (2005) Transplantation of 2 partially HLA-matched umbilical cord blood units to enhance engraftment in adults with hematologic malignancy. Blood 105(3):1343–1347.

Chapter 5
Mesenchymal Stem Cells: Applications in Cell and Gene Therapy

Pablo Bosch and Steven L. Stice

Mesenchymal stem cells (MSCs) are one of the most extensively studied adult stem cells. These cells are believed to reside in tissues of mesenchymal origin, particularly, in the bone marrow but they have also been found in many other tissues including cord blood. Both in vivo and in vitro, these cells can differentiate down the adipogenic, chondrogenic, and osteogenic lineages. MSCs also play an important role in hematopoiesis since they form part of the bone marrow microenvironment that promotes hematopoietic stem cell proliferation and differentiation. In addition to the accepted orthodox plasticity of MSCs, several laboratories have reported a broader differentiation spectrum for MSCs, including cell phenotypes from other embryonic germ layers such as neuron-like cells. Due to their stem cell nature, MSCs exhibit extensive proliferative potential in vitro ($\sim$40 cell doublings) while retaining multipotential differentiation capacity. Local administration of ex vivo expanded MSCs alone or in matrices has proven to be useful for the treatment of bone and cartilage defects in a number of animal models and humans. Another approach envisions the use of genetically modified MSCs as in vivo mini-pumps for delivery of various therapeutic factors. The successful clinical applications of these and other MSC-based gene therapy approaches will depend greatly on our ability to efficiently deliver the gene of interest into MSCs. We will review the MSCs isolation, proliferation, differentiation, and some of the therapeutic applications, alone and in combination with gene therapy.

Introduction

In addition to hematopoietic stem cells, it has been long recognized that the postnatal bone marrow in mammals is populated by a distinct stem cell population known as mesenchymal stem cells (MSCs) also referred as marrow somatic cells

P. Bosch (✉)
Instituto Technológico de Chascomús (IIB-INTECH), CONICET-Universidad Nacional de General San Martín, Camino de Circunvalación Laguna Km. 6 CC 164, (B7130IWA) Chascomús, Provincia de Buenos Aires, Argentina
e-mail: boschp@gmail.com

N. Bhattacharya, P. Stubblefield (eds.), *Frontiers of Cord Blood Science*,
DOI 10.1007/978-1-84800-167-1_5, © Springer-Verlag London Limited 2009

or colony forming unit fibroblastic (CFU-F) cells. In vivo, MSCs and other non-hematopoietic cells (e.g., macrophages, reticular cells, endothelial cells, smooth muscle cells, adipocytes) in combination with the extracellular matrix form what is known as "hematopoietic inductive microenvironment." This complex bone marrow microenvironment provides support for hematopoiesis, i.e., process of formation of new blood cells, through cell-to-cell interactions and soluble clues. However, MSCs are not exclusively located in the bone marrow and were found in various other tissues, including the cord blood, fetal blood and liver, amniotic fluid and, in some circumstances, in adult peripheral blood. Although MSCs can be isolated from several tissues, they are a fairly rare and unique cell type, at most 0.01% of adult human bone marrow [1]. This is true for cord blood as well [2]. However, more MSCs exist within the umbilical vein endothelial/subendothelial layer [3].

Mesenchymal stem cells are considered pluripotent cells with capacity to differentiate into mesodermal lineages, such as adipocytes, osteoblasts, and chondrocytes both in vivo and in vitro. Several studies have demonstrated that these pluripotent stem cells derived from the marrow stroma can be easily isolated from bone marrow specimens, proliferate extensively ex vivo to originate relatively homogeneous cell populations [1, 4] and are endowed with the capacity to differentiate into mesodermal [1, 5] and non-mesodermal [6, 7] cell types. Due to their multipotentiality and extensive self-renewal capacity, MSCs hold great promise as source of cells for many cell-based strategies for the treatment of human diseases. The aim of the present review is to present an in-depth description of the biology, isolation, characterization, and potential therapeutic applications of MSCs.

Isolation and Culture of Mesenchymal Stem Cells

Cells with features of mesenchymal precursors have been isolated from the bone marrow of many mammals including laboratory rodents [8, 9], humans [1], monkeys [10], cats [11], dogs [12], and pigs [5, 13]. In humans, MSCs are normally isolated from bone marrow aspirates collected from the superior iliac crest of the pelvis [1, 14], tibial or femoral compartment [15, 16] or thoracic and lumbar vertebra [17]. In non-rodent animals, bone marrow can be harvested from the iliac crest, sternum or head of long bones like the humerus using similar aspiration techniques adapted from humans [18, 19, 20]. Alternatively, in dead animals, bone marrow can be harvested from spongy bone present in the epiphysis of long bones [13]. Unlike in large animals, in laboratory rodents, bone marrow is flushed out from the mid-diaphysis of the tibia or femur [21, 22, 23].

Bone marrow specimens (aspirates or biopsies) are composed of a mixture of hematopoietic and stromal components from the bone marrow plus a variable amount of contaminating blood. It has been estimated that approximately 1 in every 10,000 nucleated cells present in bone marrow is a MSC [1]. Therefore, in order to eliminate the bulk of unwanted cells, including erythrocytes and platelets, a common practice during isolation of MSCs is to subject the bone marrow sample to fractionation in a density gradient such as Percoll. Mononuclear cells are recovered from the interface and plated on plastic dishes or flasks in a basal medium such as Dulbecco's modified Eagle's medium with 10–20% fetal bovine serum (FBS). MSCs are selected from other cells present in the mixture (e.g., macrophages, endothelial cells, lymphocytes, and smooth muscle cells) based on their strong adherence to the plastic surface. Within 24–48 h from plating, MSCs have attached to plastic and non-adherent cells are removed with culture medium exchanges. Discrete colonies of adherent fibroblastic cells can be observed as early as 4–5 days of culture. These colonies originated from a single cell eventually coalesce to form a near-confluent culture by day 14 (Fig. 5.1) when cells can be trypsinized and expanded by sequential passages to confluence. Theoretically, if the right culture

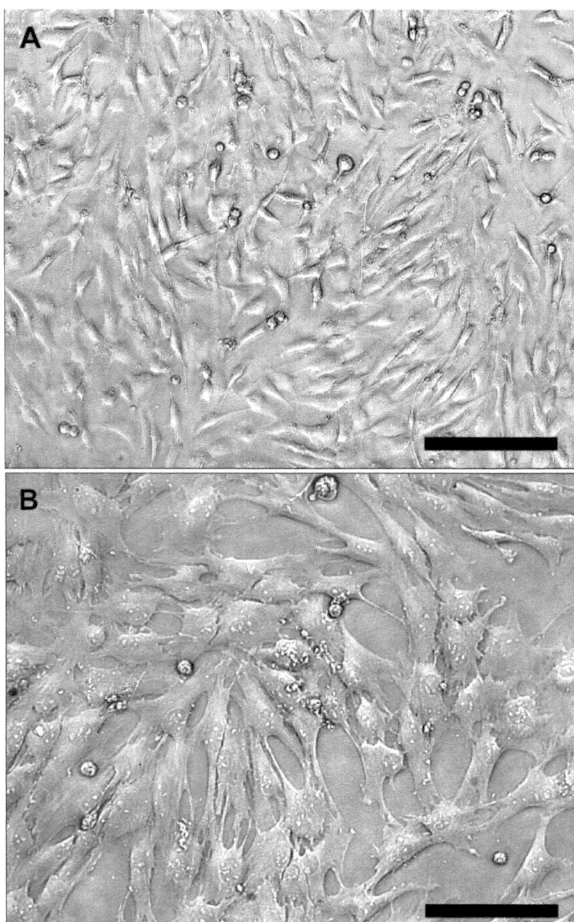

Fig. 5.1 Morphology of adherent fibroblast-like cells, later identified as MSCs, isolated from pig bone marrow after 14 days from initial plating (**A**). Same cell line at higher magnification showing detailed fibroblastic morphology of pMSCs (**B**). Bar = 200 μm (**A**) and 100 μm (**B**). (Reproduced from Ref [5] with permission from the Society for the Study of Reproduction, Inc.)

conditions are met, stem cells would have unlimited proliferative capacity in vitro. Despite their long life span in vitro, MSCs would eventually senesce during in vitro culture [24]. For instance, multi-colony-derived (non-clonal) MSC lines cultured under optimal conditions can undergo about 25 passages, representing more than 50 cell doublings before senescence [25]. In another study, human MSC clonal lines completely stopped growing at about 22 cell doublings after approximately 80 days in culture [4], showing a significant, although limited lifespan in vitro. Species-specific differences in lifespan of MSCs exist since senescence in rat MSCs has not been observed [21]. It is plausible that by adjusting some environmental variables during MSC in vitro culture, such as oxygen tension or growth factors, it might be possible to promote self-renewal capacity of these adult stem cells. For instance, higher populations doublings (>50) have been achieved by the incorporation of fibroblast growth factor 2 (FGF-2) to the basal culture medium [25, 26]. However, the absolute self-renewal capacity of MSCs in vivo and in vitro remains an open question that needs to be experimentally addressed.

An important property of MSCs is the clonal expansion capability when they are plated at low densities or sorted as single cells. This colony-forming feature of MSCs was first described by the pioneering work of Friedenstein et al. [27, 28], who reported for the first time the isolation of bone marrow stromal fibroblastic cells capable of osteogenic differentiation. The number and size of individual MSC colonies can be objectively studied when cells are plated at low densities in the CFU-F assay providing a mean to estimate the frequency of MSCs in bone marrow aspirates and investigate the effect of different culture conditions on MSCs. Analysis of colonies originated from the CFU-F assay has revealed a great heterogeneity in terms of cell morphology (size and shape) and differentiation potential among colonies derived from the same bone marrow specimen [14, 29, 30]. It has been clearly established through the analysis of the progeny originated from a single cell that in a given MSC population, there are cells with different differentiation potential and expansion capacity [14]. A small proportion of cells has tripotential differentiation capacity (adipogenic, chondrogenic, and osteogenic) while most of the cells possess only bi- or even unipotential capacity [14]. Furthermore, Muraglia et al. [4] have documented a gradual loss of differentiation potential with passaging. In conjunction, these data could be interpreted as MSC populations isolated by culture of adherent cells as described in this review are in fact mixture of stem cells and progenitors with different degree of commitment to specific lineages supporting a hierarchal model in MSC cultures [31] similar to that described for hematopoietic cells.

Isolation and ex vivo expansion of MSCs depend entirely on the growth factors present in FBS used as supplement of the basal medium [32]. Development of serum-free defined culture system that support ex vivo expansion of MSCs while retaining the pluripotential capacity would be highly desirable not only to study the effect of particular molecules (e.g., growth factors, cytokines, etc.) on MSC function, but also for future therapy strategies, which will require cells derived from xeno-free culture conditions. It is currently known that proliferation of MSCs is enhanced by several mitogenic factors including platelet-derived growth factor

(PDGF), epidermal growth factor (EGF), basic FGF, transforming growth factor beta (TGF-β) and insulin-like growth factor-I (IGF-I) [33]. Addition of FGF-2 to the culture medium of MSCs has been associated with increased lifespan and increased telomere length, indicating that this growth factor may select for cell populations with extended proliferation capacity [25]. In addition to cell proliferation and cell longevity, growth factors may influence different aspects of in vitro and in vivo differentiation pathways in MSCs. For instance, FGF-2 added to the culture medium of MSCs led to enhanced osteogenic [34] and chondrogenic [35] potential in cultured human MSCs. More research in this area will provide the tools for the development of defined growth media for MSCs to achieve more reproducible culture protocols and safety in future clinical use.

Despite the fact that MSCs have been primarily derived from bone marrow, other tissue sources of MSCs have been identified [36]. Using methodologies similar to that originally described by Friedenstein et al. to isolate stromal fibroblastic cells from rat bone marrow [37], cells with analogous properties to MSCs have been isolated from compact bone, adipose tissue, cord blood, amniotic fluid, fetal tissues and blood [38, 39, 40, 41, 42, 43, 44, 45, 46, 47, 48]. It is not known at this point, however, whether the stromal precursors isolated from those tissues are truly the same MSCs originally isolated from bone marrow or the use of similar techniques for isolation and culture make them appear the same cell type in vitro. A major limitation in these studies has been the lack of specific MSC surface markers to prospectively identify mesenchymal cells.

A long-lasting hypothesis has been that bone marrow-derived MSCs are a source of undifferentiated cells for maintenance and regeneration of normal or injured peripheral tissues. Central to this hypothesis is the transit of MSCs from the bone marrow to mesenchymal tissues through circulation. Several studies have been carried out in human and animals in search of circulating MSCs, which resulted in successful isolation of circulating mesenchymal progenitor cells from fetal and adult peripheral blood [2, 38, 43, 49, 50, 51, 52]. However, Lazarus et al. [53] and Wexler et al. [54] were unable to reproduce these results in similar studies. Differences in the mobilization procedures and cell preparation may account for these conflicting data. Interestingly, large numbers of MSC-like cells are present in the fetal circulation from the 7th to approximately 12th week of gestation [38]. These cells are phenotypically similar to the adult MSCs, and as expected, they have greater proliferative potential and a broader differentiation capacity compared with the adult counterparts [38]. This finding suggests a surge of circulating stromal pluripotent cells during the early fetal life aimed to populate the stromal compartment of hematopoietic and other tissues. Whether these pluripotent stromal cells present during the fetal life persist throughout life and whether they represent the ancestors of the well-characterized MSC from bone marrow are currently unknown. Another piece of evidence that supports the hypothesis of MSC involvement in tissue repair and regeneration is the engraftment of systemically infused MSCs in multiple mesenchymal tissues [55, 56]. After infusion, donor-derived MSCs have been detected in peripheral tissues at very low frequency (usually detected by PCR) [57] and definitive evidence that the grafted cells differentiate in participatory cells of the host tissue has not been definitely provided. Furthermore, engraftment of systemically administered MSCs does not imply that marrow-derived MSCs naturally mobilize in response to tissue injury. The complete understanding of the role of MSCs in peripheric tissue maintenance and repair will certainly depend on the development of methodologies to study MSC function in vivo.

Another cell type that is believed to be distinct from, but somehow related to bone marrow MSCs is the multipotent adult progenitor cell (MAPC) more recently isolated and characterized by Verfaillie et al. [58, 59, 60]. MAPCs have been isolated from human, rat, and mouse bone marrow as a subpopulation of CD45/glycophorin-A depleted bone marrow-derived mononuclear cells that selectively attach to laminin-coated plates and grow in serum-low or serum-free conditions with EGF and PDGF-BB. MAPCs, which have also been isolated from muscle and brain, are much more plastic than the "classic" bone marrow MSC since they can differentiate not only in mesenchymal derivatives (osteoblasts, chondrocytes, adipocytes, and fibroblasts), but also in almost all mesodermal cell lineages [61, 62]. There is also evidence that MAPCs can be induced to differentiate into neuroectodermal and endodermal lineages [63]. When injected as single cell into mouse blastocysts, MAPCs contributed to the formation of all tissues, including all cell types of the central nervous system (CNS) [61]. Furthermore, MAPCs possess vast proliferative capacity in vitro (>100 cell doublings) without the evidence of replicative senescence or loss of differentiation potential. Although it has been suggested that MAPCs represent a more primitive pluripotent progenitor of MSCs, the relationship between these two cell types has not been established.

Phenotypic Characterization of Mesenchymal Stem Cells

Considerable effort has been invested to characterize the antigenic profile of cultured MSCs. Identification of appropriate cell markers for selection, isolation, and testing of MSCs would be of utmost importance to study MSC biology and future practical applications. However, none of the several markers described so far, alone or in combination, have been useful to unequivocally identify MSC populations. There is consensus among different reports that MSCs are devoid of the following hematopoietic surface markers: CD45, CD14, CD31, CD133, and CD11b [1]. Species-specific differences have been observed for the hematopoietic marker CD34, which is not expressed in human and rat MSCs but it is variably expressed in murine MSCs [21, 64, 65]. MSCs express a number of cell adhesion molecules such as CD44, CD49e, CD62, and several integrins, which are certainly very important in hematopoietic-stroma cell interactions (reviewed by Verfaillie [66]). Different laboratories have reported variable expression of CD90 (Thy 1.1), CD117 (c-kit), CD105 (endoglin), and CD73. These discrepancies are probably originated in differences in isolation method, culture conditions and origin of MSCs.

Several monoclonal antibodies have been raised against antigenic determinants present on the cell membrane of MSCs. Stro 1 is a monoclonal antibody, which is expressed at high levels in MSCs [67] though some populations of hematopoietic cells express low levels of Stro 1 [68]. Gronthos et al. [69] have reported the use of Stro 1 to isolate a fairly pure population of non-cycling bone marrow stromal progenitor cell populations, which exhibited telomerase activity and multilineage potential. SH-2 antibody described by Haynesworth et al. [70], which recognizes an epitope present on the TGF-β receptor, has been used to immunomagnetically select populations of MSCs [71]. SH-3 and SH-4 are two distinct monoclonal antibodies that apparently react with epitopes on the membrane-bound ecto-5'-nucleotidase (CD73) present on the surface of MSCs [72]. There is, however, no agreement on which of these monoclonal antibodies is most useful for characterization and isolation of bone marrow MSCs.

Differentiation Potential of MSCs

The ability of cultured expanded MSC populations from different species to differentiate into mesenchymal tissues like bone, cartilage, and fat (in vivo and in vitro) has been described and extensively characterized. In vivo grafting followed by demonstration of differentiation has been used as the gold standard to establish pluripotency of MSCs. In addition, several studies have reported differentiation of MSCs into other pathways, including differentiation into cell types from unrelated tissues such as neurons [7, 73, 74]. Most of these studies claim differentiation of MSCs based on morphologic, gene expression and/or phenotypic data. However, in most of these reports, the functional criterion has not been satisfied. Until these data are confirmed and the functional criteria are satisfied, differentiation into non-mesodermal cell types cannot be considered a hallmark characteristic of MSCs.

Osteogenic Differentiation

In vitro bone formation is normally induced by exposing MSC monolayers to serum-containing medium supplemented with β-glycerol-phosphate, ascorbic acid-2-phosphate, and dexamethasone [1, 21]. MSCs cultured under these conditions acquired an osteoblastic morphology, expressed osteogenic genes and deposited mineralized extracellular matrix. Assessment of differentiation is accomplished by histochemical stains, patterns of gene expression and/or phenotypic characteristic. Accumulation of phosphates and carbonates, indicative of osteogenic differentiation or calcium deposits are commonly demonstrated by the von Kossa silver reduction method (Fig. 5.2) [1, 5] or alizarin red method, respectively. Along with histochemical stains, upregulation of osteogenic genes like ostocalcin, osteopontin, and osteonectin have been used as an indication of osteogenic induction. Alkaline phosphatase activity is also upregulated in MSCs undergoing osteogenesis. Friedenstein et al. [27, 75] were the first to demonstrate that in vitro expanded stromal precursors transplanted in closed systems (diffusion chambers) or open systems (under the renal capsule, or subcutaneously) not only could reconstitute the hematopoietic supporting stroma, but also originate bone tissue. This initial demonstration

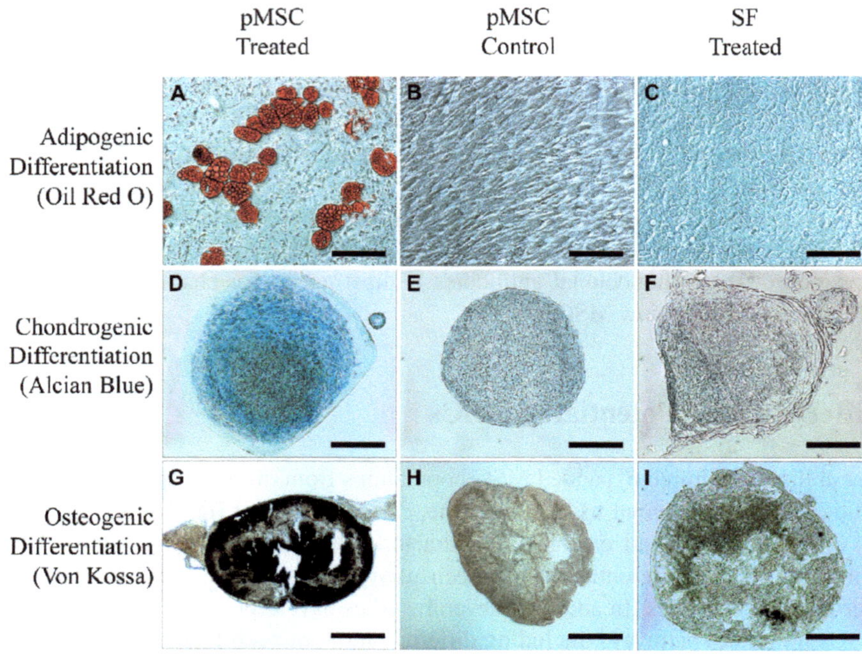

Fig. 5.2 Histochemical stains of SFs and pMSCs exposed to lipogenic, chondrogenic, osteogenic or control media. pMSCs underwent lipogenic (**A**), chondrogenic (**D**), and osteogenic differentiation when exposed to specific induction media. pMSCs cultured in control medium (**B, E,** and **H**) and isogenic SFs (**C, F,** and **I**) exposed to differentiation conditions failed to differentiate. Bar = 100 μm (**A–C**) and 0.5 mm (**D–I**). (Reproduced from Ref [5] with permission from the Society for the Study of Reproduction, Inc.)

was later confirmed by numerous reports of MSC osteogenic differentiation upon grafting in appropriate animal models [18, 76, 77] and set the stage for the use of cultured expanded MSCs in future therapeutic applications for skeletal repair.

Chondrogenic Differentiation

The following in vitro culture conditions are normally required to induce cartilage formation in MSC cultures: (1) a three-dimensional culture system (e.g., micromass culture); (2) a serum-free environment and (3) incorporation of a member of the TGF-β super-family [1, 78]. Under these conditions, a profound change of morphology of fibroblastic MSCs is accompanied by secretion of a number of cartilage-specific extracellular matrix components such as glycosaminoglycan [79], which stain positive with alcian blue (Fig. 5.2). Interestingly, the patterns of sulfation of chondroitin sulfate during in vitro cartilage formation are similar to those observed in maturation of human articular cartilage [80]. Chondrogenic differentiation is seldom observed in monolayer cultures of MSCs; some kind of three-dimensional culture system is required. By far, the most common approach utilizes micromass, a culture system in which, MSCs are pelleted on the bottom of a tube where they form a round mass of cells within ∼24 h of culture. It is believed that this system provides low oxygen tension permissive for chondrogenesis. In addition, in vitro cartilage formation by MSCs is induced by TGF-β1, TGF-β2 or TGF-β3. However, TGF-β2 and TGF-β3 seem to be more effective than TGF-β1 in inducing differentiation of MSC cultures down the chondrogenic pathway [79]. The chondrogenic potential of MSCs has been also demonstrated in vivo by transplantation of MSCs loaded in diffusion chambers [81] or fibronectin-coated hydroxyapatite cubes [82].

Adipogenic Differentiation

A variable proportion of MSCs growing in monolayers can differentiate into adipocytes when exposed to substances that induce elevation of intracellular cyclic AMP. Isobutylmethylxanthine alone or in combination with dbcAMP has been reported to elicit differentiation of MSCs in adipocyte-like cells with large lipid-filed vacuoles which stain positive with lipid-specific dyes like oil O red (Fig. 5.2) or Nile red. In addition to morphological changes, induced cells upregulate genes involved in lipogenesis, including peroxisome proliferator-activated receptor-gamma and fatty acid synthetase. Release of leptin into the culture medium has been used as an indicator of lipogenic differentiation of MSCs [83, 84].

Therapeutic Applications of MSCs

Due to the ability of MSCs to proliferate extensively ex vivo, while maintaining their pluripotent differentiation capabilities (in vivo and in vitro), they are regarded as a particularly attractive cell type for many cell-based therapies in humans. For these applications, autologous or allogenic ex vivo expanded MSCs can be locally or systemically delivered into patients (Fig. 5.3). This setting opens the possibility of genetic manipulation (transient or stable) of MSCs during in vitro expansion previous to transplantation. Another feature of MSCs that enhance their therapeutic appeal is the alleged capacity of these cells to suppress immune responses and their particular immunophenotype that could render them hypoimmunogenic or non-immunogenic upon allotransplantation. In vitro studies indicated that MSCs can suppress T-lymphocyte proliferation induced by irradiated allogeneic blood lymphocytes, dendritic cells, or phytohemaglutinin [85]. Le Blanc [86] has reported that MSCs can inhibit the formation of cytotoxic lymphocytes and can escape lysis by cytotoxic lymphocytes and natural killer cells. Cultured MSCs express HLA Class I antigen but are negative for HLA Class II, CD40, CD80, and CD86 [87, 88]. This immunophenotype is considered as non-immunogenic and suggests that MSCs could induce immunotolerance after transplantation to HLA-mismatched individuals. In line with these in vitro findings, systemic administration of

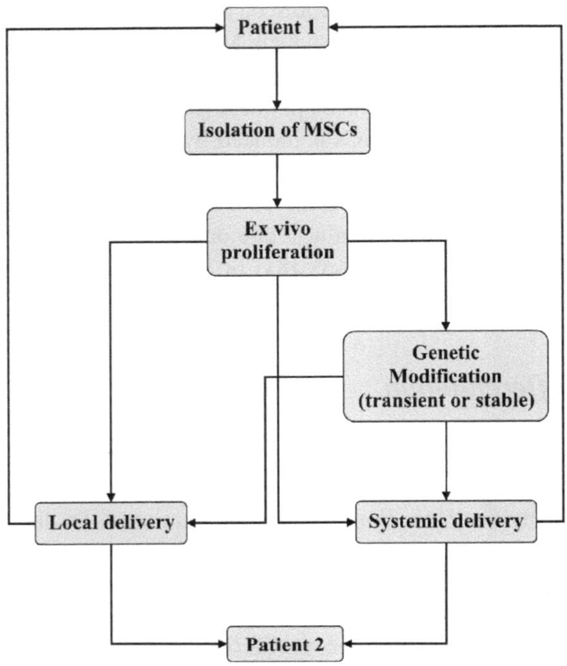

Fig. 5.3 Flowchart showing different therapeutic alternatives of MSCs. Cells are harvested from a donor (Patient 1) and expanded in vitro. Intact or genetically manipulated cells are locally or systemically grafted into the same patient 1 (autologous transplantation) or different patient (patient 2; allogeneic transplantation)

HLA-mismatched MSCs prolonged the survival of skin allografts in immunocompetent baboons [89]. Another study showed that mouse tumoral cells injected subcutaneously in allogeneic hosts formed tumors only when coinjected with MSCs [90]. Furthermore, transplantation of allogeneic MSCs in human trials has resulted in good tolerance to grafted cells with no evidence of graft-versus-host disease [91, 92, 93]. Immunomodulatory properties of MSCs make them a strong candidate cell for many therapeutic applications, especially acute conditions that require immediate cell-based treatment. Based on these alleged immunologic properties, MSCs could be used "off the shelf" for conditions like myocardial infarction, in which, cellular therapy needs to be performed before scar tissue develops.

Local Transplantation

In this approach, the cells are directly placed in the damaged tissue, avoiding cell losses associated with the systemic route. Local administration of cells alone or loaded in different matrices has been the method of choice for the treatment of bone and cartilage defects [94, 95, 96]. Preclinical studies conducted in animal models have unequivocally demonstrated the benefits of using MSC grafts for orthopedic purposes [18, 97, 98, 99, 100]. Quarto et al. [101] have reported successful treatment of long bone defects in patients with defective fracture healing by local injection of autologous, in vitro expanded MSCs. Site-directed administration of MSCs has been also used to repair focal defects in articular cartilage [102, 103] and tendon [104]. In a caprine model of osteoarthritis, autologous MSCs injected in the knee joint were capable of engraftment and repair of the damaged tissues [19]. MSCs engineered to produce growth factors such as those involved in bone and cartilage formation hold great promise in the area of orthopedic medicine [105, 106]. Despite positive results, much work lays ahead in order to optimize these procedures. For instance, determination of the ideal culture conditions for ex vivo expansion of MSCs, optimal composition and structure of the cell carriers and appropriate cell doses to achieve bone/cartilage formation are some areas that will need further study.

Systemic Transplantation

Infusion of MSCs into the general circulation has been attempted in the context of bone marrow transplantation (BMT) or for the treatment of generalized skeletal diseases in which local delivery would not be practical. Since during oncological or hematological BMT, the stroma (containing MSC populations) is not commonly transplanted along with hematopoietic tissue [107, 108], it has been proposed that cotransplantation of MSCs during BMT might hasten hematopoietic recovery [109, 110]. A second rationale for the inclusion of MSCs in BMT is based on the immunological properties of MSCs, which might favor engraftment and reduce the risk of graft-versus-host disease [109]. Based on these unproven but intuitive concepts, several clinical trials aimed to assess the effects of MSCs cotransplantation with hematopoietic cells have been carried out. In general, these studies have reported well tolerance of transplanted cells but low engraftment of donor MSCs and short-term persistence of donor stromal cells [111, 112, 113, 114]. However, in other study, cotransplantation of human ex vivo expanded MSCs with hematopoietic stem cells ($CD34^+$) into NOD-SCID mice induced a 10- to 20-fold increase in engraftment compared with that in animals receiving $CD34^+$ cells alone [115]. Therefore, the benefits and extent of stromal cell or MSC engraftment following standard myeloablative BMT is still a source of controversy.

The ability of MSCs infused into circulation to colonize other tissues has been the focus of many studies. It is clear that infusion of large numbers of MSCs systemically results in non-specific sequestration of cells in capillary beads of different organs specially lung [57, 116, 117]. Low numbers of systemically infused MSCs are found distributed in different tissues, providing evidence for donor cell survival, but stringent criteria to determine engraftment has not been normally provided. Convincing clinical improvements were seen after allogeneic BMT in patients with osteogenesis imperfecta despite the low engraftment observed (only 1.5–2% of osteoblasts were from donor origin) [92, 118]. On the other hand, there is some experimental evidence that suggests specific homing of infused MSCs to sites of injury or tumoral tissue [119, 120, 121]. The mechanisms that guide implanted MSCs to wounded areas or tumors are not clear. One study indicated that inflammatory chemotactic agents and cytokines released during cerebral ischemic damage are responsible for selective migration of infused MSCs into the injured brain [122]. Additional evidence for MSC homing has been provided by Rombouts and Ploemacher [123] in a syngeneic mouse model. The authors reported that homing and engraftment of MSCs to bone marrow in sublethally irradiated mice was much higher than that in unirradiated counterparts. This study also demonstrated that in vitro culture of MSCs previous to transplantation hinders their ability to home and engraft in the bone marrow. The capacity of MSCs infused intravenously to seek out the site of tissue damage has been also demonstrated in animal models of myocardial infarction [124, 125]. A better understanding of the mechanisms governing homing of MSCs will certainly lead to improved MSC-based therapeutic protocols.

Myocardial Repair

Much attention has attracted the application of systemic or site-directed cell-based therapies for future treatment of myocardial damage. Using animal models of acute myocardial infarction, improvements in myocardial function have been reported after administration of cells from a number of sources: fibroblasts, skeletal myoblasts, cardiomyoblasts, unprocessed bone marrow cells, hematopoietic stem cells, and MSCs [125, 126, 127, 128, 129, 130, 131, 132, 133, 134, 135, 136, 137]. Several studies have documented that enriched populations of MSCs when placed in the hearts of adult laboratory rodents engraft in the myocardium and undergo cardiomyocyte differentiation [125, 137, 138]. Despite the fact that MSCs usually integrate at low rates, they exhibited a cardiomyocyte phenotype as evidenced by expression of sarcomeric myosin heavy chain, cardiac troponin I, desmin, and α-actin. In addition to cardiomyocyte replacement, alternative mechanisms to explain improved cardiac and hemodynamic function in these animal models have been postulated, including inhibition of apoptosis, induction of angiogenesis and increased collagen production [139]. Which cell type will be ultimately superior or more practical than the others for cell-based myocardial regeneration remains to be established.

Central Nervous System and Spinal Injury

Central nervous system and spinal injuries are other promising experimental targets for MSC-based therapy strategies. Several laboratories have reported induction of MSC differentiation along the neurogenic pathway under different in vitro culture conditions [7, 73, 74, 140, 141, 142]. Following the demonstration of in vitro neurogenic plasticity, the beneficial effect of local administration of MSCs in animal models of CNS and spinal damage has been documented [143, 144, 145, 146]. In addition to replacing cellular components, it is believed that transplanted MSCs could release trophic factors which in turn might improve the neurologic outcome.

Genetically Modified MSCs for Gene Therapy

Bone marrow-derived MSCs are emerging as an attractive cell type for many cell-based gene therapy strategies. These adult stem cells possess characteristics that make them ideal vehicles for gene delivery: they are relatively easy to obtain from bone marrow aspirates, can be expanded extensively in culture while maintaining their pluripotent differentiation capabilities [1] and are amenable to genetic manipulation to elicit efficient transgene expression [147].

Depending on the final objective, transient or permanent gene modification of cultured MSCs is the desired outcome. When a short-lived effect is necessary, such as for skeletal regeneration, transient transduction can be achieved using DNA plasmids in combination with electroporation or chemical methods like lipofection or calcium phosphate.

An alternative method to obtain transient transfection is the use of adenovirus vectors which can carry double-stranded linear DNA of up to ~36 kb in length in the last generation vectors [148, 149]. Adenoviruses are particularly attractive vectors for ex vivo gene transfer due to their ability to infect a wide range of cell types including quiescent cells, accommodate large pieces of exogenous DNA, and the possibility of production of stocks with high viral titers [150]. Since adenovirus very rarely integrates into the host genome by non-homologous recombination, replication-defective recombinant adenoviral vectors are used as efficient expression vectors particularly for those applications in which high transgene expression for a limited period of time are required.

In replication deficient adenovirus vectors, some or all of the viral genes can be removed (reviewed in [151]). In the first generation adenoviral vectors, the E1 and/or E3 viral genes were deleted, making space for the introduction of up to 6.5 kb of foreign DNA, usually under the control of a heterologous promoter. In second generation adenovectors, some or all of the E2 genes were removed [152, 153], leading to vectors without the capacity to replicate their DNA and to produce replication-competent adenovirus. In a later generation of adenovirus vectors (third generation), more viral genes were removed [154]. In the latest versions, nearly the entire viral DNA but all the inverted terminal repeats (ITRs) and packaging sequences were excised ("gutless" vectors) [148, 149], making enough space to accommodate transgenes of up to ~36 kb in length.

Efficiency of adenovirus-mediated gene deliver is largely limited by the availability of specific viral receptors on target cells. Adenovirus serotype 5-based vectors cell entry is mediated through a receptor-mediated biphasic process. First, the vector recognizes the target cells through attachment of the knob domain of the viral fiber capsid protein to the cellular coxsackie and adenovirus receptor (CAR) [155]. The second step involves the internalization of the vector particle via interaction of the capsid penton protein with $\alpha_V\beta$ integrins present in target cells [156]. Therefore, infectivity of a particular cell type depends largely on the density of CAR and integrins [157, 158]. Despite the broad adenoviral tropism, many cell types are refractory to adenoviral infection due to the lack of or low expression of adenovirus-specific receptors. For instance, adenoviral receptors are expressed at low levels in primitive hematopoietic stem cells [159, 160] and human MSCs [161, 162], leading to poor transduction efficiency by type 5 adenovirus vectors. Consequently, several approaches have been undertaken in order to circumvent this problem. The use of fiber-modified adenovectors or Ad5 vectors possessing fiber proteins from a different adenovirus serotype has become an increasingly popular approach to achieve infection of cells via CAR-independent mechanisms. One of such chimeric vectors is the Ad5/F35, in which, the Ad5 fiber has been replaced by the fiber of Ad35 serotype. In this way, the tropism of Ad5 can be retargeted to that of Ad35, which utilizes cofactor protein CD46 as cellular receptor [163] and thereby can infect CAR-deficient target cells such as human primitive hematopoietic cells [164] and human MSCs [162]. However, CD46 appear to be preferentially expressed in eyes and testes in rodent species [165, 166, 167], limiting the versatility of chimeric Ad5/F35 vectors in these species.

In addition to methods that abrogate CAR tropism, combination of various compounds with adenovirus has been reported to enhance transduction of target cells likely via a receptor-independent pathway. Polycations and cationic lipids form complexes with adenoviral particles facilitating in vitro transduction of refractory tumor cell lines [168, 169] and primary and established cell lines [170, 171, 172, 173]. Similarly, adenoviral infection of primitive human hematopoietic cells can be strongly enhanced by several cationic lipids [174]. Therefore, by using adenovirus vector complexed with polycations, it is possible to combine the advantages of each system to achieve high transduction efficiencies: excellent cellular uptake contributed by the polycation [175] with endosomal escape and nuclear targeting function provided by the vector [176]. We have recently reported that adenoviral infection of human and porcine MSCs in the presence of the polyamine-based transfection reagent GeneJammer (Stratagene, La Jolla, CA, USA) can greatly enhance transduction efficiency of these primary cell lines with replication-defective adenovectors as demonstrated by high-level transgene expression [GFP and bone morphogenetic protein (BMP); Fig. 5.4] [177, 178]. Evidence supports a receptor-independent mechanism for GeneJammer positive effect on adenoviral transduction [178] as it has been demonstrated for cationic molecules [172, 173].

One promising application is the autografting or allografting of genetically modified MSCs as vehicles for local delivery of therapeutic gene products [121, 162, 179, 180]. For instance, MSC delivery system that can produce high levels of active BMP2 and induce bone formation in vivo [105, 106, 162, 179, 181] may prove to be of use for the treatment of several skeletal injuries and diseases. Another particularly interesting application is the use of genetically engineered MSCs as platform for delivery of chemotherapeutics into tumors [121, 182, 183]. The feasibility of this approach has been recently demonstrated in a xenogeneic mouse model (i.e., human MSCs, human tumors grown in immunodeficient mice) [121, 180, 183]. Systemic administration of human MSCs engineered to express human interferon-β (IFN-β), a biological agent with known antiproliferative activity, preferentially homed to tumors where they induced tumor regression presumably through local delivery of IFN-β [121, 183]. More recently, successful delivery of other antitumor agents by MSCs has been reported [182, 184]. Based on these promising results, the use of

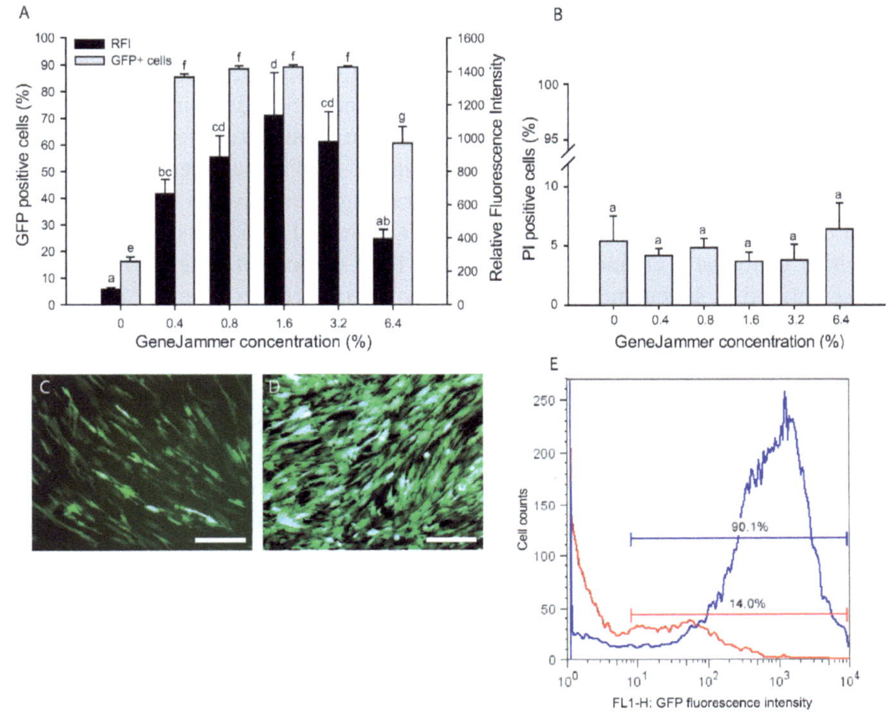

Fig. 5.4 Effect of GeneJammer on transduction efficiency of pMSCs with Ad5F35eGFP (13.8 MOI). pMSC cultures were transduced without (control) or with increasing concentrations of GeneJammer. Twenty-four hours after the induced infection, the percentage of pMSCs expressing GFP and relative fluorescence intensity were analyzed via flow cytometry (**A**). GeneJammer treatment did not affect the percentage of non-viable cells (**B**). Photomicrographs of pMSC cultures 24 h after transduction in absence (**C**) or presence (**D**) of GeneJammer (1.6%). Representative distribution of GFP negative/positive cells from non-treated (red curve; 14.0% of positive cells) and GeneJammer-treated cells (1.6 μL/100 μL; blue curve, 90.1% of positive cells) (**E**). [a,b,c,d,e,f,g]Bars with different letters denote significant differences ($P < 0.05$; ANOVA) within each variable studied. Results are expressed as mean ± SEM from three independent replicates. Bar = 200 μm. (Reproduced from Ref [177] with permission of Wiley-Liss, Inc.)

MSCs as vehicle for delivery of biological agents might prove to be a novel strategy for cancer therapy.

For diseases in which a biological activity is impaired or absent, long-lasting or stable genetic modification of MSCs is usually required for effective treatment. To achieve permanent genetic changes in target cells, virus vectors with intrinsic ability to intercalate in the host genome are chosen. These include: retrovirus, lentivirus, adeno-associated virus and a number of hybrid vectors between adenovirus (non-integrating) with retrovirus, adeno-associated or Epstein-Barr virus. Each of the individual vectors has advantages and disadvantages; the election of a particular one ultimately depends on the specific application. Many studies have documented in vitro transduction of MSCs with different viral vectors (retrovirus, adeno-associated or lentivirus vectors) or a combination of ex vivo viral transduction followed by transplantation into animal models to investigate in vivo gene expression [185, 186, 187, 188, 189, 190, 191, 192, 193, 194, 195, 196, 197, 198, 199, 200, 201, 202]. Generation of genetically engineered MSCs directing the synthesis of reporter molecules, interleukin 3, erythropoietin, coagulation factor VIII, tyrosine hydroxylase, or 3,4-dihydroxyphenylalanine (L-DOPA) has been reported [185, 187, 190, 191, 193, 198, 200, 202]. An interesting alternative to the systemic or local delivery of transduced cells is the implantation of a matrix (e.g., Matrigel), in which genetically engineered MSCs have been embedded. These MSC-matrix masses placed in subcutaneous spaces are neovascularized to form an "organoid," which releases transgenic protein into the bloodstream [193]. These studies demonstrate the great therapeutic potential of these strategies, but at the same time they underscore the hurdles to overcome before this technology is available for clinical use. One obstacle is the development of methods to achieve optimal ex vivo transduction of MSCs. The second problem relates to the relatively short-lived protein expression in the recipient (no more than 4 months) [192]. Loss of transplanted cells and methylation-dependent gene silencing were implicated as major factors responsible for the transitory in vivo transgene expression [185, 191]. Finally, short- and long-term safety concerns associated with the use of vector transduced cells (e.g., neoplastic transformation) must be addressed in appropriate animal models before these technologies can move to the clinical setting.

List of Abbreviations

Ad	Adenovirus
bFGF	Basic fibroblast growth factor
BMP	Bone morphogenetic protein
BMT	Bone marrow transplantation
CAR	Coxsackie and adenovirus receptor
CNS	Central nervous system
EGF	Epidermal growth factor
FBS	Fetal bovine serum
FGF	Fibroblast growth factor
GFP	Green fluorescent protein
IFN	Interferon
IGF-I	Insulin-like growth factor one
ITR	Inverted terminal repeat
L-DOPA	Tyrosine hydroxylase, or 3,4-dihydroxyphenylalanine
MAPC	Multipotent adult progenitor cell
MSC	Mesenchymal stem cell
NOD-SCID	Non-obese diabetic severe combined immunodeficient
PDGF	Platelet derived growth factor
pMSC	Porcine mesenchymal stem cell
PPAR-γ	Peroxisome proliferator-activated receptor-gamma
TGF	Transforming growth factor

References

1. Pittenger MF, Mackay AM, Beck SC et al. (1999) Multilineage potential of adult human mesenchymal stem cells. Science 284:143–147.
2. Erices A, Conget P Minguell JJ (2000) Mesenchymal progenitor cells in human umbilical cord blood. Br J Haematol 109:235–242.
3. Romnov YA, Svintsitskaya VA Smirnov VN (2003) Searching for alternative sources of postnatal human mesenchymal stem cells: Candidate MSC-like cells from umbilical cord. Stem Cells 21:105–110.
4. Muraglia A, Cancedda R Quarto R (2000) Clonal mesenchymal progenitors from human bone marrow differentiate in vitro according to a hierarchical model. J Cell Sci 113 (Pt 7):1161–1166.
5. Bosch P, Pratt SL Stice SL (2006) Isolation, characterization, gene modification and nuclear reprogramming of porcine mesenchymal stem cells. Biol Reprod 74:46–57.
6. Kohyama J, Abe H, Shimazaki T et al. (2001) Brain from bone: Efficient "meta-differentiation" of marrow stroma-derived mature osteoblasts to neurons with noggin or a demethylating agent. Differentiation 68:235–244.
7. Woodbury D, Schwarz EJ, Prockop DJ et al. (2000) Adult rat and human bone marrow stromal cells differentiate into neurons. J Neurosci Res 61:364–370.
8. Friedenstein AJ, Gorskaja JF Kulagina NN (1976) Fibroblast precursors in normal and irradiated mouse hematopoietic organs. Exp Hematol 4:267–274.
9. Simmons DJ, Seitz P, Kidder L et al. (1991) Partial characterization of rat marrow stromal cells. Calcif Tissue Int 48:326–334.
10. Mendelow B, Grobicki D, de la Hunt M et al. (1980) Characterization of bone marrow stromal cells in suspension and monolayer cultures. Br J Haematol 46:15–22.
11. Martin DR, Cox NR, Hathcock TL et al. (2002) Isolation and characterization of multipotential mesenchymal stem cells from feline bone marrow. Exp Hematol 30:879–886.
12. Huss R, Hoy CA Deeg HJ (1995) Contact- and growth factor-dependent survival in a canine marrow-derived stromal cell line. Blood 85:2414–2421.
13. Ringe J, Kaps C, Schmitt B et al. (2002) Porcine mesenchymal stem cells. Induction of distinct mesenchymal cell lineages. Cell Tissue Res 307:321–327.
14. Digirolamo CM, Stokes D, Colter D et al. (1999) Propagation and senescence of human marrow stromal cells in culture: A simple colony-forming assay identifies samples with the greatest potential to propagate and differentiate. Br J Haematol 107:275–281.
15. Murphy JM, Dixon K, Beck S et al. (2002) Reduced chondrogenic and adipogenic activity of mesenchymal stem cells from patients with advanced osteoarthritis. Arthritis Rheum 46:704–713.
16. Oreffo RO, Bord S Triffitt JT (1998) Skeletal progenitor cells and ageing human populations. Clin Sci (Lond) 94:549–555.
17. D'Ippolito G, Schiller PC, Ricordi C et al. (1999) Age-related osteogenic potential of mesenchymal stromal stem cells from human vertebral bone marrow. J Bone Miner Res 14:1115–1122.
18. Kadiyala S, Young RG, Thiede MA et al. (1997) Culture expanded canine mesenchymal stem cells possess osteochondrogenic potential in vivo and in vitro. Cell Transplant 6: 125–134.
19. Murphy JM, Fink DJ, Hunziker EB et al. (2003) Stem cell therapy in a caprine model of osteoarthritis. Arthritis Rheum 48:3464–3474.
20. Shake JG, Gruber PJ, Baumgartner WA et al. (2002) Mesenchymal stem cell implantation in a swine myocardial infarct model: Engraftment and functional effects. Ann Thorac Surg 73:1919–1925; discussion 1926.
21. Javazon EH, Colter DC, Schwarz EJ et al. (2001) Rat marrow stromal cells are more sensitive to plating density and expand more rapidly from single-cell-derived colonies than human marrow stromal cells. Stem Cells 19:219–225.

22. Kuznetsov SA, Friedenstein AJ Robey PG (1997) Factors required for bone marrow stromal fibroblast colony formation in vitro. Br J Haematol 97:561–570.
23. Phinney DG, Kopen G, Isaacson RL et al. (1999) Plastic adherent stromal cells from the bone marrow of commonly used strains of inbred mice: Variations in yield, growth, and differentiation. J Cell Biochem 72:570–585.
24. Banfi A, Bianchi G, Notaro R et al. (2002) Replicative aging and gene expression in long-term cultures of human bone marrow stromal cells. Tissue Eng 8:901–910.
25. Bianchi G, Banfi A, Mastrogiacomo M et al. (2003) Ex vivo enrichment of mesenchymal cell progenitors by fibroblast growth factor 2. Exp Cell Res 287:98–105.
26. Ito T, Sawada R, Fujiwara Y et al. (2007) FGF-2 suppresses cellular senescence of human mesenchymal stem cells by down-regulation of TGF-beta2. Biochem Biophys Res Commun 359:108–114.
27. Friedenstein AJ, Chailakhjan RK Lalykina KS (1970) The development of fibroblast colonies in monolayer cultures of guinea-pig bone marrow and spleen cells. Cell Tissue Kinet 3:393–403.
28. Friedenstein AJ, Deriglasova UF, Kulagina NN et al. (1974) Precursors for fibroblasts in different populations of hematopoietic cells as detected by the in vitro colony assay method. Exp Hematol 2:83–92.
29. Kuznetsov SA, Krebsbach PH, Satomura K et al. (1997) Single-colony derived strains of human marrow stromal fibroblasts form bone after transplantation in vivo. J Bone Miner Res 12:1335–1347.
30. Owen M Friedenstein AJ (1988) Stromal stem cells: Marrow-derived osteogenic precursors. Ciba Found Symp 136:42–60.
31. Minguell JJ, Erices A Conget P (2001) Mesenchymal stem cells. Exp Biol Med (Maywood) 226:507–520.
32. Castro-Malaspina H, Gay RE, Resnick G et al. (1980) Characterization of human bone marrow fibroblast colony-forming cells (CFU-F) and their progeny. Blood 56:289–301.
33. Gronthos S Simmons PJ (1995) The growth factor requirements of STRO-1-positive human bone marrow stromal precursors under serum-deprived conditions in vitro. Blood 85: 929–940.
34. Martin I, Muraglia A, Campanile G et al. (1997) Fibroblast growth factor-2 supports ex vivo expansion and maintenance of osteogenic precursors from human bone marrow. Endocrinology 138:4456–4462.
35. Solchaga LA, Penick K, Porter JD et al. (2005) FGF-2 enhances the mitotic and chondrogenic potentials of human adult bone marrow-derived mesenchymal stem cells. J Cell Physiol 203:398–409.
36. da Silva Meirelles L, Chagastelles PC Nardi NB (2006) Mesenchymal stem cells reside in virtually all post-natal organs and tissues. J Cell Sci 119:2204–2213.
37. Friedenstein AJ, Chailakhyan RK, Latsinik NV et al. (1974) Stromal cells responsible for transferring the microenvironment of the hemopoietic tissues. Cloning in vitro and retransplantation in vivo. Transplantation 17:331–340.
38. Campagnoli C, Roberts IA, Kumar S et al. (2001) Identification of mesenchymal stem/progenitor cells in human first-trimester fetal blood, liver, and bone marrow. Blood 98:2396–2402.
39. Charbord P, Oostendorp R, Pang W et al. (2002) Comparative study of stromal cell lines derived from embryonic, fetal, and postnatal mouse blood-forming tissues. Exp Hematol 30:1202–1210.
40. Gronthos S, Franklin DM, Leddy HA et al. (2001) Surface protein characterization of human adipose tissue-derived stromal cells. J Cell Physiol 189:54–63.
41. In't Anker PS, Noort WA, Scherjon SA et al. (2003) Mesenchymal stem cells in human second-trimester bone marrow, liver, lung, and spleen exhibit a similar immunophenotype but a heterogeneous multilineage differentiation potential. Haematologica 88: 845–852.

42. In't Anker PS, Scherjon SA, Kleijburg-van der Keur C et al. (2003) Amniotic fluid as a novel source of mesenchymal stem cells for therapeutic transplantation. Blood 102: 1548–1549.
43. Kuznetsov SA, Mankani MH, Gronthos S et al. (2001) Circulating skeletal stem cells. J Cell Biol 153:1133–1140.
44. Luria EA, Panasyuk AF Friedenstein AY (1971) Fibroblast colony formation from monolayer cultures of blood cells. Transfusion 11:345–349.
45. Nakahara H, Dennis JE, Bruder SP et al. (1991) In vitro differentiation of bone and hypertrophic cartilage from periosteal-derived cells. Exp Cell Res 195:492–503.
46. O'Donoghue K, Choolani M, Chan J et al. (2003) Identification of fetal mesenchymal stem cells in maternal blood: Implications for non-invasive prenatal diagnosis. Mol Hum Reprod 9:497–502.
47. Roufosse CA, Direkze NC, Otto WR et al. (2004) Circulating mesenchymal stem cells. Int J Biochem Cell Biol 36:585–597.
48. Zuk PA, Zhu M, Ashjian P et al. (2002) Human adipose tissue is a source of multipotent stem cells. Mol Biol Cell 13:4279–4295.
49. Fernandez M, Simon V, Herrera G et al. (1997) Detection of stromal cells in peripheral blood progenitor cell collections from breast cancer patients. Bone Marrow Transplant 20: 265–271.
50. Huss R, Lange C, Weissinger EM et al. (2000) Evidence of peripheral blood-derived, plastic-adherent CD34(-/low) hematopoietic stem cell clones with mesenchymal stem cell characteristics. Stem Cells 18:252–260.
51. Wu GD, Nolta JA, Jin YS et al. (2003) Migration of mesenchymal stem cells to heart allografts during chronic rejection. Transplantation 75:679–685.
52. Zvaifler NJ, Marinova-Mutafchieva L, Adams G et al. (2000) Mesenchymal precursor cells in the blood of normal individuals. Arthritis Res 2:477–488.
53. Lazarus HM, Haynesworth SE, Gerson SL et al. (1997) Human bone marrow-derived mesenchymal (stromal) progenitor cells (mpcs) cannot be recovered from peripheral blood progenitor cell collections. J Hematother 6:447–455.
54. Wexler SA, Donaldson C, Denning-Kendall P et al. (2003) Adult bone marrow is a rich source of human mesenchymal 'stem' cells but umbilical cord and mobilized adult blood are not. Br J Haematol 121:368–374.
55. Pereira RF, Halford KW, O'Hara MD et al. (1995) Cultured adherent cells from marrow can serve as long-lasting precursor cells for bone, cartilage, and lung in irradiated mice. Proc Natl Acad Sci U S A 92:4857–4861.
56. Prockop DJ (1997) Marrow stromal cells as stem cells for nonhematopoietic tissues. Science 276:71–74.
57. Gao J, Dennis JE, Muzic RF et al. (2001) The dynamic in vivo distribution of bone marrow-derived mesenchymal stem cells after infusion. Cells Tissues Organs 169:12–20.
58. Reyes M, Lund T, Lenvik T et al. (2001) Purification and ex vivo expansion of postnatal human marrow mesodermal progenitor cells. Blood 98:2615–2625.
59. Reyes M Verfaillie CM (2001) Characterization of multipotent adult progenitor cells, a subpopulation of mesenchymal stem cells. Ann N Y Acad Sci 938:231–233; discussion 233–235.
60. Ulloa-Montoya F, Kidder BL, Pauwelyn KA et al. (2007) Comparative transcriptome analysis of embryonic and adult stem cells with extended and limited differentiation capacity. Genome Biol 8:R163.
61. Jiang Y, Jahagirdar BN, Reinhardt RL et al. (2002) Pluripotency of mesenchymal stem cells derived from adult marrow. Nature 418:41–49.
62. Schwartz RE, Reyes M, Koodie L et al. (2002) Multipotent adult progenitor cells from bone marrow differentiate into functional hepatocyte-like cells. J Clin Invest 109:1291–1302.
63. Reyes M, Dudek A, Jahagirdar B et al. (2002) Origin of endothelial progenitors in human postnatal bone marrow. J Clin Invest 109:337–346.

64. Colter DC, Class R, DiGirolamo CM et al. (2000) Rapid expansion of recycling stem cells in cultures of plastic-adherent cells from human bone marrow. Proc Natl Acad Sci U S A 97:3213–3218.
65. Peister A, Mellad JA, Larson BL et al. (2004) Adult stem cells from bone marrow (MSCs) isolated from different strains of inbred mice vary in surface epitopes, rates of proliferation, and differentiation potential. Blood 103:1662–1668.
66. Verfaillie CM (1998) Adhesion receptors as regulators of the hematopoietic process. Blood 92:2609–2612.
67. Simmons PJ Torok-Storb B (1991) Identification of stromal cell precursors in human bone marrow by a novel monoclonal antibody, STRO-1. Blood 78:55–62.
68. Gronthos S, Graves SE, Ohta S et al. (1994) The STRO-1+ fraction of adult human bone marrow contains the osteogenic precursors. Blood 84:4164–4173.
69. Gronthos S, Zannettino AC, Hay SJ et al. (2003) Molecular and cellular characterisation of highly purified stromal stem cells derived from human bone marrow. J Cell Sci 116: 1827–1835.
70. Haynesworth SE, Baber MA Caplan AI (1992) Cell surface antigens on human marrow-derived mesenchymal cells are detected by monoclonal antibodies. Bone 13:69–80.
71. Barry FP, Boynton RE, Haynesworth S et al. (1999) The monoclonal antibody SH-2, raised against human mesenchymal stem cells, recognizes an epitope on endoglin (CD105). Biochem Biophys Res Commun 265:134–139.
72. Barry FP, Boynton RE, Murphy M et al. (2001) The SH-3 and SH-4 antibodies recognize distinct epitopes on CD73 from human mesenchymal stem cells. Biochem Biophys Res Commun 289:519–524.
73. Deng W, Obrocka M, Fischer I et al. (2001) In vitro differentiation of human marrow stromal cells into early progenitors of neural cells by conditions that increase intracellular cyclic AMP. Biochem Biophys Res Commun 282:148–152.
74. Sanchez-Ramos J, Song S, Cardozo-Pelaez F et al. (2000) Adult bone marrow stromal cells differentiate into neural cells in vitro. Exp Neurol 164:247–256.
75. Friedenstein AJ, Piatetzky S II, Petrakova KV (1966) Osteogenesis in transplants of bone marrow cells. J Embryol Exp Morphol 16:381–390.
76. Goshima J, Goldberg VM Caplan AI (1991) The origin of bone formed in composite grafts of porous calcium phosphate ceramic loaded with marrow cells. Clin Orthop Relat Res 269:274–283.
77. Krebsbach PH, Kuznetsov SA, Satomura K et al. (1997) Bone formation in vivo: Comparison of osteogenesis by transplanted mouse and human marrow stromal fibroblasts. Transplantation 63:1059–1069.
78. Mackay AM, Beck SC, Murphy JM et al. (1998) Chondrogenic differentiation of cultured human mesenchymal stem cells from marrow. Tissue Eng 4:415–428.
79. Barry FP, Boynton RE, Liu B et al. (2001) Chondrogenic differentiation of mesenchymal stem cells from bone marrow: Differentiation-dependent gene expression of matrix components. Exp Cell Res 268:189–200.
80. Bayliss MT (1990) Proteoglycan structure and metabolism during maturation and ageing of human articular cartilage. Biochem Soc Trans 18:799–802.
81. Ashton BA, Allen TD, Howlett CR et al. (1980) Formation of bone and cartilage by marrow stromal cells in diffusion chambers in vivo. Clin Orthop Relat Res 151:294–307.
82. Barry FP Murphy JM (2004) Mesenchymal stem cells: Clinical applications and biological characterization. Int J Biochem Cell Biol 36:568–584.
83. Janderova L, McNeil M, Murrell AN et al. (2003) Human mesenchymal stem cells as an in vitro model for human adipogenesis. Obes Res 11:65–74.
84. Ryden M, Dicker A, Gotherstrom C et al. (2003) Functional characterization of human mesenchymal stem cell-derived adipocytes. Biochem Biophys Res Commun 311:391–397.
85. Di Nicola M, Carlo-Stella C, Magni M et al. (2002) Human bone marrow stromal cells suppress T-lymphocyte proliferation induced by cellular or nonspecific mitogenic stimuli. Blood 99:3838–3843.

86. Le Blanc K (2003) Immunomodulatory effects of fetal and adult mesenchymal stem cells. Cytotherapy 5:485–489.
87. Majumdar MK, Keane-Moore M, Buyaner D et al. (2003) Characterization and functionality of cell surface molecules on human mesenchymal stem cells. J Biomed Sci 10: 228–241.
88. Tse WT, Pendleton JD, Beyer WM et al. (2003) Suppression of allogeneic T-cell proliferation by human marrow stromal cells: Implications in transplantation. Transplantation 75:389–397.
89. Bartholomew A, Sturgeon C, Siatskas M et al. (2002) Mesenchymal stem cells suppress lymphocyte proliferation in vitro and prolong skin graft survival in vivo. Exp Hematol 30:42–48.
90. Djouad F, Plence P, Bony C et al. (2003) Immunosuppressive effect of mesenchymal stem cells favors tumor growth in allogeneic animals. Blood 102:3837–3844.
91. Fouillard L, Bensidhoum M, Bories D et al. (2003) Engraftment of allogeneic mesenchymal stem cells in the bone marrow of a patient with severe idiopathic aplastic anemia improves stroma. Leukemia 17:474–476.
92. Horwitz EM, Prockop DJ, Fitzpatrick LA et al. (1999) Transplantability and therapeutic effects of bone marrow-derived mesenchymal cells in children with osteogenesis imperfecta. Nat Med 5:309–313.
93. Koc ON, Day J, Nieder M et al. (2002) Allogeneic mesenchymal stem cell infusion for treatment of metachromatic leukodystrophy (MLD) and hurler syndrome (MPS-IH). Bone Marrow Transplant 30:215–222.
94. Diduch DR, Jordan LC, Mierisch CM et al. (2000) Marrow stromal cells embedded in alginate for repair of osteochondral defects. Arthroscopy 16:571–577.
95. Mankani MH, Kuznetsov SA, Fowler B et al. (2001) In vivo bone formation by human bone marrow stromal cells: Effect of carrier particle size and shape. Biotechnol Bioeng 72: 96–107.
96. Tsuchida H, Hashimoto J, Crawford E et al. (2003) Engineered allogeneic mesenchymal stem cells repair femoral segmental defect in rats. J Orthop Res 21:44–53.
97. Bruder SP, Fink DJ Caplan AI (1994) Mesenchymal stem cells in bone development, bone repair, and skeletal regeneration therapy. J Cell Biochem 56:283–294.
98. Bruder SP, Kraus KH, Goldberg VM et al. (1998) The effect of implants loaded with autologous mesenchymal stem cells on the healing of canine segmental bone defects. J Bone Joint Surg Am 80:985–996.
99. Kon E, Muraglia A, Corsi A et al. (2000) Autologous bone marrow stromal cells loaded onto porous hydroxyapatite ceramic accelerate bone repair in critical-size defects of sheep long bones. J Biomed Mater Res 49:328–337.
100. Ohgushi H, Goldberg VM Caplan AI (1989) Repair of bone defects with marrow cells and porous ceramic. Experiments in rats. Acta Orthop Scand 60:334–339.
101. Quarto R, Mastrogiacomo M, Cancedda R et al. (2001) Repair of large bone defects with the use of autologous bone marrow stromal cells. N Engl J Med 344:385–386.
102. Ponticiello MS, Schinagl RM, Kadiyala S et al. (2000) Gelatin-based resorbable sponge as a carrier matrix for human mesenchymal stem cells in cartilage regeneration therapy. J Biomed Mater Res 52:246–255.
103. Solchaga LA, Gao J, Dennis JE et al. (2002) Treatment of osteochondral defects with autologous bone marrow in a hyaluronan-based delivery vehicle. Tissue Eng 8:333–347.
104. Young RG, Butler DL, Weber W et al. (1998) Use of mesenchymal stem cells in a collagen matrix for Achilles tendon repair. J Orthop Res 16:406–413.
105. Gazit D, Turgeman G, Kelley P et al. (1999) Engineered pluripotent mesenchymal cells integrate and differentiate in regenerating bone: A novel cell-mediated gene therapy. J Gene Med 1:121–133.
106. Riew KD, Wright NM, Cheng S et al. (1998) Induction of bone formation using a recombinant adenoviral vector carrying the human BMP-2 gene in a rabbit spinal fusion model. Calcif Tissue Int 63:357–360.

107. Laver J, Jhanwar SC, O'Reilly RJ et al. (1987) Host origin of the human hematopoietic microenvironment following allogeneic bone marrow transplantation. Blood 70: 1966–1968.
108. Ma DD, Da WM, Purvis-Smith S et al. (1987) Chromosomal analysis of bone marrow stromal fibroblasts in allogeneic HLA compatible sibling bone marrow transplantations. Leuk Res 11:661–663.
109. Deans RJ Moseley AB (2000) Mesenchymal stem cells: Biology and potential clinical uses. Exp Hematol 28:875–884.
110. Fan TX, Hisha H, Jin TN et al. (2001) Successful allogeneic bone marrow transplantation (BMT) by injection of bone marrow cells via portal vein: Stromal cells as BMT-facilitating cells. Stem Cells 19:144–150.
111. Agematsu K Nakahori Y (1991) Recipient origin of bone marrow-derived fibroblastic stromal cells during all periods following bone marrow transplantation in humans. Br J Haematol 79:359–365.
112. Awaya N, Rupert K, Bryant E et al. (2002) Failure of adult marrow-derived stem cells to generate marrow stroma after successful hematopoietic stem cell transplantation. Exp Hematol 30:937–942.
113. Simmons PJ, Przepiorka D, Thomas ED et al. (1987) Host origin of marrow stromal cells following allogeneic bone marrow transplantation. Nature 328:429–432.
114. Stute N, Fehse B, Schroder J et al. (2002) Human mesenchymal stem cells are not of donor origin in patients with severe aplastic anemia who underwent sex-mismatched allogeneic bone marrow transplant. J Hematother Stem Cell Res 11:977–984.
115. Brandt JE, Galy AH, Luens KM et al. (1998) Bone marrow repopulation by human marrow stem cells after long-term expansion culture on a porcine endothelial cell line. Exp Hematol 26:950–961.
116. Hou Z, Nguyen Q, Frenkel B et al. (1999) Osteoblast-specific gene expression after transplantation of marrow cells: Implications for skeletal gene therapy. Proc Natl Acad Sci U S A 96:7294–7299.
117. Pereira RF, O'Hara MD, Laptev AV et al. (1998) Marrow stromal cells as a source of progenitor cells for nonhematopoietic tissues in transgenic mice with a phenotype of osteogenesis imperfecta. Proc Natl Acad Sci U S A 95:1142–1147.
118. Horwitz EM, Prockop DJ, Gordon PL et al. (2001) Clinical responses to bone marrow transplantation in children with severe osteogenesis imperfecta. Blood 97:1227–1231.
119. Herrera MB, Bussolati B, Bruno S et al. (2007) Exogenous mesenchymal stem cells localize to the kidney by means of CD44 following acute tubular injury. Kidney Int 72: 430–441.
120. Komarova S, Kawakami Y, Stoff-Khalili MA et al. (2006) Mesenchymal progenitor cells as cellular vehicles for delivery of oncolytic adenoviruses. Mol Cancer Ther 5:755–766.
121. Studeny M, Marini FC, Champlin RE et al. (2002) Bone marrow-derived mesenchymal stem cells as vehicles for interferon-beta delivery into tumors. Cancer Res 62:3603–3608.
122. Wang L, Li Y, Chen X et al. (2002) MCP-1, MIP-1, IL-8 and ischemic cerebral tissue enhance human bone marrow stromal cell migration in interface culture. Hematology 7: 113–117.
123. Rombouts WJ Ploemacher RE (2003) Primary murine MSC show highly efficient homing to the bone marrow but lose homing ability following culture. Leukemia 17:160–170.
124. Nagaya N, Fujii T, Iwase T et al. (2004) Intravenous administration of mesenchymal stem cells improves cardiac function in rats with acute myocardial infarction through angiogenesis and myogenesis. Am J Physiol Heart Circ Physiol 287:H2670–H2676.
125. Toma C, Pittenger MF, Cahill KS et al. (2002) Human mesenchymal stem cells differentiate to a cardiomyocyte phenotype in the adult murine heart. Circulation 105:93–98.
126. Barbash IM, Chouraqui P, Baron J et al. (2003) Systemic delivery of bone marrow-derived mesenchymal stem cells to the infarcted myocardium: Feasibility, cell migration, and body distribution. Circulation 108:863–868.

127. Gandy KL Weissman IL (1998) Tolerance of allogeneic heart grafts in mice simultaneously reconstituted with purified allogeneic hematopoietic stem cells. Transplantation 65: 295–304.
128. Jackson KA, Majka SM, Wang H et al. (2001) Regeneration of ischemic cardiac muscle and vascular endothelium by adult stem cells. J Clin Invest 107:1395–1402.
129. Mangi AA, Noiseux N, Kong D et al. (2003) Mesenchymal stem cells modified with Akt prevent remodeling and restore performance of infarcted hearts. Nat Med 9:1195–1201.
130. Min JY, Sullivan MF, Yang Y et al. (2002) Significant improvement of heart function by cotransplantation of human mesenchymal stem cells and fetal cardiomyocytes in postinfarcted pigs. Ann Thorac Surg 74:1568–1575.
131. Orlic D, Kajstura J, Chimenti S et al. (2001) Transplanted adult bone marrow cells repair myocardial infarcts in mice. Ann N Y Acad Sci 938:221–229; discussion 229–230.
132. Orlic D, Kajstura J, Chimenti S et al. (2003) Bone marrow stem cells regenerate infarcted myocardium. Pediatr Transplant 7 Suppl 3:86–88.
133. Saito T, Kuang JQ, Lin CC et al. (2003) Transcoronary implantation of bone marrow stromal cells ameliorates cardiac function after myocardial infarction. J Thorac Cardiovasc Surg 126:114–123.
134. Sakai T, Li RK, Weisel RD et al. (1999) Fetal cell transplantation: A comparison of three cell types. J Thorac Cardiovasc Surg 118:715–724.
135. Tambara K, Sakakibara Y, Sakaguchi G et al. (2003) Transplanted skeletal myoblasts can fully replace the infarcted myocardium when they survive in the host in large numbers. Circulation 108 Suppl 1:II259–II263.
136. Thompson RB, Emani SM, Davis BH et al. (2003) Comparison of intracardiac cell transplantation: Autologous skeletal myoblasts versus bone marrow cells. Circulation 108 Suppl 1:II264–II271.
137. Tomita S, Li RK, Weisel RD et al. (1999) Autologous transplantation of bone marrow cells improves damaged heart function. Circulation 100:II247–II256.
138. Wang JS, Shum-Tim D, Galipeau J et al. (2000) Marrow stromal cells for cellular cardiomyoplasty: Feasibility and potential clinical advantages. J Thorac Cardiovasc Surg 120: 999–1005.
139. Hou M, Yang KM, Zhang H et al. (2007) Transplantation of mesenchymal stem cells from human bone marrow improves damaged heart function in rats. Int J Cardiol 115:220–228.
140. Black IB Woodbury D (2001) Adult rat and human bone marrow stromal stem cells differentiate into neurons. Blood Cells Mol Dis 27:632–636.
141. Krampera M, Marconi S, Pasini A et al. (2007) Induction of neural-like differentiation in human mesenchymal stem cells derived from bone marrow, fat, spleen and thymus. Bone 40:382–390.
142. Mareschi K, Novara M, Rustichelli D et al. (2006) Neural differentiation of human mesenchymal stem cells: Evidence for expression of neural markers and eag K+ channel types. Exp Hematol 34:1563–1572.
143. Hofstetter CP, Schwarz EJ, Hess D et al. (2002) Marrow stromal cells form guiding strands in the injured spinal cord and promote recovery. Proc Natl Acad Sci U S A 99:2199–2204.
144. Lu D, Li Y, Wang L et al. (2001) Intraarterial administration of marrow stromal cells in a rat model of traumatic brain injury. J Neurotrauma 18:813–819.
145. Wu S, Suzuki Y, Ejiri Y et al. (2003) Bone marrow stromal cells enhance differentiation of cocultured neurosphere cells and promote regeneration of injured spinal cord. J Neurosci Res 72:343–351.
146. Zhang H, Huang Z, Xu Y et al. (2006) Differentiation and neurological benefit of the mesenchymal stem cells transplanted into the rat brain following intracerebral hemorrhage. Neurol Res 28:104–112.
147. Hung SC, Lu CY, Shyue SK et al. (2004) Lineage differentiation-associated loss of adenoviral susceptibility and coxsackie-adenovirus receptor expression in human mesenchymal stem cells. Stem Cells 22:1321–1329.

148. Morsy MA, Gu M, Motzel S et al. (1998) An adenoviral vector deleted for all viral coding sequences results in enhanced safety and extended expression of a leptin transgene. Proc Natl Acad Sci U S A 95:7866–7871.
149. Steinwaerder DS, Carlson CA Lieber A (1999) Generation of adenovirus vectors devoid of all viral genes by recombination between inverted repeats. J Virol 73:9303–9313.
150. Amalfitano A (2004) Utilization of adenovirus vectors for multiple gene transfer applications. Methods 33:173–178.
151. Russell WC (2000) Update on adenovirus and its vectors. J Gen Virol 81:2573–2604.
152. Lusky M, Grave L, Dieterle A et al. (1999) Regulation of adenovirus-mediated transgene expression by the viral e4 gene products: Requirement for E4 ORF3. J Virol 73:8308–8319.
153. Moorhead JW, Clayton GH, Smith RL et al. (1999) A replication-incompetent adenovirus vector with the preterminal protein gene deleted efficiently transduces mouse ears. J Virol 73:1046–1053.
154. Amalfitano A, Hauser MA, Hu H et al. (1998) Production and characterization of improved adenovirus vectors with the E1, E2b, and E3 genes deleted. J Virol 72:926–933.
155. Bergelson JM, Cunningham JA, Droguett G et al. (1997) Isolation of a common receptor for coxsackie b viruses and adenoviruses 2 and 5. Science 275:1320–1323.
156. Wickham TJ, Mathias P, Cheresh DA et al. (1993) Integrins alpha v beta 3 and alpha v beta 5 promote adenovirus internalization but not virus attachment. Cell 73:309–319.
157. Goldman M, Su Q Wilson JM (1996) Gradient of RGD-dependent entry of adenoviral vector in nasal and intrapulmonary epithelia: Implications for gene therapy of cystic fibrosis. Gene Ther 3:811–818.
158. Wickham TJ, Roelvink PW, Brough DE et al. (1996) Adenovirus targeted to heparan-containing receptors increases its gene delivery efficiency to multiple cell types. Nat Biotechnol 14:1570–1573.
159. Rebel VI, Hartnett S, Denham J et al. (2000) Maturation and lineage-specific expression of the coxsackie and adenovirus receptor in hematopoietic cells. Stem Cells 18:176–182.
160. Thoma SJ, Lamping CP Ziegler BL (1994) Phenotype analysis of hematopoietic CD34+ cell populations derived from human umbilical cord blood using flow cytometry and CDNA-polymerase chain reaction. Blood 83:2103–2114.
161. Conget PA Minguell JJ (2000) Adenoviral-mediated gene transfer into ex vivo expanded human bone marrow mesenchymal progenitor cells. Exp Hematol 28:382–390.
162. Olmsted-Davis EA, Gugala Z, Gannon FH et al. (2002) Use of a chimeric adenovirus vector enhances BMP2 production and bone formation. Hum Gene Ther 13:1337–1347.
163. Gaggar A, Shayakhmetov DM Lieber A (2003) CD46 is a cellular receptor for group b adenoviruses. Nat Med 9:1408–1412.
164. Yotnda P, Onishi H, Heslop HE et al. (2001) Efficient infection of primitive hematopoietic stem cells by modified adenovirus. Gene Ther 8:930–937.
165. Miwa T, Nonaka M, Okada N et al. (1998) Molecular cloning of rat and mouse membrane cofactor protein (MCP, CD46): Preferential expression in testis and close linkage between the mouse Mcp and Cr2 genes on distal chromosome 1. Immunogenetics 48:363–371.
166. Sohn JH, Kaplan HJ, Suk HJ et al. (2000) Chronic low level complement activation within the eye is controlled by intraocular complement regulatory proteins. Invest Ophthalmol Vis Sci 41:3492–3502.
167. Tsujimura A, Shida K, Kitamura M et al. (1998) Molecular cloning of a murine homologue of membrane cofactor protein (CD46): Preferential expression in testicular germ cells. Biochem J 330 (Pt 1):163–168.
168. Clark PR, Stopeck AT, Brailey JL et al. (1999) Polycations and cationic lipids enhance adenovirus transduction and transgene expression in tumor cells. Cancer Gene Ther 6: 437–446.
169. Lee EM, Hong SH, Lee YJ et al. (2004) Liposome-complexed adenoviral gene transfer in cancer cells expressing various levels of coxsackievirus and adenovirus receptor. J Cancer Res Clin Oncol 130:169–177.

170. Arcasoy SM, Latoche JD, Gondor M et al. (1997) Polycations increase the efficiency of adenovirus-mediated gene transfer to epithelial and endothelial cells in vitro. Gene Ther 4:32–38.
171. Dodds E, Piper TA, Murphy SJ et al. (1999) Cationic lipids and polymers are able to enhance adenoviral infection of cultured mouse myotubes. J Neurochem 72:2105–2112.
172. Fasbender A, Zabner J, Chillon M et al. (1997) Complexes of adenovirus with polycationic polymers and cationic lipids increase the efficiency of gene transfer in vitro and in vivo. J Biol Chem 272:6479–6489.
173. Qiu C, De Young MB, Finn A et al. (1998) Cationic liposomes enhance adenovirus entry via a pathway independent of the fiber receptor and alpha(v)-integrins. Hum Gene Ther 9:507–520.
174. Byk T, Haddada H, Vainchenker W et al. (1998) Lipofectamine and related cationic lipids strongly improve adenoviral infection efficiency of primitive human hematopoietic cells. Hum Gene Ther 9:2493–2502.
175. Zabner J, Fasbender AJ, Moninger T et al. (1995) Cellular and molecular barriers to gene transfer by a cationic lipid. J Biol Chem 270:18997–19007.
176. Seth P (1994) Mechanism of adenovirus-mediated endosome lysis: Role of the intact adenovirus capsid structure. Biochem Biophys Res Commun 205:1318–1324.
177. Bosch P, Fouletier-Dilling C, Olmsted-Davis EA et al. (2006) Efficient adenoviral-mediated gene delivery into porcine mesenchymal stem cells. Mol Reprod Dev 73: 1393–1403.
178. Fouletier-Dilling CM, Bosch P, Davis AR et al. (2005) Novel compound enables high-level adenovirus transduction in the absence of an adenovirus-specific receptor. Hum Gene Ther 16:1287–1297.
179. Cheng SL, Lou J, Wright NM et al. (2001) In vitro and in vivo induction of bone formation using a recombinant adenoviral vector carrying the human BMP-2 gene. Calcif Tissue Int 68:87–94.
180. Nakamizo A, Marini F, Amano T et al. (2005) Human bone marrow-derived mesenchymal stem cells in the treatment of gliomas. Cancer Res 65:3307–3318.
181. Chang SC, Wei FC, Chuang H et al. (2003) Ex vivo gene therapy in autologous critical-size craniofacial bone regeneration. Plast Reconstr Surg 112:1841–1850.
182. Kanehira M, Xin H, Hoshino K et al. (2007) Targeted delivery of nk4 to multiple lung tumors by bone marrow-derived mesenchymal stem cells. Cancer Gene Ther 14:894–903.
183. Studeny M, Marini FC, Dembinski JL et al. (2004) Mesenchymal stem cells: Potential precursors for tumor stroma and targeted-delivery vehicles for anticancer agents. J Natl Cancer Inst 96:1593–1603.
184. Xin H, Kanehira M, Mizuguchi H et al. (2007) Targeted delivery of CX3CL1 to multiple lung tumors by mesenchymal stem cells. Stem Cells 25:1618–1626.
185. Allay JA, Dennis JE, Haynesworth SE et al. (1997) LacZ and interleukin-3 expression in vivo after retroviral transduction of marrow-derived human osteogenic mesenchymal progenitors. Hum Gene Ther 8:1417–1427.
186. Anjos-Afonso F, Siapati EK Bonnet D (2004) In vivo contribution of murine mesenchymal stem cells into multiple cell-types under minimal damage conditions. J Cell Sci 117: 5655–5664.
187. Bartholomew A, Patil S, Mackay A et al. (2001) Baboon mesenchymal stem cells can be genetically modified to secrete human erythropoietin in vivo. Hum Gene Ther 12:1527–1541.
188. Brouard N, Chapel A, Thierry D et al. (2000) Transplantation of gene-modified human bone marrow stromal cells into mouse-human bone chimeras. J Hematother Stem Cell Res 9: 175–181.
189. Bulabois CE, Yerly-Motta V, Mortensen BT et al. (1998) Retroviral-mediated marker gene transfer in hematopoiesis-supportive marrow stromal cells. J Hematother 7:225–239.
190. Chan J, O'Donoghue K, de la Fuente J et al. (2005) Human fetal mesenchymal stem cells as vehicles for gene delivery. Stem Cells 23:93–102.

191. Chuah MK, Van Damme A, Zwinnen H et al. (2000) Long-term persistence of human bone marrow stromal cells transduced with factor VIII-retroviral vectors and transient production of therapeutic levels of human factor VIII in nonmyeloablated immunodeficient mice. Hum Gene Ther 11:729–738.
192. Ding L, Lu S, Batchu R et al. (1999) Bone marrow stromal cells as a vehicle for gene transfer. Gene Ther 6:1611–1616.
193. Eliopoulos N, Al-Khaldi A, Crosato M et al. (2003) A neovascularized organoid derived from retrovirally engineered bone marrow stroma leads to prolonged in vivo systemic delivery of erythropoietin in nonmyeloablated, immunocompetent mice. Gene Ther 10: 478–489.
194. Gordon EM, Skotzko M, Kundu RK et al. (1997) Capture and expansion of bone marrow-derived mesenchymal progenitor cells with a transforming growth factor-beta1-von Willebrand's factor fusion protein for retrovirus-mediated delivery of coagulation factor IX. Hum Gene Ther 8:1385–1394.
195. Kumar S, Mahendra G, Nagy TR et al. (2004) Osteogenic differentiation of recombinant adeno-associated virus 2-transduced murine mesenchymal stem cells and development of an immunocompetent mouse model for ex vivo osteoporosis gene therapy. Hum Gene Ther 15:1197–1206.
196. Lee CI, Kohn DB, Ekert JE et al. (2004) Morphological analysis and lentiviral transduction of fetal monkey bone marrow-derived mesenchymal stem cells. Mol Ther 9:112–123.
197. Li KJ, Dilber MS, Abedi MR et al. (1995) Retroviral-mediated gene transfer into human bone marrow stromal cells: Studies of efficiency and in vivo survival in SCID mice. Eur J Haematol 55:302–306.
198. Lu L, Zhao C, Liu Y et al. (2005) Therapeutic benefit of TH-engineered mesenchymal stem cells for Parkinson's disease. Brain Res Brain Res Protoc 15:46–51.
199. Oyama M, Tatlock A, Fukuta S et al. (1999) Retrovirally transduced bone marrow stromal cells isolated from a mouse model of human osteogenesis imperfecta (oim) persist in bone and retain the ability to form cartilage and bone after extended passaging. Gene Ther 6: 321–329.
200. Schwarz EJ, Alexander GM, Prockop DJ et al. (1999) Multipotential marrow stromal cells transduced to produce L-DOPA: Engraftment in a rat model of Parkinson disease. Hum Gene Ther 10:2539–2549.
201. Totsugawa T, Kobayashi N, Okitsu T et al. (2002) Lentiviral transfer of the LacZ gene into human endothelial cells and human bone marrow mesenchymal stem cells. Cell Transplant 11:481–488.
202. Zhang XY, La Russa VF, Bao L et al. (2002) Lentiviral vectors for sustained transgene expression in human bone marrow-derived stromal cells. Mol Ther 5:555–565.

Chapter 6
Non-hematopoietic Stem and Progenitor Cells Derived From Human Umbilical Cord Blood

Karen Bieback and Harald Kluter

Introduction

Regenerative medicine is of growing interest in biomedical research [1]. The role of stem cells in this context is under intense scrutiny, on the one hand to define principles of organ regeneration and on the other to develop innovative methods to treat organ failure [2]. In general, organ injuries, or defects induce a mobilization of immature progenitor cells either locally or systemically. Triggered by the milieu, regulated by factors of the extracellular matrix, cellular components, or soluble mediators, the progenitor cells differentiate along a hierarchy of committed to mature cells to functionally regenerate the cellular compartment of the organ [3]. Utilizing stem and progenitor cells for therapeutic organ regeneration has been the practice for many years when performing hematopoietic stem cell (HSC) transplantation [4].

Since the early beginnings of transplanting whole bone marrow (BM), more and more knowledge has been gained, leading to mobilizing HSCs to allow a more convenient and less invasive way of HSC isolation by peripheral blood (PB) aphaeresis. Umbilical cord or placental blood (CB) came into focus as a third source for HSC transplantation after the first successful transplantation performed by E. Gluckman et al. in 1989 [5]. With respect to cord blood transplantation, CB offers substantial logistic and clinical advantages [6, 7]:

1. CB contains the highest number of HSC when compared to BM and PB, but the absolute number is limited to the one-time harvest of a defined volume of CB.
2. CB contains highly immature cells providing a high proliferative capacity.
3. CB provides a fast availability of cryopreserved and pre-tested CB units.
4. The donor pool is extended, as a 1–2 mismatch in the HLA (Human Leukocyte Antigen) system is well tolerated. The long-term storage after pre-testing can select for higher frequency of rare haplotypes.

K. Bieback (✉)
Institute for Transfusion Medicine and Immunology, Germany Red Cross Blood Donor Service Baden-Württemberg - Hessen gGmbH

N. Bhattacharya, P. Stubblefield (eds.), *Frontiers of Cord Blood Science*,
DOI 10.1007/978-1-84800-167-1_6, © Springer-Verlag London Limited 2009

5. CB transplantation induces a lower incidence in severity in graft-versus-host disease (GvHD), which might be related to the immunological immaturity of CB cells.
6. CB displays a lower contamination with infectious agents.
7. In contrast to BM or PB procurement, there is no risk for the donor during CB procurement.

However, despite the various advantages, two major disadvantages have hampered the use of CB in HSC transplantation so far:

1. The absolute number of HSC is limited by the volume of CB to be procured, approximately 100 ml. The low HSC number increases the risk of graft failure and delayed engraftment.
2. Since a CB harvest can only be performed once post-natal, no donor lymphocyte immunotherapy is impossible.

Since the cell dose of a CB graft is the major determinant for engraftment and survival in unrelated CB transplantation, attempts to increase the cell dose are under intense scrutiny to enable CB transplantation also in adults [8, 9]. Besides the optimization of CB processing, new protocols for transplantation are investigated: double cord blood transplants, ex vivo progenitor expansion, facilitation of homing by intraossic infusion as well as co-transplantation with stromal cells have been the subject of discussions [6].

In addition to the hematopoietic aspects, UCB is becoming increasingly interesting for tissue engineering approaches to regenerate solid organs. This is based on reports of solid organ engraftment after experimental or clinical whole CB transplantation (reviewed in [10]). For example, in models of experimental liver damage, human CB cells led to hepatocyte generation, regeneration of liver tissue and reduced mortality [11, 12, 13]. In these approaches, lineage-depleted or CD34(+)-enriched stem cell preparations were marked to track the migration of the CB cells. Within a mouse model of chemically induced liver damage, not only the intravenously infused CB cells homed to the BM, but also few cells were incorporated into the liver [14]. However, it is significant in this context that the number of human cells attaining a hepatocyte phenotype was low with about 12 per 1×10^5 cells. Interestingly, human cells were only detected in the liver after injury, which simultaneously enhanced the homing to the BM. Within the liver, closer examination of the human hepatocytes revealed that they were formed by fusion events [14]. In non-obese diabetic (NOD) mice with autoimmune diabetes, administration of human umbilical cord blood T cell-depleted mononuclear cells has been shown to improve both the animals' blood glucose levels and survival accompanied by differentiation of CB cells into insulin-producing cells [15]. In this study, both fusion-dependent and -independent mechanisms leading to insulin-producing cells were observed. Importantly, the production of c-peptide was detectable, indicating that human insulin was generated through the physiological degeneration of proinsulin produced by the human donor cells.

In addition, CB mononuclear cells have been used pre-clinically in animal models of brain and spinal cord injuries, in which functional recovery was achieved (reviewed in [16]). The CB cells migrated primarily to the boundary of the ischemic tissue and few of them expressed neuronal tissue-specific markers like glial-fibrillary-acidic protein, neuronal nuclear protein, and neuronal microtubule-associated protein 2 (MAP-2). The treatment window which enabled functional recovery was discovered to be optimal between 24 and 72 hours after inducing brain ischemia. Within this period, the chemoattractant proteins secreted by the injured tissue were the highest and induced migration of CB cells. So, compared to the recent very short time window of approximately 3 hours for treatment in stroke, CB transplantation may offer a cellular therapy for patients at later stages after stroke. Similar observations were made in models of myocardial infarction. CB cells caused reduced infarction and lesion sizes accompanied by a reduced infiltration of inflammatory cells [17, 18].

In clinical sex-mismatched CB and BM transplant settings, donor cells co-expressing tissue lineage markers have been identified as gastrointestinal epithelial cells. This may indicate that CB cells as well as BM cells may become interesting also in clinical settings to treat gastrointestinal disorders, such as Crohn's disease or ulcerative colitis [19].

There is evidence that beyond (or amongst, see below) the HSC, other stem or progenitor populations exist in umbilical cord blood which might be responsible for regenerating non-hematopoietic organs. A plethora of different stem and progenitor cell populations have been postulated, with potential ranging from embryonal-like to lineage-committed progenitor cells (described in detail in the final chapter). Whether or not these differentially named cells refer to similar cell populations obtained by different isolation or culture methods, whether these cells relate to a common (hematopoietic) ancestor [20, 21], are in constant (epi)genetical transition enabling them to shift to different phenotypes [22], emerge upon in vitro culture or even by dedifferentiation effects [23] remains unidentified and represents a major challenge for the future.

Based on the current extremely confusing data, it is not possible to clearly define any of these stem or progenitor populations. Consequently, this chapter mainly focuses on two populations: in the first, a human cord-blood-derived, plastic adherent fibroblastoid population expressing a similar set of markers like BM-derived mesenchymal stromal cells (MSC) and in the second, endothelial progenitor cells (EPC), characterized by the expression of CD133, CD34 and vascular endothelial growth factor 2 (VEGFR-2).

Mesenchymal Stromal Cells

Classically, mesenchymal stromal cells (MSC) have been isolated from the BM; however, alternative tissues have been identified, including adipose tissue, cutaneous tissues, fetal tissues, dental pulp, hair follicle, synovium, blood as well as CB [24, 25, 26].

The BM stroma comprises various cell types, including reticular endothelial cells, fibroblasts, adipocytes, and osteogenic progenitor cells to provide the basis for hematopoiesis. This has been shown by Dexter et al., who developed long-term BM cultures [27]. The fibroblastic compartment has been described by Friedenstein as colony-forming-unit fibroblastoid (CFU-F) [28]. These colonies consisting of fibroblastoid cells were derived by plating BM in cell cultures containing only medium and fetal bovine serum (FBS). Interestingly, following ectopic transplantation, these cells were reported to give rise to a spectrum of connective tissue lineages and it has been proposed that a common precursor existed in the CFU-F population, which has been named in analogy to the HSCs, mesenchymal stem cells (MSC) [29]. MSC exhibit an enormous in vitro expansion potential and more importantly a broad differentiation potential into not only mesodermal (including osteoblasts, adipocytes, and chondrocytes), but also endodermal (hepatocyte-like cells), and ectodermal cells (neuronal, neuroglial cells) [30, 31, 32]. BM-derived MSC engraft in numerous organs and differentiate to some extent along tissue-specific lineages when transplanted into a fetal sheep model, which mimics the developing organism and thus provides a milieu to assess stem cell capacities [33]. Admittedly, the true definition of a stem cell has not been fulfilled with MSC so far: it has not been demonstrated that a single implanted MSC can regenerate and maintain a whole tissue compartment, as this has been shown for HSC [24]. In addition, MSC grown in culture do not exert an unlimited self-renewal capacity associated by a lack of telomerase activity and telomere shortening upon proliferation [34]. This is in contrast to embryonic stem cells, which display no replicative senescence in culture [35]. Hence, there is a trend toward redefining this cells as "mesenchymal stromal cells" (MSC) [36].

Nevertheless, MSC have become increasingly interesting in the entire field of cellular therapies. This is not only based on their auspicious differentiative capacities, but currently particularly on their immunomodulatory characteristics [37]. In vitro analyses provide a multiplicity of data demonstrating that MSC, despite the constitutive expression of HLA class I and the interferon gamma (IFN γ)-inducible expression of HLA class II, can not only suppress allogeneic T, NK, and B cell responses, but also can affect dendritic cell functions and tumor cell growth [38]. Neither T-cell apoptosis nor anergy cause this effect, which is dependent on the presence but not necessarily on direct contact of the MSC and T cells. MSC seem to alter the cytokine expression profile of immune cells, including dendritic cells, toward an anti-inflammatory/tolerance inducing milieu [39]. Based on these in vitro data and observations made in vivo where a co-transplantation of BM-derived MSC did not facilitate engraftment but rather reduced the rate of acute and chronic GvHD, led to the clinical exploitation of using MSC to treat GvHD [37, 40, 41]. This indeed proved to be effective and initiated large international clinical trials [42].

Although currently BM represents the main source of MSC for both experimental and clinical studies, some authors speculate that the clinical value might be diminished as the number of MSC and their differentiation capacity decline with age [43, 44]. Alternative tissue sources giving rise to cells with both extensive potency of proliferation and differentiation would therefore represent an optimal tool for future cell-based therapeutic applications [45].

Isolation, Expansion and in vitro Characterization of CB-MSC

Although MSC seem to be present in any tissue analyzed so far, the presence of circulating MSC has been controversially discussed [46, 47, 48, 49, 50, 51, 52, 53]. Indeed, MSC can circulate in PB and CB but at much lower frequencies than their hematopoietic counterparts, which makes them difficult to isolate and culture [49, 54, 55]. The first reports dealing with issues of mesenchymal cells in CB claimed that a population of either stromal feeder cells [46, 47] or osteoprogenitors can be cultured from CB [56]. Later on, Goodwin et al. and Erices et al. showed that cells capable of differentiating into bone, cartilage and adipose tissue could in fact be derived from the fibroblastic monolayer after adherence culture in FBS-supplemented media [48, 49]. This encouraging data was neglected by a number of authors who tried but failed to isolate MSC from CB, but succeeded with BM [52, 53, 57]. Analyzing factors which might influence the unpredictable isolation success in full-term umbilical cord blood ranging between 20 and 40% of utilized cord blood units [48, 49, 58, 59, 60], it has been demonstrated that by selecting units with decreased storage time and a high volume of cell-rich cord blood, the isolation success was enhanced toward 60% [54]. This suggested that selecting CB units with high quality predicts higher isolation success and that CB units stored in CB banks may be well suitable also for isolating MSC. Contrariwise, a correlation of the isolation success of the unrestricted somatic stem cells (USSC) (see below) with the quality of the used CB units or the number of mononucleated cells after gradient centrifugation and MSC growth has not been observed [56, 61]. The infrequent isolation suggests that either not every cord blood contains MSC in sufficient quantities to establish cultures or that a reliable medium equivalent to the one used to generate MSC cultures from BM has yet to be defined. One can also consider it is possible that those factors, which have been described affecting the frequency of HSC, such as maternal age, mode of delivery, birth weight, hemoglobin levels, and placental size may also relate to MSC frequency [62, 63].

Evidence has been reported suggesting that at least the gestation time and frequency of circulating MSC correlate inversely, as preterm CB contained MSC at much higher levels than full-term CB [49, 50, 52, 64]. This finding has been attributed to the sequence of fetal hematopoiesis, which initiates in the yolk sac before moving to the aorta gonad mesonephros region, the fetal liver and finally homing to the adult BM as major site of adult hematopoiesis [65]. Symmetric division of HSC to reproduce the hematopoietic system is dependent on close contact with the stromal compartment providing extracellular matrices as well as soluble factors [66, 67]. Therefore, as MSC supply all necessary factors for hematopoiesis, it is postulated that MSC co-circulate with HSC during early embryonic hematopoiesis and subsequently home to the BM in the adult organism [45, 64, 68].

Interestingly, for clinical use, MSC can even be isolated from cryopreserved UCB [69, 70]. Despite their low frequency and difficulties in isolation, these cells are highly interesting for therapeutic interventions, since they combine all the advantages of cord blood discussed for HSC (young and immature cells, no risk for the donors during harvesting, high proliferative potential) with a multi-differentiative capacity into meso-, endo-, and ectodermal cell types [55].

In expansion culture of CB, one major problem is the contamination with hematopoietic mononuclear cells. Monocytes especially adhere to the plastic surfaces and tend to fuse to form large syncytia, resembling osteoclasts (Fig. 6.1) [49, 54].

Many controversies remain with respect to the phenotype of the MSC in vivo correlate: most data indicate that these cells reside within a CD45-low expressing population, challenging the concept of a non-hematopoietic origin [71, 72]. Thus, various attempts to enrich MSC and to remove contaminating cells have been reported: for example, the depletion of cells expressing lineage markers, the selection of subpopulations expressing CD133 [55, 73] or culturing the cells onto extracellular matrices to change the adherence kinetics of the monocytic cells [54, 63].

In CB, if at all, a few fusiform fibroblast-like cells appear after 10–16 days in culture forming colonies, similar to what is observed in BM cultures. After repetitive change of medium and passaging, contaminating cells disappear and a monolayer of fibroblastoid cells develops [54]. The morphology of cells can differ slightly, ranging from very elongated and thin fibroblast-like cells to more spherical cells (Fig. 6.1). Interestingly, these morphologically distinct populations seem to exert different proliferation and differentiation capacities, suggesting that they may represent different maturation stages [74, 75].

Despite the low frequency, CB-MSC display a tremendous expansion capacity which exceeds BM- and adipose tissue-derived MSC to generate cell numbers required for clinical application [76, 77]. CB-MSC proliferate faster and can be propagated in culture for a prolonged time compared to BM-MSC [48, 54, 76]. This is supported by enhanced telomerase activity and longer telomere length [78].

At present, no unique phenotype, comparable to CD34 for HSC [79], has been identified, which allows a standardized prospective isolation of MSC with

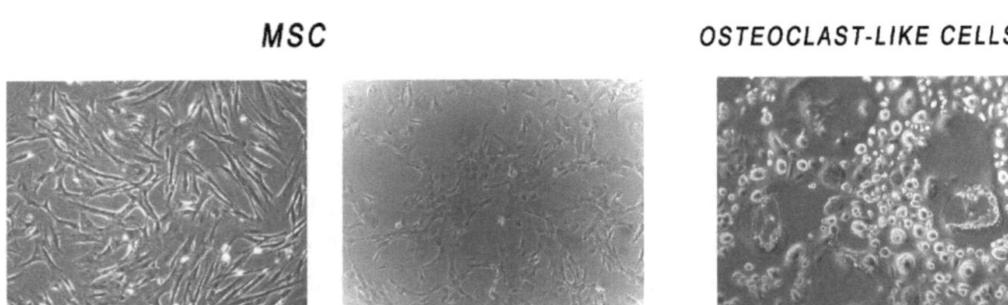

Fig. 6.1 Morphology of CB derived adherent cells displaying a fibroblastoid, MSC typical, or an osteoclast-like- morphology. CB derived fibroblastoid cells display either a consistent spindle-shaped (left) or a more spherical, less spindle-shaped morphology (middle). The morphology of CB-derived osteoclast-like cells in primary culture at day 16 is shown in the right

predictable differentiative potential [26, 35]. Given that a cell surface marker exclusively defining MSC has yet to be determined, the expression profile of culture-expanded MSC consists of a variety of markers typical for other cell lineages; so a combination of expressed and not-expressed (most importantly, all hematopoietic lineage) markers is currently used to define MSC [36]. Classically, MSC express CD44, CD73 (SH-3, SH-4), CD90 (Thy-1), CD105 (SH-2, Endoglin), CD106 (VCAM-1), HLA class I but lack the expression of CD14, CD34, CD45 (Leukocyte Common Antigen) and HLA class II [80]. Thus, the term non-hematopoietic obviously rather describes the phenotype after ex vivo expansion than the in vivo situation.

Since currently the immunophenotype is insufficient to define MSC, the demanded assay to characterize MSC is to analyze their differentiative capacity at least toward the mesodermal lineage as summarized (Fig. 6.2). MSC respond to osteogenic stimuli like β-glycerophosphate and dexamethasone with the upregulation of osteogenic markers, assessed either by PCR, immuno- or histochemical staining (reviewed in e.g. in [81]). When assessed quantitatively, CB-MSC seem to have a stronger osteogenic potential in vitro compared to BM-MSC [78]. The differentiation into the chondrogenic lineage can be induced by using a micromass culture and various growth factors [82]. CB-MSC form cartilage as well as BM-MSC

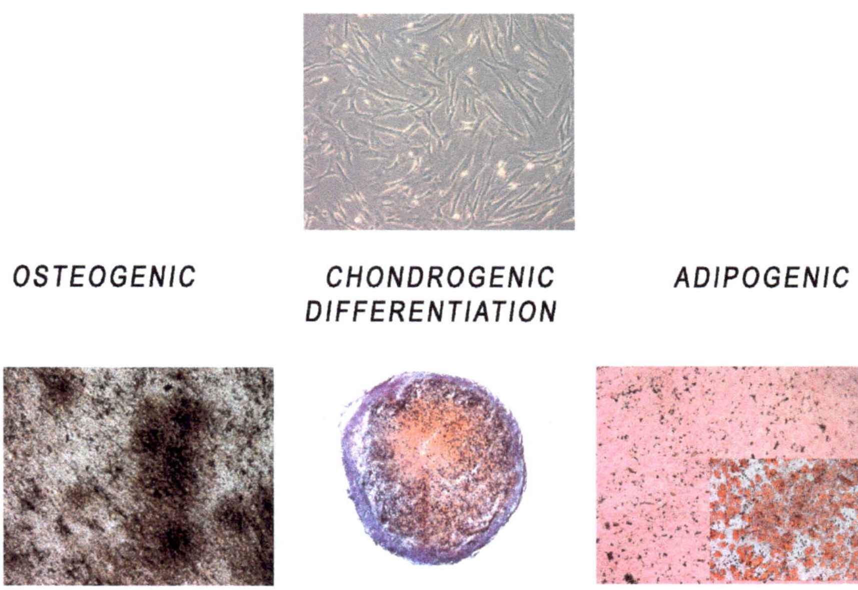

Fig. 6.2 Differentiation capacity of CB-MSC. CB-MSC differentiate appropriately to the osteogenic lineage (calcium mineralization detected by von Kossa stain) and to the chondrogenic lineage (cryosection of a MSC-derived mini-cartilage stained with safranin-o to stain sulphated glycosaminoglycans). Adipogenic differentiation is only rarely induced in CB-MSC, whereas in contrast BM-MSC as depicted in the inserted photomicrograph, produce a mass of lipid-rich vacuoles stainable with Oil-Red-O

[54, 55, 76, 83]. Differing observations have been published regarding the adipogenic differentiation capacity of CB-MSC. In some studies, CB-MSC demonstrate none to only low-level adipogenic differentiation after culture in media containing 3-isobutyl-1-methyl-xanthine, insulin, dexamethasone, and indomethacin [54, 74, 76]. Here, cells with lipid-filled vacuoles were only sporadically apparent in CB-MSC, indicating a markedly reduced sensitivity toward adipogenic differentiation when compared to BM and adipose tissue-derived MSC. Since other authors report no limited adipogenic potential [48, 49, 55, 75], the differing data may either relate to variable differentiation protocols, or as suggested by Chang et al., are caused by different subpopulations [74]. Although Markov et al. similarly have identified the two different populations of CB-MSC, they have not observed the differential adipogenic differentiation potential [75]. Thus, there remains the speculation that a subsequent gain in responsiveness toward specific differentiative inductors upon development exists. This theory is based on the observations that stromal layers derived from fetal in comparison to adult hematopoietic tissues do not form fat despite the expression of corticosteroid receptors on all stromal cells [84, 85].

A variety of data support the idea that there is no mesodermal germ-layer restricted differentiation potential in CB-MSC. Depending on the in vitro stimulus, CB-MSC can differentiate in addition also into neural cells [48, 86, 87, 88, 89], neuroglial and hepatocyte-like cells [55, 90], endothelial cells [91, 92], skeletal myoblasts [93, 94], respiratory epithelial cells [95] and cardiomyogenic cells [96]. Importantly, Lee et al. showed that a single clonally expanded population of MSC, cultured under neurogenic conditions, produced cells positive for neuroglial markers, and vitally voltage-sensitive calcium-channels, which are critical for the functioning of neuronal cells [55]. Cells derived from the same clonally expanded population acquired a cuboidal morphology under hepatogenic conditions and expressed a variety of hepatic markers accompanied by functional uptake of low-density lipoproteins. This strongly suggests that rather a single CB-derived cell exhibits multilineage differentiation capacity than different subpopulations of precursors for the respective lineage. Compared to BM-MSC, Goodwin et al. observed a variety of markers indicative for osteblastic and neural lineages already expressed on BM-MSC but induced in CB-MSC upon induction, suggesting a commitment of BM-MSC in contrast to CB-MSC [48]. The inducible expression, as well as differing responsiveness to differentiative stimuli may therefore relate to a more primitive cell population contained in CB.

As mentioned above, CB-MSC share many similarities with BM-MSC; however, whether the MSC populations derived from the different tissues like adipose tissue, muscle, dental pulp, placenta etc. are the same as BM-MSC and represent tissue-specific reservoirs is yet unknown [97]. Comparative analysis of genomic and proteomic expression profiles in comparison to mature lineages as well as embryonic stem cells revealed shared patterns but also marked differences, which however, might result from differing isolation and culture conditions and may have to be re-evaluated after adjusting to common or standardized protocols [98, 99, 100, 101, 102, 103, 104, 105].

Therapeutic Potential

Regenerative Medicine

MSC are promising candidates for use in regenerative medicine due to their differentiative and expansion capacity. Regarding the clinical use of MSC, most studies have been conducted using BM-derived MSC [106, 107]. Basically, these studies can be divided into two kinds: site and tissue-directed or systemic administration of MSC [24]. The site-directed administration appears to result in engraftment and integration of the MSC once a danger signal by, for example, tissue injury is provided [108]. The question remains open as to whether the incorporation of MSC is due to true engraftment accompanied by differentiation to obtain a mature lineage-specific phenotype or whether donor-derived cells result from fusion events [109].

Owing to problems in quantifying engraftment, MSC biodistribution and assessing the therapeutic outcome, the published results vary enormously. Up to the present, the verified biological effects seem to be more related to the local production of growth factors rather than to their direct participation in tissue repair [24].

The systemic administration, in contrast, seems to result in general in even less persistence of tissue-localized MSC. After infusion, MSC remain in the circulation for no more than 1 hour [110]. Thereafter, MSC are detectable primarily in the lungs and then secondarily in the liver and other organs, depending on the injury stimulus [111, 112, 113]. Specific homing to and survival in the BM have been shown not only for BM-derived MSC, but also for CB-MSC after transplantation into immunodeficient nude mice without conditioning pre-treatment [114]. In this study, CB-MSC have been as well demonstrated in other tissues including cardiac muscle, teeth and spleen, suggesting a mesenchymal-directed fate of engrafting cells.

Although currently the question regarding the physiological function of MSC in situ cannot be answered, there is no doubt about their therapeutic potential, which lies at present also in the hypo-immunogenic nature of MSC allowing for a HLA-incompatible transplantation (see below).

One of the first examples of the clinical utility of MSC has been for osteogenesis imperfecta (OI) [115, 116]. OI patients suffer from a genetic defect affecting the body's production of type I collagen, which severely affects the stability of bone. Patients receiving allogeneic BM transplants improved significantly associated by the production of normal collagen type I [117]. Whereas in the first trial whole BM was transplanted, a second trial employed culture-expanded MSC. An induced acceleration of growth velocity, accompanied by reduced bone fracture frequencies during the first 6 months post-infusion was observed in this study as well [118]. Systemically administered allogeneic MSC showed some effect in patients with Hurlers syndrome, metachromatic leukodystrophy and severe aplastic anemia [119, 120]. In patients with these lysosomal or peroxisomal storage diseases, MSC showed some benefit probably because the cells secrete several enzymes of therapeutic value [121]. Summarized, these studies have demonstrated that MSC transplantation is safe and feasible.

The probably most successful application has been the site-directed repair of skeletal tissues. MSC have been used to accelerate bone and cartilage formation when implanted on a variety of matrices or engineered to produce growth factors [122, 123, 124, 125]. Currently, the only study reporting on CB-MSC in this context, however, has demonstrated that CB-MSC might be deficient compared to BM. Rosada et al. observed reduced bone formation in vivo with CB-MSC transplanted in a hydroxyapaite/tricalcium phosphate matrix [56].

A few investigations have documented wholesome effects of MSC injection in diseases of the central nervous system, like amyotrophic lateral sclerosis or chronic spinal cord injury [126, 127, 128, 129]. Preliminary studies demonstrated the beneficial effects of canine CB-MSC injection in spinal cord injury [130]. As again only very few cells co-expressing neuronal markers were identified, the most likely effect was the production of trophic factors which recruited endogenous repair mechanisms [131]. One patient suffering from chronic spinal cord injury clinically improved after transplantation of HLA-matched CB-MSC associated with sensory perception, slight moving improvement, and regeneration at the injured site [132].

Early results indicate safety and efficacy of using MSC in patients with vascular disease, peripheral artery disease, coronary artery disease, or non-healing chronic wounds [133, 134, 135]. With respect to ischemic diseases, CB-MSC have been already applied successfully in four patients with Buerger's disease (thromboangiitis obliterans), a non-atherosclerotic vascular disease. In these patients, CB-MSC transplantation led to the disappearance of rest pain and healing of the gangrenes within 4 weeks post injection [136].

In the context of cellular therapies in vascular medicine, the probably most intensely investigated target is the damaged myocardium. A variety of cell sources including myoblasts, cardiomyoblasts, unprocessed BM cells, HSC-enriched for CD34(+)or CD133(+) and EPCs have already been applied and interestingly, all improved myocardial functions, elusive of the mechanistic effect [137]. In vitro, MSC can be induced to express a cardiac phenotype and, once transplanted migrate, survive, and improve cardiac function after myocardial infarction [112, 138, 139]. Within a rat model, the bioluminescence imaging of marked CB-MSC revealed their homing to the myocardium [140].

Hematopoietic Support

In cord-blood transplantation, the cell dose as a major determinant of rate and incidence of hematopoietic recovery is limited to the volume which can be collected from one placenta. With the body weight as a limiting factor, this often restricts its use to pediatric patients [8]. Strategies to improve engraftment are under investigation and include, for instance, ex vivo expansion of HSCs and co-infusion of MSC [6]. Both approaches aim at utilizing the capacities of MSC to provide necessary signals for HSC maintenance and differentiation.

Ex vivo expansion of CB-HSC has been achieved on monolayers of MSC, either derived from BM or CB; indeed, as mentioned above, the first attempts aimed at isolating stromal layers from CB [46, 47]. In fact CB-MSC constitutively secrete a variety of growth factors affecting HSCs [141, 142]. Thus, stromal layers derived from CB-MSC, as well as from BM-MSC, were capable of maintaining and amplifying colony-forming cells over a prolonged period of time [47].

In the context of co-transplantation, it is questioned whether enough culture-expanded MSC can home and engraft to the BM after systemic administration. Although the majority of cells are sequestered in the lung and later on degraded in the liver, a variety of experimental studies demonstrate that MSC can home and engraft to the BM [113, 143, 144]. CB-MSC as well as BM-MSC express the chemokine receptor CXCR-4 (receptor for stromal-derived factor-1 (SDF-1)) and the receptor for hepatocyte growth factor (HGH or scatter factor), which can attract MSC to specific tissue sites or stem cell niches [70, 145].

On the contrary, when trying to identify long-term persisting donor cells in the host after standard BM transplantation, the data are conflicting. Since HSC transplantation in general includes a pre-conditioning regime to eradicate the patient's disease prior to the infusion of HSC, most likely the stroma becomes injured, leaving space to be replaced by donor stromal cells [146]. The majority of studies failed to document long-term persisting donor stromal cells [121, 147]. On the contrary, Pozzi et al. analyzed patients who underwent either allogeneic BM or CB transplantation. Within cultured recipient BM-MSC, they could observe in both groups a few preparations with mixed chimerism with donor cells [148].

Thus, although the actual number of MSC capable of homing and engrafting to the BM seems to be considerably low, the therapeutic effect of facilitating CB-HSC engraftment has been demonstrated not only in a variety of experimental settings but also in early clinical reports suggesting that co-transplanting MSC can enhance engraftment [149, 150, 151, 152]. The co-transplantation of CB-MSC can lead to an enhanced and accelerated engraftment of CB-HSC within the murine NOD/SCID (NOD/severe combined immune deficiency) transplantation model [153, 154]. Although no homing and engraftment of the MSC was reported in the previously mentioned publications, CB-MSC have been shown to home to the BM and to facilitate engraftment of CB-HSC in NOD/SCID mice [114]. It can be supposed that either homing of MSC to the BM may not be required or that the number of cells effective in promoting engraftment is at or beneath the detection limit. Again, the release of cytokines might be sufficient to promote HSC homing and/or proliferation.

Immune Modulation

Several studies based on initial reports by Le Blanc et al. report that MSC play a role in modulating immune responses [155, 156]. BM-MSC seem to be poor antigen-presenting cells in vitro and hypo-immunogenic in vivo. The phenotypic characteristic is the lack of HLA class II expression as well as of the costimulatory molecules CD40, CD80, and CD86. Despite the expression of HLA class I and an IFNγ-induced expression of HLA class II, they do not activate allogeneic T cell responses and are even capable of suppressing ongoing alloreactions [157]. This has been attributed to a modulation of host dendritic and T cell function, the activation of suppressor and regulatory T cells [39, 158]. In experimental models, injection of MSC resulted in prolonged graft survival as well as decreased tumor rejection [159, 160, 161].

Immunological responses elicited by fetal and adult MSC seem to be comparable and also CB-MSC have been shown to act anti-proliferative on T cells [77, 162]. More recent data, however, suggest that under certain circumstances, MSC have immunogenic properties eliciting a host-anti-donor immune response by inducing a memory T cell response [163, 164].

Translating these observations into the clinic, early case studies have suggested that BM-MSC are effective in preventing and treating severe steroid resistant GvHD: Lee et al. demonstrated this in a patient with acute myeloid leukemia, treated with HSC and MSC from a haplo-identical family donor, who benefited from rapid engraftment and strikingly no acute or chronic GvHD, indicating that MSC may suppress GvHD [165]. In analogy, Le Blanc et al. reported a leukemia patient who had developed a steroid-resistant grade IV acute GvHD after allogeneic HSC transplantation [165]. He received two replicate MSC infusions, which stimulated a prompt recovery of the gastrointestinal symptoms, demonstrating the efficacy of MSC for treating GvHD.

Gene Therapy

The genetic modification of stem cells attracted interest because of their long-term survival and proliferative capacity compared to mature somatic cells. MSC can be easily transduced by a variety of viral vectors [106, 166]. Non-viral methods for transgene delivery in contrast have shown little effect and afforded optimization but worked well thereafter. Therefore, MSC are envisioned as vehicles for short- and long-term gene transfer. The secretion of growth factors, as stated above, has already been effective in bone disorders, when MSC were engineered to secrete bone morphogenic proteins [167]. Progress has also been made when using rodent models of neurodegenerative disorders, like for example, Parkinson's-Disease [168]. Other inherited disorders, including hemophilia A and B, have been targeted using human erythropoietin-secreting engineered MSC [169].

MSC, as being adults' stem cells, lack telomerase activity and therefore exhibit a finite life span, reaching senescence in ex vivo culture after approximately 50 cumulative population doublings and gradually losing the differentiation potential [26]. The ectopic expression of human telomerase reverse transcriptase has been shown to extend the lifespan of MSC and to maintain their differentiative capacity [170]. The prosurvival gene Akt overexpressed in MSC was highly effective in repairing the infarcted myocardium [171].

Cancer gene therapy seems to be a highly promising field in gene therapy. As safety is a prerequisite, tumor-specific targeting is essential. The specific homing of MSC to tumor stroma led to the idea to utilize MSC to deliver anti-tumor drugs. MSC genetically manipulated to express IFNβ were effective in inducing tumor regression in a xenogeneic mouse model [172]. Equivalent to BM-MSC, genetically modified CB-MSC displayed maintained transgene expression and stem cell properties [173, 174, 175, 176].

Another application is the insertion of reporter genes to allow in vivo tracking of the transplanted cells [140]. It is important for assessing the potential effect, as also the risk of stem cell transplantation to follow the biodistribution of injected cells in vivo. The most abundantly used proteins in experimental settings are beta-galactosidase and green fluorescent protein. Data on using transgenic MSC indicate that MSC distribute to a variety of tissues and that a few cells can acquire a tissue-specific morphology [177].

Clinical Manufacturing of CB-MSC

Initially, all media used for isolating and expanding MSC were supplemented with FBS [30, 178]. However, FBS contains xenogeneic proteins which are internalized by MSC [179]. Consequently, a host of potential problems can arise, such as viral and prion transmission or immunological reactions [180, 181]. These risks have initiated the search for alternative substitutes: recently, either serum, plasma or platelet-derived substitutes have been introduced enabling the FBS-free propagation of MSC [182, 183]. Obviously, the same holds true for CB-MSC: very recently, human platelet lysate has been established as supplement to expand CB-MSC for clinical applications, paving its way to the clinic [77].

Endothelial Progenitor Cells

Two processes are responsible for the formation of new blood vessels: vasculogenesis and angiogenesis. Until recently, it was believed that vasculogenesis, the formation of the fetal capillary network from migrating EPC, was restricted to early embryonic development, while the blood vessels in an adult organism are derived from pre-existing endothelial cells (angiogenesis) [184]. However, new evidence suggests that EPC mobilized from niches in the BM may play an important role in post-natal neo-vascularization [185, 186, 187]. Whereas in healthy vessels, there is only a low turnover of endothelial cell replacement, stress injury induces the migration and proliferation of mature endothelial cells. But as these are terminally differentiated cells, the lifelong substitution to vessel repair is more probably maintained by circulating BM-derived EPC [188]. According to this assumption, BM-derived cells have been shown to induce new vessel formation after ischemia in myocardium, limbs, and retina, in wound healing, in atherosclerosis and by endothelialization of graft material [189, 190, 191]. Therefore, intensive investigations are currently being focussed on defining the role of circulating EPC in the repair of damaged vascular endothelium and in tumor angiogenesis [192, 193, 194]. The main thrust is to try to translate experimental findings into clinical protocols for repair of vascular injury, ischemic tissues or for anticancer therapy. However, this is being hampered by the complexity of defining EPCs as described below.

Isolation, Expansion, and in vitro Characterization of CB-EPC

The identification and isolation of EPCs has proved to be difficult due to the absence of specific markers and functional assays to distinguish migrating EPCs from circulating mature endothelial cells or even endothelial microparticles [195]. Based on the recent publications, at least three populations of circulating endothelial-lineage committed precursor cells can be isolated from PB mononuclear cells: short-time culture-adapted mononuclear cells are spindle-shaped cells that uniformly express CD14 and other myeloid markers. Importantly, these cells do not proliferate substantially in cell culture [196]. In contrast, in growth factor-supplemented long-term culture of CB or PB, outgrowing cells develop as morphologically mature endothelial cells, which however expand rapidly (Fig. 6.3). This proliferation capacity indicates that they may be derived from an EPC [197]. The third protocol which can be performed using a commercially available kit (EndoCult®, Stem Cell Technologies Inc.) is based on the depletion of early adhering monocytes and mature endothelial cells. Non-adherent cells are transferred and replated onto fibronectin-coated plastic to form endothelial colonies [198]. Given the complexity in nomenclature, heterogeneity, differences, or even deficits in characterizing cell populations, it is striking that all cell populations demonstrated angiogenic potential in vitro and in vivo [199, 200]. One important step toward re-defining EPC is provided by Prater et al. [201]. Thus the following should be read with reservations due to the applied cell populations.

By comparing cord blood with adult PB, it became clear that in CB, the number of late-outgrowing endothelial cell colonies was increased 15-fold and that the proliferative potential significantly exceeded that of adult blood-derived cells with approximately 100 populations doublings in CB compared to 30 in adult PB [197]. Actually, mature endothelial cell proliferation has been considered to be low. But, blood vessel-derived endothelial cells, e.g., the well-defined Human Umbilical Vein Endothelial Cells (HUVEC) or Human Aortic Endothelial Cells, can be cultured for various passages, with high proliferative capacity in vitro. This has been attributed to the presence of resident EPC within these tissues. Ingram et al. postulated –

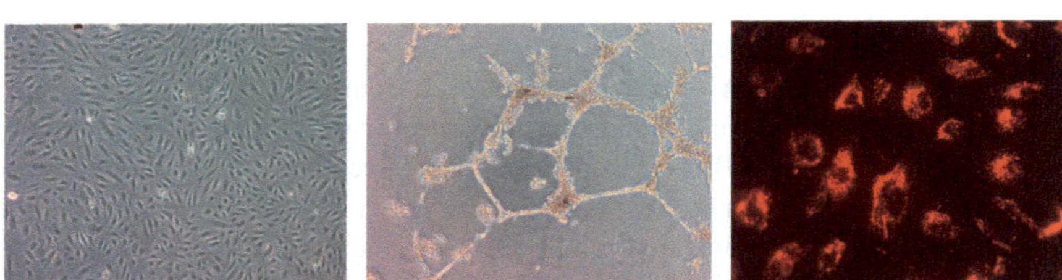

Fig. 6.3 *Characteristics of late outgrowing CB-EPC*. The photomicrograph in the left depicts the typical cobblestone-like morphology of CB-EPC resembling mature endothelial cells. The formation of vessel-like structures can be induced after culture on Matrigel in these cells as shown in the middle picture. The incorporation of acetylated low density-lipoprotein is presented on the right as representative endothelial marker

based on their clonogenic and proliferative potential – a hierarchy of EPC within the endothelial lineage, similar to the differentiation charts drawn to describe hematopoiesis [202].

It is likely that both growth factors and the adhesion on specific extracellular matrix substrates exhibit a stimulus to induce differentiation of cultured EPC populations [185]. Bompais et al. thus introduced the term endothelial progenitor-derived cell to describe a population derived after adherence and growth factor-mediated expansion culture [200]. For mononuclear cells expressing CD14, it has been shown that the culture step is mandatory for the gain of function. Only culture-modified CD14+ or CD14− cells were capable of improving neovascularization in a model of hind-limb ischemia whereas freshly isolated CD14+ cells did not exert these angiogenic properties [203].

As indicated initially, flow cytometric identification of EPC is confounded by the overlap of markers expressed as well on hematopoietic cells and the absence of a discriminatory marker between EPC and circulating endothelial cells [204]. Commonly used markers to describe EPC are CD34, c-kit (CD117), VE-cadherin (CD144), VEGFR-2 (synonym: KDR), CD146, CXCR4, von Willebrand Factor, CD31 (PECAM; platelet/endothelial cell adhesion molecule-1), bound acetylated low-density-lipoprotein and lectin from Ulex Europaeus (Fig. 6.3). The only marker which seems to be suitable in distinguishing immature from mature endothelial cells so far is the novel stem cell marker CD133 (or AC133), which is expressed on progenitor cells but absent on matured endothelial cells [205, 206]. Pure populations of CD34(+), CD133(+), VEGFR-2(+) circulating EPCs can be isolated from fetal liver, CB, and adult PB [205]. It is important to mention that the frequency of these cells is extremely low, with the highest numbers found in CB. With a low percentage of CD34(+) cells (approximately 1% of all mononucleated cells in CB) and only about the half co-expressing CD133, frequency of true EPC expressing CD34, CD133, and VEGFR-2 is estimated to be as low as 0.01%.

It is not to forget to mention, that some publications report that within CB, EPC can also reside in the CD34(−), CD133(−) compartment, although most studies allocate EPC to the hematopoietic CD34(+) population [207, 208]. It has been speculated that the close relationship between endothelial and hematopoietic stem/progenitor cells is ontogenetically based: both hematopoietic and endothelial cells are thought to arise from one common precursor, the hemangioblast. Here, the ontogenic development of hematopoietic and endothelial lineages is linked to VEGFR-2 [209]. Knockout of the VEGFR-2 gene causes a combined defect of hematopoiesis and endothelial cell growth, possibly mediated by a defect of the embryonic hemangioblast [210]. Challenging the concept of EPC marked by the co-expression of CD34, CD133, and VEGFR-2 is the current finding from Ingram's laboratory: by simultaneously analyzing hematopoietic and endothelial capacities in clonogenic assays, they observed that triple-positive cells exerted merely hematopoietic activities, but no endothelial. The yield of endothelial progeny was restricted to populations defined by the expression of CD34 in line with the absence of CD45 [211].

Therapeutic Potential

Neovascularization

Ischemic diseases such as coronary artery disease, cerebrovascular disease and peripheral vascular thrombosis have burgeoning socio-economic implications. As the natural mechanisms of arterio- and angiogenesis which are induced by ischemia are progressively lost with ageing, therapeutic interventions base on the pro-angiogenic function of EPC [212, 213]. A variety of pre-clinical and clinical studies have shown that BM- or PB-derived mononucleated cells, HSC or cultured EPC seem to be effective in enhancing angiogenesis in ischemic tissues [137]. Since CB has been shown to contain the highest number of EPC, the feasibility to use CB as a source for allogeneic pro-angiogenic therapies seems obvious [214, 215].

At present, however, CB-derived EPC transplantation is still at the experimental stage. Within the model of hind-limb ischemia, numerous data demonstrated augmentation of neovascularization and blood flow attained by injecting CB cells [133, 214, 216, 217, 218]. Incorporation of the transplanted cells into capillary networks of the ischemic limb was detected. The elevated expression of VEGF and SDF-1α has shown to exploit chemoattractant stimuli for the recruitment of the systemically injected EPC. P- and E-Selectin, upregulated on the ischemic endothelium, interacted with the ligand PSGL-1 (P-selectin glycoprotein ligand 1) expressed on the EPC to promote homing and adhesion [219]. A direct comparison of CB- and BM-derived EPC, has indicated that both equivalently induced neovascularization within a model of hind-limb ischemia. Both controls of mononucleated cells however were not effective in enhancing capillary densities [133]. By comparing CB- and BM-derived CD133(+) cells, however, only the BM-CD133(+) cells led to the formation of myocardial contractile tissue, although both populations improved mortality, reduced the infarct size and induced capillary formation [220]. Although obviously further investigations are demanded, these data may indicate that CB-CD133(+) display differing capacities compared to BM-CD133(+) in inducing muscle tissue formation. However, interestingly, within these studies neither of both populations differentiated in vitro into myoblasts, leaving these observations open to further speculations.

Complete angiogenesis necessitates the interaction of EPC with perivascular cells, like smooth muscle cells or pericytes, which provide maturation signals to the EPC [221]. Freshly isolated CB-CD34(+) cells injected into ischemic muscles have been shown to gain phenotypes of both cell types: endothelial as well as skeletal muscle cells [222]. To translate this into tissue-engineering approaches, replacement material like living patches can be engineered successfully from CB endothelial cells and cord stroma MSC or myofibroblasts to provide an autologous replacement material for congenital heart surgery [223]. In children with pre-natally diagnosed congenital heart malformations, these cells may be utilized to tissue-engineer heart valves, which then are ready for use immediately after birth.

Approaches to overcome the low frequency of circulating EPC for therapeutic interventions include the use of CB-EPC, the cytokine-induced mobilization of endogenous BM-EPC into the circulation and the ex vivo gene transfer to attract EPC. Intramuscular or intramyocardial gene transfer of proangiogenic cytokines like VEGF or SDF into the target tissues already has been shown to enhance the mobilization of endogenous EPC [224, 225]. But also pharmacological substances like statins were effective in augmenting not only EPC mobilization, but also homing by modulating the expression of adhesion molecules on the circulating EPC [196, 226]. The transfection of EPC by the human VEGF gene or immortalization with a retroviral vector encoding the simian virus 40 large T (SV40T) antigen efficiently participated in neovascularization and augmented blood flow in the ischemic hind-limb model [227, 228]. Likewise, CB-EPC transduced to express either VEGF or coagulation factor VIII showed promising results [229, 230].

To sum up, despite the obvious rapid progress in clinical application, research seems to be lagging behind in one sense. The biology and origin of EPC is still ill-defined; so more stringent criteria in nomenclature defining "EPC" are needed to allow the translation into routine therapies. It should be borne in mind that it took 20 years of research and translational studies to develop HSC transplantation from a highly experimental to a routinely performed cell therapy.

Targeting Tumors

The systemic delivery of therapeutic genes to tumors is one challenge in anti-tumor therapy [231]. To engage cells, which are targeted to the tumor neo-endothelium, as potent gene factories, is a matter of debate as already mentioned above. Since growing tumors are largely dependent on tumor neo-angiogenesis, growth requires active endothelial proliferation. So, either endothelial migration and sprouting of pre-existing endothelial cells or recruitment of EPC from the circulation is induced by the tumor milieu. In fact, vasculogenesis accompanied by remodelling of the extracellular matrix appears to be the crucial step in the tumor progression from a few malignant cells to tumor growth and metastasis [232, 233]. Although some tumors may be vascularized by sprouting of pre-existing vessels without signs of neo-angiogenesis [234, 235, 236], in others it is still a matter of debate, whether and to what extent EPC contribute to tumor angiogenesis: whereas some authors failed to demonstrate a significant contribution of BM-derived EPC to tumor vascularization [237], others clearly demonstrated that endogenously mobilized BM cells incorporate to the tumor vasculature, albeit at a frequency below 1% [238, 239]. In contrast to this data, other workers reported that significant amounts of BM-EPC home and incorporate to tumor vasculature and differentiate into mature endothelial cells and that in some tumors, BM-derived EPC are an essential component for tumor development [240, 241, 242].

CB-derived EPC as well have been shown to specifically home to the tumor vasculature whereas control cells, like HUVEC, showed no tropism [243, 244, 245]. The mobilization and recruitment of EPC to ischemic sites and tumors, seem to resemble closely those steps postulated for leukodiapedesis [189, 190, 191]. Vajkoczy et al. proposed a model where the recruitment of embryonal EPC is characterized by a multi-step nature, including initial activation of the tumor endothelium, capture and firm adhesion of circulating progenitor cells, secondary cytokine activation of the captured cell, extravasation, interstitial trafficking within the tumor stroma, and differentiation [246]. This process very closely resembles what is known from leukocyte recruitment to inflamed endothelium, giving rise to a variety of therapeutic options to block this sequence.

As outlined, the amount of recruited and incorporated progenitor cells varies considerably among different experimental situations. Numerous variables, like tumor type and size, cell population, site of implantation, and parameters of analysis, time point of analysis and type of marker used for detection, can significantly influence the outcome of experiments [247, 248]. This heterogeneity was impressively demonstrated by Duda et al., who employed genetically tagged BM cells in different tumor type-bearing mice. The incorporation of BM-derived endothelial cells to the tumor vasculature varied strikingly with tumor model and mice strain between 1.3 and 58.4% [249].

Although the overall contribution of progenitor cells to the formation of new tumor vessels has to be estimated on the basis of all published data to be relatively low, the feasibility of targeting endothelial or EPCs by transgene expression to angiogenic tumor vessels has already been demonstrated [250, 251]. A better knowledge of the biology and the mechanisms underlying EPC recruitment are of interest for anti-tumor therapy. EPC may also be used as cellular vehicles to deliver toxins, as they are specifically recruited to the tumor: genetically modified CD34(+) cells transduced with a thymidine kinase-encoding herpes virus induced, when combined with ganciclovir, the killing of a high proportion of the transduced cells [252]. This, in concordance, resulted in an abrogation of tumor growth.

In conclusion, a better understanding of the molecular pathways leading to mobilization, homing, recruitment, and homing of adult EPC will be helpful for developing novel strategies to target tumor growth.

Embryonic Stem Cell-like Cells Derived from CB

A cell type displaying extensive proliferation capacity as well as multilineage differentiation capacity has been described by the group of C. Verfaillie and is termed multipotent adult progenitor cells (MAPC) [253]. These cells are isolated by depleting CD45(+) and Glycophorin A(+) cells by immunomagnetic labeling. A single cell of this cell type, which might either be completely different from MSC or a subpopulation of MSC, has been shown to contribute when injected into a murine blastocyst to most somatic cell types, indicating a multipotent differentiation potential similar to embryonic stem cells [253]. Although this cell type has been isolated from a variety of normal human, rodent, and possibly other mammalian post-natal tissues, it has never been identified in umbilical cord blood [254].

A population with comparable differentiation potential, when assessed in the in utero sheep model, however, has been identified solely in umbilical cord blood, which therefore may be the cord blood equivalent to the MAPC – called USSC [61].

Supplementing the culture medium with 30% FCS and Dexamethasone yielded cells with a fibroblastoid phenotype similar to MSC. Also, the frequency data of USSC resembled MSC, as they have been isolated from only 40% of CB collections with a frequency of mean four colonies per $2\text{–}20 \times 10^8$ mononucleated cells. Comparable to MSC, these cells could differentiate into osteoblasts, adipocytes, chondrocytes, endothelial cells, hepatocytes, cardiomyocytes, and neuronal cells, but in contrast these cells showed also plasticity toward hematopoietic differentiation, as assessed either in vitro or in the non-injury pre-immune sheep model [255]. The transplantation into the instructive milieu of the developing brain, however, revealed no differentiation into neural cells, in contrast to primary neural cells [256]. Using a model of myocardial infarction, an independent group demonstrated pre-clinically a therapeutic effect of USSC. The improvement of regional and global heart function, however, has been described in every cell transplantation study so far [257]. Within the study of Koegler et al., it was demonstrated that in contrast to BM-MSC, the USSC were able to differentiate not only into Purkinje fibers but also cardiomyocytes [61].

Interestingly, when aiming at improving ex vivo expansion of HSC is that USSC have been shown to provide growth factors, cytokines, and cell–cell contacts necessary for hematopoiesis [258]. In expanding the long-term culture-initiating cells as primitive hematopoietic progenitors and CD34(+) cells, they were superior to BM-MSC.

Embryonic stem cell-like properties have been attributed by a variety of groups to CB: one population is already termed cord-blood-derived embryonic-like stem cells (CBE) [259]. In contrast to what has been described above, these cells are lineage-restricted immunomagnetically-separated cells cultured under different culture conditions, by adding thrombopoietin, flt-3 ligand, and c-kit ligand. Within these conditions the adherent cell clustered to form embryoid body-like colonies, that are positive for a variety of stage-specific embryonic antigens: SSEA-3 and 4 (but not SSEA-1), the tumor-rejection antigens Tra 1-60, Tra 1-81, and the transcription factor Oct-4. For these cells at least the potential of hepatic progenitor cells production within a 3-dimensional tissue-engineering approach has been demonstrated [259, 260].

Very small embryonic-like CXCR4(+)SSEA-1(+)Oct-4+ stem cells isolated by erythrocyte lysis followed by multiparametric flow-cytometric sorting yielded an interesting population with probably similar pluripotent stem cell properties as their BM counterpart [261, 262].

Another lineage marker negative population, additionally lacking the expression of CD45, CD34, and CD133, which can be prospectively isolated without any need for culture, displayed chondrogenic and strikingly also hematopoietic differentiation capacity [263].

CB mononuclear-derived cells described by Zhao et al. also exhibited capacity toward hematopoiesis as well as differentiation into endothelial, neuronal, and endodermal insulin-producing cells [264].

Although the above-mentioned cell types have to be accepted as being highly interesting as closest-related alternatives to the ethically restricted ES cells, these adult ES-like cells in most cases lack the verification and reproduction by independent research groups. A closer examination is therefore demanded to assess their true therapeutic potential.

Conclusion

According to NETCORD, more than 100,000 CB units have been collected, frozen and stored worldwide in anticipation of their potential use to treat hematopoietic disorders [265]. As summarized in this chapter, increasing knowledge regarding their non-hematopoietic counterparts may be used for developing future therapeutic strategies. Since aspirating BM from the patient is a highly invasive procedure, and in addition, the quality (number and proliferative capacity) decreases with age, alternative sources are acquired and CB might prove to be a reasonably good one. The autologous application of stem cells collected at birth necessitates a large amount of technical and financial resources for storing the frozen cell samples throughout the period of life of their potential user. Although such a procedure seems possible from a technical point of view, the current view is that the possible benefits do not justify it [266].

For allogeneic use, the primitive umbilical cord-blood-derived non-HSC population provides perhaps the most readily accessible and, at the same time, underutilized stem cell source with little ethical conflict and a number of advantages. The question as to whether CB progenitor cells will prove to be superior or more practical in terms of an alleviating allogeneic use when compared to other adult tissue-derived progenitor cells, remains open at this time. Nevertheless, efficient and reproducible methods to isolate, expand and differentiate CB progenitor cells are required. When extrapolated to the developments in HSC transplantation, where within 10 years CB has become a more and more accepted alternative source for HSC, probably as many years will pass by until the eventual use of CB-derived non-hematopoietic stem cells in clinical therapy.

References

1. Lagasse E, Shizuru JA, Uchida N, Tsukamoto A, Weissman IL. Toward regenerative medicine. Immunity 2001; 14: 425–436.
2. Rando TA. Stem cells, ageing and the quest for immortality. Nature 2006; 441: 1080–1086.
3. Ding S, Schultz PG. A role for chemistry in stem cell biology. Nat Biotechnol 2004; 22: 833–840.
4. Storb R. Allogeneic hematopoietic stem cell transplantation – yesterday, today, and tomorrow. Exp Hematol 2003; 31: 1–10.
5. Gluckman E, Broxmeyer HA, Auerbach AD, Friedman ×HS, Douglas GW, Devergie A, Esperou H, Thierry D, Socie G, Lehn P. Hematopoietic reconstitution in a patient with Fanconi's anemia by means of umbilical-cord blood from an HLA-identical sibling. N Engl J Med 1989; 321: 1174–1178.
6. Brunstein CG, Setubal DC, Wagner JE. Expanding the role of umbilical cord blood transplantation. Br J Haematol 2007; 137: 20–35.

7. Broxmeyer HE. Biology of cord blood cells and future prospects for enhanced clinical benefit. Cytotherapy 2005; 7: 209–218.
8. Migliaccio AR, Adamson JW, Stevens CE, Dobrila NL, Carrier CM, Rubinstein P. Cell dose and speed of engraftment in placental/umbilical cord blood transplantation: graft progenitor cell content is a better predictor than nucleated cell quantity. Blood 2000; 96: 2717–2722.
9. de Lima M, Shpall E. Strategies for widening the use of cord blood in hematopoietic stem cell transplantation. Haematologica 2006; 91: 584–587.
10. Korbling M, Robinson S, Estrov Z, Champlin R, Shpall E. Umbilical cord blood-derived cells for tissue repair. Cytotherapy 2005; 7: 258–261.
11. Sharma AD, Cantz T, Richter R, Eckert K, Henschler R, Wilkens L, Jochheim-Richter A, Arseniev L, Ott M. Human cord blood stem cells generate human cytokeratin 18-negative hepatocyte-like cells in injured mouse liver. Am J Pathol 2005; 167: 555–564.
12. Kakinuma S, Asahina K, Okamura K, Teramoto K, Tateno C, Yoshizato K, Tanaka Y, Yasumizu T, Sakamoto N, Watanabe M, Teraoka H. Human cord blood cells transplanted into chronically damaged liver exhibit similar characteristics to functional hepatocytes. Transplant Proc 2007; 39: 240–243.
13. Newsome PN, Johannessen I, Boyle S, Dalakas E, McAulay KA, Samuel K, Rae F, Forrester L, Turner ML, Hayes PC, Harrison DJ, Bickmore WA, Plevris JN. Human cord blood-derived cells can differentiate into hepatocytes in the mouse liver with no evidence of cellular fusion. Gastroenterology 2003; 124: 1891–1900.
14. Kashofer K, Siapati EK, Bonnet D. In vivo formation of unstable heterokaryons after liver damage and hematopoietic stem cell/progenitor transplantation. Stem Cells 2006; 24: 1104–1112.
15. Yoshida S, Ishikawa F, Kawano N, Shimoda K, Nagafuchi S, Shimoda S, Yasukawa M, Kanemaru T, Ishibashi H, Shultz LD, Harada M. Human cord blood–derived cells generate insulin-producing cells in vivo. Stem Cells 2005; 23: 1409–1416.
16. Sanberg PR, Willing AE, Garbuzova-Davis S, Saporta S, Liu G, Sanberg CD, Bickford PC, Klasko SK, El Badri NS. Umbilical cord blood-derived stem cells and brain repair. Ann N Y Acad Sci 2005; 1049: 67–83.
17. Henning RJ, Abu-Ali H, Balis JU, Morgan MB, Willing AE, Sanberg PR. Human umbilical cord blood mononuclear cells for the treatment of acute myocardial infarction. Cell Transplant 2004; 13: 729–739.
18. Ma N, Ladilov Y, Kaminski A, Piechaczek C, Choi YH, Li W, Steinhoff G, Stamm C. Umbilical cord blood cell transplantation for myocardial regeneration. Transplant Proc 2006; 38: 771–773.
19. Ishikawa F, Yasukawa M, Yoshida S, Nakamura K, Nagatoshi Y, Kanemaru T, Shimoda K, Shimoda S, Miyamoto T, Okamura J, Shultz LD, Harada M. Human cord blood- and bone marrow-derived CD34+ cells regenerate gastrointestinal epithelial cells. FASEB J 2004; 18: 1958–1960.
20. Ebihara Y, Masuya M, Larue AC, Fleming PA, Visconti RP, Minamiguchi H, Drake CJ, Ogawa M. Hematopoietic origins of fibroblasts: II. In vitro studies of fibroblasts, CFU-F, and fibrocytes. Exp Hematol 2006; 34: 219–229.
21. Ogawa M, Larue AC, Drake CJ. Hematopoietic origin of fibroblasts/myofibroblasts: Its pathophysiologic implications. Blood 2006; 108: 2893–2896.
22. Zipori D. The nature of stem cells: state rather than entity. Nat Rev Genet 2004; 5: 873–878.
23. Prindull GA, Fibach E. Are postnatal hemangioblasts generated by dedifferentiation from committed hematopoietic stem cells? Exp Hematol 2007; 35: 691–701.
24. Javazon EH, Beggs KJ, Flake AW. Mesenchymal stem cells: paradoxes of passaging. Exp Hematol 2004; 32: 414–425.
25. Baksh D, Song L, Tuan RS. Adult mesenchymal stem cells: characterization, differentiation, and application in cell and gene therapy. J Cell Mol Med 2004; 8: 301–316.
26. Kassem M. Mesenchymal stem cells: biological characteristics and potential clinical applications. Cloning Stem Cells 2004; 6: 369–374.

27. Lanotte M, Allen TD, Dexter TM. Histochemical and ultrastructural characteristics of a cell line from human bone-marrow stroma. J Cell Sci 1981; 50: 281–297.
28. Friedenstein AJ, Gorskaja JF, Kulagina NN. Fibroblast precursors in normal and irradiated mouse hematopoietic organs. Exp Hematol 1976; 4: 267–274.
29. Caplan AI. Mesenchymal stem cells. J Orthop Res 1991; 9: 641–650.
30. Pittenger MF, Mackay AM, Beck SC, Jaiswal RK, Douglas R, Mosca JD, Moorman MA, Simonetti DW, Craig S, Marshak DR. Multilineage potential of adult human mesenchymal stem cells. Science 1999; 284: 143–147.
31. Lee KD, Kuo TK, Whang-Peng J, Chung YF, Lin CT, Chou SH, Chen JR, Chen YP, Lee OK. In vitro hepatic differentiation of human mesenchymal stem cells. Hepatology 2004; 40: 1275–1284.
32. Zhao LR, Duan WM, Reyes M, Keene CD, Verfaillie CM, Low WC. Human bone marrow stem cells exhibit neural phenotypes and ameliorate neurological deficits after grafting into the ischemic brain of rats. Exp Neurol 2002; 174: 11–20.
33. Liechty KW, Mackenzie TC, Shaaban AF, Radu A, Moseley AM, Deans R, Marshak DR, Flake AW. Human mesenchymal stem cells engraft and demonstrate site-specific differentiation after in utero transplantation in sheep. Nat Med 2000; 6: 1282–1286.
34. Baxter MA, Wynn RF, Jowitt SN, Wraith JE, Fairbairn LJ, Bellantuono I. Study of telomere length reveals rapid aging of human marrow stromal cells following in vitro expansion. Stem Cells 2004; 22: 675–682.
35. Keating A. Mesenchymal stromal cells. Curr Opin Hematol 2006; 13: 419–425.
36. Dominici M, Le Blanc K, Mueller I, Slaper-Cortenbach I, Marini F, Krause D, Deans R, Keating A, Prockop D, Horwitz E. Minimal criteria for defining multipotent mesenchymal stromal cells. The International Society for Cellular Therapy position statement. Cytotherapy 2006; 8: 315–317.
37. Le Blanc K, Ringden O. Mesenchymal stem cells: properties and role in clinical bone marrow transplantation. Curr Opin Immunol 2006; 18: 586–591.
38. Tyndall A, Walker UA, Cope A, Dazzi F, De Bari C, Fibbe W, Guiducci S, Jones S, Jorgensen C, Le Blanc K, Luyten F, McGonagle D, Martin I, Bocelli-Tyndall C, Pennesi G, Pistoia V, Pitzalis C, Uccelli A, Wulffraat N, Feldmann M. Immunomodulatory properties of mesenchymal stem cells: a review based on an interdisciplinary meeting held at the Kennedy Institute of Rheumatology Division, London, UK, 31 October 2005. Arthritis Res Ther 2007; 9: 301.
39. Aggarwal S, Pittenger MF. Human mesenchymal stem cells modulate allogeneic immune cell responses. Blood 2005; 105: 1815–1822.
40. Ringden O, Le Blanc K. Allogeneic hematopoietic stem cell transplantation: state of the art and new perspectives. APMIS 2005; 113: 813–830.
41. Le Blanc K, Rasmusson I, Sundberg B, Gotherstrom C, Hassan M, Uzunel M, Ringden O. Treatment of severe acute graft-versus-host disease with third party haploidentical mesenchymal stem cells. Lancet 2004; 363: 1439–1441.
42 http://clinicaltrials.gov. http://clinicaltrials.gov. 2007. Ref Type: Internet Communication
43 D'Ippolito G, Schiller PC, Ricordi C, Roos BA, Howard GA. Age-related osteogenic potential of mesenchymal stromal stem cells from human vertebral bone marrow. J. Bone Miner Res 1999; 14: 1115–1122.
44. Nishida S, Endo N, Yamagiwa H, Tanizawa T, Takahashi HE. Number of osteoprogenitor cells in human bone marrow markedly decreases after skeletal maturation. J Bone Miner Metab 1999; 17: 171–177.
45. Pojda Z, Machaj EK, Oldak T, Gajkowska A, Jastrzewska M. Nonhematopoietic stem cells of fetal origin – how much of today's enthusiasm will pass the time test? Folia Histochem Cytobiol 2005; 43: 209–212.
46. Prindull G, Ben Ishay Z, Ebell W, Bergholz M, Dirk T, Prindull B. CFU-F circulating in cord blood. Blut 1987; 54: 351–359.

47. Ye ZQ, Burkholder JK, Qiu P, Schultz JC, Shahidi NT, Yang NS. Establishment of an adherent cell feeder layer from human umbilical cord blood for support of long-term hematopoietic progenitor cell growth. Proc Natl Acad Sci USA 1994; 91: 12140–12144.
48. Goodwin HS, Bicknese AR, Chien SN, Bogucki BD, Quinn CO, Wall DA. Multilineage differentiation activity by cells isolated from umbilical cord blood: expression of bone, fat, and neural markers. Biol Blood Marrow Transplant 2001; 7: 581–588.
49. Erices A, Conget P, Minguell JJ. Mesenchymal progenitor cells in human umbilical cord blood. Br J Haematol 2000; 109: 235–242.
50. Campagnoli C, Roberts IA, Kumar S, Bennett PR, Bellantuono I, Fisk NM. Identification of mesenchymal stem/progenitor cells in human first-trimester fetal blood, liver, and bone marrow. Blood 2001; 98: 2396–2402.
51. Quesenberry PJ, Dooner G, Colvin G, Abedi M. Stem cell biology and the plasticity polemic. Exp Hematol 2005; 33: 389–394.
52. Yu M, Xiao Z, Shen L, Li L. Mid-trimester fetal blood-derived adherent cells share characteristics similar to mesenchymal stem cells but full-term umbilical cord blood does not. Br J Haematol 2004; 124: 666–675.
53. Mareschi K, Biasin E, Piacibello W, Aglietta M, Madon E, Fagioli F. Isolation of human mesenchymal stem cells: bone marrow versus umbilical cord blood. Haematologica 2001; 86: 1099–1100.
54. Bieback K, Kern S, Kluter H, Eichler H. Critical parameters for the isolation of mesenchymal stem cells from umbilical cord blood. Stem Cells 2004; 22: 625–634.
55. Lee OK, Kuo TK, Chen WM, Lee KD, Hsieh SL, Chen TH. Isolation of multipotent mesenchymal stem cells from umbilical cord blood. Blood 2004; 103: 1669–1675.
56. Rosada C, Justesen J, Melsvik D, Ebbesen P, Kassem M. The human umbilical cord blood: a potential source for osteoblast progenitor cells. Calcif Tissue Int 2003; 72: 135–142.
57. Wexler SA, Donaldson C, Denning-Kendall P, Rice C, Bradley B, Hows JM. Adult bone marrow is a rich source of human mesenchymal 'stem' cells but umbilical cord and mobilized adult blood are not. Br J Haematol 2003; 121: 368–374.
58. Yang SE, Ha CW, Jung M, Jin HJ, Lee M, Song H, Choi S, Oh W, Yang YS. Mesenchymal stem/progenitor cells developed in cultures from UC blood. Cytotherapy 2004; 6: 476–486.
59. Kang TJ, Yeom JE, Lee HJ, Rho SH, Han H, Chae GT. Growth kinetics of human mesenchymal stem cells from bone marrow and umbilical cord blood. Acta Haematol 2004; 112: 230–233.
60. Kang XQ, Zang WJ, Bao LJ, Li DL, Xu XL, Yu XJ. Differentiating characterization of human umbilical cord blood-derived mesenchymal stem cells in vitro. Cell Biol Int 2006; 30: 569–575.
61. Kogler G, Sensken S, Airey JA, Trapp T, Muschen M, Feldhahn N, Liedtke S, Sorg RV, Fischer J, Rosenbaum C, Greschat S, Knipper A, Bender J, Degistirici O, Gao J, Caplan AI, Colletti EJ, Almeida-Porada G, Muller HW, Zanjani E, Wernet P. A new human somatic stem cell from placental cord blood with intrinsic pluripotent differentiation potential. J Exp Med 2004; 200: 123–135.
62. Nakagawa R, Watanabe T, Kawano Y, Kanai S, Suzuya H, Kaneko M, Watanabe H, Okamoto Y, Kuroda Y, Nakayama T. Analysis of maternal and neonatal factors that influence the nucleated and CD34+ cell yield for cord blood banking. Transfusion 2004; 44: 262–267.
63. Hutson EL, Boyer S, Genever PG. Rapid isolation, expansion, and differentiation of osteoprogenitors from full-term umbilical cord blood. Tissue Eng 2005; 11: 1407–1420.
64. Mendes SC, Robin C, Dzierzak E. Mesenchymal progenitor cells localize within hematopoietic sites throughout ontogeny. Development 2005; 132: 1127–1136.
65. Baron MH, Fraser ST. The specification of early hematopoiesis in the mammal. Curr Opin Hematol 2005; 12: 217–221.
66. Muller-Sieburg CE, Deryugina E. The stromal cells' guide to the stem cell universe. Stem Cells 1995; 13: 477–486.

67. Eaves CJ, Cashman JD, Sutherland HJ, Otsuka T, Humphries RK, Hogge DE, Lansdorp PL, Eaves AC. Molecular analysis of primitive hematopoietic cell proliferation control mechanisms. Ann N Y Acad Sci 1991; 628: 298–306.
68. Guillot PV, O'Donoghue K, Kurata H, Fisk NM. Fetal stem cells: betwixt and between. Semin Reprod Med 2006; 24: 340–347.
69. Lee MW, Yang MS, Park JS, Kim HC, Kim YJ, Choi J. Isolation of mesenchymal stem cells from cryopreserved human umbilical cord blood. Int J Hematol 2005; 81: 126–130.
70. Lee MW, Choi J, Yang MS, Moon YJ, Park JS, Kim HC, Kim YJ. Mesenchymal stem cells from cryopreserved human umbilical cord blood. Biochem Biophys Res Commun 2004; 320: 273–278.
71. Tondreau T, Lagneaux L, Dejeneffe M, Delforge A, Massy M, Mortier C, Bron D. Isolation of BM mesenchymal stem cells by plastic adhesion or negative selection: phenotype, proliferation kinetics and differentiation potential. Cytotherapy 2004; 6: 372–379.
72. Jones EA, English A, Kinsey SE, Straszynski L, Emery P, Ponchel F, McGonagle D. Optimization of a flow cytometry-based protocol for detection and phenotypic characterization of multipotent mesenchymal stromal cells from human bone marrow. Cytometry B Clin Cytom 2006; 70: 391–399.
73. Tondreau T, Meuleman N, Delforge A, Dejeneffe M, Leroy R, Massy M, Mortier C, Bron D, Lagneaux L. Mesenchymal stem cells derived from CD133-positive cells in mobilized peripheral blood and cord blood: proliferation, Oct4 expression, and plasticity. Stem Cells 2005; 23: 1105–1112.
74. Chang YJ, Tseng CP, Hsu LF, Hsieh TB, Hwang SM. Characterization of two populations of mesenchymal progenitor cells in umbilical cord blood. Cell Biol Int 2006; 30: 495–499.
75. Markov V, Kusumi K, Tadesse MG, William DA, Hall DM, Lounev V, Carlton A, Leonard J, Cohen RI, Rappaport EF, Saitta B. Identification of cord blood-derived mesenchymal stem/stromal cell populations with distinct growth kinetics, differentiation potentials, and gene expression profiles. Stem Cells Dev 2007; 16: 53–73.
76. Kern S, Eichler H, Stoeve J, Kluter H, Bieback K. Comparative analysis of mesenchymal stem cells from bone marrow, umbilical cord blood, or adipose tissue. Stem Cells 2006; 24: 1294–1301.
77. Reinisch A, Bartmann C, Rohde E, Schallmoser K, Bjelic-Radisic V, Lanzer G, Linkesch W, Strunk D. Humanized system to propagate cord blood-derived multipotent mesenchymal stromal cells for clinical application. Regen Med 2007; 2: 371–382.
78. Chang YJ, Shih DT, Tseng CP, Hsieh TB, Lee DC, Hwang SM. Disparate mesenchyme-lineage tendencies in mesenchymal stem cells from human bone marrow and umbilical cord blood. Stem Cells 2006; 24: 679–685.
79. Gratama JW, Kraan J, Keeney M, Sutherland DR, Granger V, Barnett D. Validation of the single-platform ISHAGE method for CD34(+) hematopoietic stem and progenitor cell enumeration in an international multicenter study. Cytotherapy 2003; 5: 55–65.
80. Majumdar MK, Keane-Moore M, Buyaner D, Hardy WB, Moorman MA, McIntosh KR, Mosca JD. Characterization and functionality of cell surface molecules on human mesenchymal stem cells. J Biomed Sci 2003; 10: 228–241.
81. Reddi AH, Ma SS, Cunningham NS. Induction and maintenance of new bone formation by growth and differentiation factors. Ann Chir Gynaecol 1988; 77: 189–192.
82. Grassel S, Ahmed N. Influence of cellular microenvironment and paracrine signals on chondrogenic differentiation. Front Biosci 2007; 12: 4946–4956.
83. Fuchs JR, Hannouche D, Terada S, Zand S, Vacanti JP, Fauza DO. Cartilage engineering from ovine umbilical cord blood mesenchymal progenitor cells. Stem Cells 2005; 23: 958–964.
84. Gimble JM, Robinson CE, Wu X, Kelly KA. The function of adipocytes in the bone marrow stroma: an update. Bone 1996; 19: 421–428.
85. Riley GP, Gordon MY. Characterization of cultured stromal layers derived from fetal and adult hemopoietic tissues. Exp Hematol 1987; 15: 78–84.

86. Jeong JA, Gang EJ, Hong SH, Hwang SH, Kim SW, Yang IH, Ahn C, Han H, Kim H. Rapid neural differentiation of human cord blood-derived mesenchymal stem cells. Neuroreport 2004; 15: 1731–1734.
87. El Badri NS, Hakki A, Saporta S, Liang X, Madhusodanan S, Willing AE, Sanberg CD, Sanberg PR. Cord blood mesenchymal stem cells: potential use in neurological disorders. Stem Cells Dev 2006; 15: 497–506.
88. Buzanska L, Machaj EK, Zablocka B, Pojda Z, Domanska-Janik K. Human cord blood-derived cells attain neuronal and glial features in vitro. J Cell Sci 2002; 115: 2131–2138.
89. Sun W, Buzanska L, Domanska-Janik K, Salvi RJ, Stachowiak MK. Voltage-sensitive and ligand-gated channels in differentiating neural stem-like cells derived from the nonhematopoietic fraction of human umbilical cord blood. Stem Cells 2005; 23: 931–945.
90. Hong SH, Gang EJ, Jeong JA, Ahn C, Hwang SH, Yang IH, Park HK, Han H, Kim H. In vitro differentiation of human umbilical cord blood-derived mesenchymal stem cells into hepatocyte-like cells. Biochem Biophys Res Commun 2005; 330: 1153–1161.
91. Gang EJ, Jeong JA, Han S, Yan Q, Jeon CJ, Kim H. In vitro endothelial potential of human UC blood-derived mesenchymal stem cells. Cytotherapy 2006; 8: 215–227.
92. Liu JW, Dunoyer-Geindre S, Serre-Beinier V, Mai G, Lambert JF, Fish RJ, Pernod G, Buehler L, Bounameaux H, Kruithof EK. Characterization of endothelial-like cells derived from human mesenchymal stem cells. J Thromb Haemost 2007; 5: 826–834.
93. Nunes VA, Cavacana N, Canovas M, Strauss BE, Zatz M. Stem cells from umbilical cord blood differentiate into myotubes and express dystrophin in vitro only after exposure to in vivo muscle environment. Biol Cell 2007; 99: 185–196.
94. Gang EJ, Jeong JA, Hong SH, Hwang SH, Kim SW, Yang IH, Ahn C, Han H, Kim H. Skeletal myogenic differentiation of mesenchymal stem cells isolated from human umbilical cord blood. Stem Cells 2004; 22: 617–624.
95. Berger MJ, Adams SD, Tigges BM, Sprague SL, Wang XJ, Collins DP, McKenna DH. Differentiation of umbilical cord blood-derived multilineage progenitor cells into respiratory epithelial cells. Cytotherapy 2006; 8: 480–487.
96. Cheng F, Zou P, Yang H, Yu Z, Zhong Z. Induced differentiation of human cord blood mesenchymal stem/progenitor cells into cardiomyocyte-like cells in vitro. J Huazhong Univ Sci Technolog Med Sci 2003; 23: 154–157.
97. Phinney DG. Building a consensus regarding the nature and origin of mesenchymal stem cells. J. Cell Biochem. Suppl 2002; 38: 7–12.
98. Panepucci RA, Siufi JL, Silva WA, Jr., Proto-Siquiera R, Neder L, Orellana M, Rocha V, Covas DT, Zago MA. Comparison of gene expression of umbilical cord vein and bone marrow-derived mesenchymal stem cells. Stem Cells 2004; 22: 1263–1278.
99. Jeong JA, Lee Y, Lee W, Jung S, Lee DS, Jeong N, Lee HS, Bae Y, Jeon CJ, Kim H. Proteomic analysis of the hydrophobic fraction of mesenchymal stem cells derived from human umbilical cord blood. Mol Cells 2006; 22: 36–43.
100. Jeong JA, Hong SH, Gang EJ, Ahn C, Hwang SH, Yang IH, Han H, Kim H. Differential gene expression profiling of human umbilical cord blood-derived mesenchymal stem cells by DNA microarray. Stem Cells 2005; 23: 584–593.
101. Feldmann RE Jr, Bieback K, Maurer MH, Kalenka A, Burgers HF, Gross B, Hunzinger C, Kluter H, Kuschinsky W, Eichler H. Stem cell proteomes: a profile of human mesenchymal stem cells derived from umbilical cord blood. Electrophoresis 2005; 26: 2749–2758.
102. Goessler UR, Bieback K, Bugert P, Heller T, Sadick H, Hormann K, Riedel F. In vitro analysis of integrin expression during chondrogenic differentiation of mesenchymal stem cells and chondrocytes upon dedifferentiation in cell culture. Int J Mol Med 2006; 17: 301–307.
103. Goessler UR, Bugert P, Bieback K, Deml M, Sadick H, Hormann K, Riedel F. In-vitro analysis of the expression of TGFbeta-superfamily-members during chondrogenic differentiation of mesenchymal stem cells and chondrocytes during dedifferentiation in cell culture. Cell Mol Biol Lett 2005; 10: 345–362.

104. Tsai MS, Hwang SM, Chen KD, Lee YS, Hsu LW, Chang YJ, Wang CN, Peng HH, Chang YL, Chao AS, Chang SD, Lee KD, Wang TH, Wang HS, Soong YK. Functional network analysis on the transcriptomes of mesenchymal stem cells derived from amniotic fluid, amniotic membrane, cord blood, and bone marrow. Stem Cells 2007; 25(10): 2511–23.
105. Wagner W, Wein F, Seckinger A, Frankhauser M, Wirkner U, Krause U, Blake J, Schwager C, Eckstein V, Ansorge W, Ho AD. Comparative characteristics of mesenchymal stem cells from human bone marrow, adipose tissue, and umbilical cord blood. Exp Hematol 2005; 33: 1402–1416.
106. Giordano A, Galderisi U, Marino IR. From the laboratory bench to the patient's bedside: an update on clinical trials with mesenchymal stem cells. J Cell Physiol 2007; 211: 27–35.
107. Vilquin JT, Rosset P. Mesenchymal stem cells in bone and cartilage repair: current status. Regen Med 2006; 1: 589–604.
108. Freyman T, Polin G, Osman H, Crary J, Lu M, Cheng L, Palasis M, Wilensky RL. A quantitative, randomized study evaluating three methods of mesenchymal stem cell delivery following myocardial infarction. Eur Heart J 2006; 27: 1114–1122.
109. Wurmser AE, Gage FH. Stem cells: cell fusion causes confusion. Nature 2002; 416: 485–487.
110. Gao J, Dennis JE, Muzic RF, Lundberg M, Caplan AI. The dynamic in vivo distribution of bone marrow-derived mesenchymal stem cells after infusion. Cells Tissues Organs 2001; 169: 12–20.
111. Viswanathan A, Painter RG, Lanson NA Jr, Wang G. Functional expression of N-formyl peptide receptors in human bone marrow-derived mesenchymal stem cells. Stem Cells 2007; 25: 1263–1269.
112. Colletti EJ, Almeida-Porada G, Chamberlain J, Zanjani ED, Airey JA. The time course of engraftment of human mesenchymal stem cells in fetal heart demonstrates that Purkinje fiber aggregates derive from a single cell and not multi-cell homing. Exp Hematol 2006; 34: 926–933.
113. Francois S, Bensidhoum M, Mouiseddine M, Mazurier C, Allenet B, Semont A, Frick J, Sache A, Bouchet S, Thierry D, Gourmelon P, Gorin NC, Chapel A. Local irradiation not only induces homing of human mesenchymal stem cells at exposed sites but promotes their widespread engraftment to multiple organs: a study of their quantitative distribution after irradiation damage. Stem Cells 2006; 24: 1020–1029.
114. Erices AA, Allers CI, Conget PA, Rojas CV, Minguell JJ. Human cord blood-derived mesenchymal stem cells home and survive in the marrow of immunodeficient mice after systemic infusion. Cell Transplant 2003; 12: 555–561.
115. Horwitz EM, Prockop DJ, Gordon PL, Koo WW, Fitzpatrick LA, Neel MD, McCarville ME, Orchard PJ, Pyeritz RE, Brenner MK. Clinical responses to bone marrow transplantation in children with severe osteogenesis imperfecta. Blood 2001; 97: 1227–1231.
116. Le Blanc K, Gotherstrom C, Ringden O, Hassan M, McMahon R, Horwitz E, Anneren G, Axelsson O, Nunn J, Ewald U, Norden-Lindeberg S, Jansson M, Dalton A, Astrom E, Westgren M. Fetal mesenchymal stem-cell engraftment in bone after in utero transplantation in a patient with severe osteogenesis imperfecta. Transplantation 2005; 79: 1607–1614.
117. Horwitz EM, Prockop DJ, Fitzpatrick LA, Koo WW, Gordon PL, Neel M, Sussman M, Orchard P, Marx JC, Pyeritz RE, Brenner MK. Transplantability and therapeutic effects of bone marrow-derived mesenchymal cells in children with osteogenesis imperfecta. Nat Med 1999; 5: 309–313.
118. Horwitz EM, Gordon PL, Koo WK, Marx JC, Neel MD, McNall RY, Muul L, Hofmann T. Isolated allogeneic bone marrow-derived mesenchymal cells engraft and stimulate growth in children with osteogenesis imperfecta: implications for cell therapy of bone. Proc Natl Acad Sci USA 2002; 99: 8932–8937.
119. Koc ON, Day J, Nieder M, Gerson SL, Lazarus HM, Krivit W. Allogeneic mesenchymal stem cell infusion for treatment of metachromatic leukodystrophy (MLD) and Hurler syndrome (MPS-IH). Bone Marrow Transplant 2002; 30: 215–222.

120. Fouillard L, Bensidhoum M, Bories D, Bonte H, Lopez M, Moseley AM, Smith A, Lesage S, Beaujean F, Thierry D, Gourmelon P, Najman A, Gorin NC. Engraftment of allogeneic mesenchymal stem cells in the bone marrow of a patient with severe idiopathic aplastic anemia improves stroma. Leukemia 2003; 17: 474–476.
121. Koc ON, Peters C, Aubourg P, Raghavan S, Dyhouse S, DeGasperi R, Kolodny EH, Yoseph YB, Gerson SL, Lazarus HM, Caplan AI, Watkins PA, Krivit W. Bone marrow-derived mesenchymal stem cells remain host-derived despite successful hematopoietic engraftment after allogeneic transplantation in patients with lysosomal and peroxisomal storage diseases. Exp Hematol 1999; 27: 1675–1681.
122. Bruder SP, Kurth AA, Shea M, Hayes WC, Jaiswal N, Kadiyala S. Bone regeneration by implantation of purified, culture-expanded human mesenchymal stem cells. J Orthop Res 1998; 16: 155–162.
123. Carstens MH, Chin M, Ng T, Tom WK. Reconstruction of #7 facial cleft with distraction-assisted in situ osteogenesis (DISO): role of recombinant human bone morphogenetic protein-2 with Helistat-activated collagen implant. J Craniofac Surg 2005; 16: 1023–1032.
124. Yamada Y, Ueda M, Hibi H, Nagasaka T. Translational research for injectable tissue-engineered bone regeneration using mesenchymal stem cells and platelet-rich plasma: from basic research to clinical case study. Cell Transplant 2004; 13: 343–355.
125. Carstanjen B, Desbois C, Hekmati M, Behr L. Successful engraftment of cultured autologous mesenchymal stem cells in a surgically repaired soft palate defect in an adult horse. Can J Vet Res 2006; 70: 143–147.
126. Mazzini L, Fagioli F, Boccaletti R, Mareschi K, Oliveri G, Olivieri C, Pastore I, Marasso R, Madon E. Stem cell therapy in amyotrophic lateral sclerosis: a methodological approach in humans. Amyotroph Lateral Scler Other Motor Neuron Disord 2003; 4: 158–161.
127. Kang SK, Shin MJ, Jung JS, Kim YG, Kim CH. Autologous adipose tissue-derived stromal cells for treatment of spinal cord injury. Stem Cells Dev 2006; 15: 583–594.
128. Kim KN, Oh SH, Lee KH, Yoon DH. Effect of human mesenchymal stem cell transplantation combined with growth factor infusion in the repair of injured spinal cord. Acta Neurochir Suppl 2006; 99: 133–136.
129. Yoon SH, Shim YS, Park YH, Chung JK, Nam JH, Kim MO, Park HC, Park SR, Min BH, Kim EY, Choi BH, Park H, Ha Y. Complete spinal cord injury treatment using autologous bone marrow cell transplantation and bone marrow stimulation with granulocyte macrophage-colony stimulating factor: phase I/II clinical trial. Stem Cells 2007; 25: 2066–2073.
130. Lim JH, Byeon YE, Ryu HH, Jeong YH, Lee YW, Kim WH, Kang KS, Kweon OK. Transplantation of canine umbilical cord blood-derived mesenchymal stem cells in experimentally induced spinal cord injured dogs. J Vet Sci 2007; 8: 275–282.
131. Phinney DG, Isakova I. Plasticity and therapeutic potential of mesenchymal stem cells in the nervous system. Curr Pharm Des 2005; 11: 1255–1265.
132. Kang KS, Kim SW, Oh YH, Yu JW, Kim KY, Park HK, Song CH, Han H. A 37-year-old spinal cord-injured female patient, transplanted of multipotent stem cells from human UC blood, with improved sensory perception and mobility, both functionally and morphologically: a case study. Cytotherapy 2005; 7: 368–373.
133. Finney MR, Greco NJ, Haynesworth SE, Martin JM, Hedrick DP, Swan JZ, Winter DG, Kadereit S, Joseph ME, Fu P, Pompili VJ, Laughlin MJ. Direct comparison of umbilical cord blood versus bone marrow-derived endothelial precursor cells in mediating neovascularization in response to vascular ischemia. Biol. Blood Marrow Transplant 2006; 12: 585–593.
134. Vojtassak J, Danisovic L, Kubes M, Bakos D, Jarabek L, Ulicna M, Blasko M. Autologous biograft and mesenchymal stem cells in treatment of the diabetic foot. Neuro Endocrinol Lett 2006; 27 Suppl 2: 134–137.
135. Katritsis DG, Sotiropoulou PA, Karvouni E, Karabinos I, Korovesis S, Perez SA, Voridis EM, Papamichail M. Transcoronary transplantation of autologous mesenchymal stem cells

and endothelial progenitors into infarcted human myocardium. Catheter Cardiovasc Interv 2005; 65: 321–329.
136. Kim SW, Han H, Chae GT, Lee SH, Bo S, Yoon JH, Lee YS, Lee KS, Park HK, Kang KS. Successful stem cell therapy using umbilical cord blood-derived multipotent stem cells for Buerger's disease and ischemic limb disease animal model. Stem Cells 2006; 24: 1620–1626.
137. Dimmeler S, Zeiher AM, Schneider MD. Unchain my heart: the scientific foundations of cardiac repair. J Clin Invest 2005; 115: 572–583.
138. Shake JG, Gruber PJ, Baumgartner WA, Senechal G, Meyers J, Redmond JM, Pittenger MF, Martin BJ. Mesenchymal stem cell implantation in a swine myocardial infarct model: engraftment and functional effects. Ann Thorac Surg 2002; 73: 1919–1925.
139. Zhang S, Ge J, Sun A, Xu D, Qian J, Lin J, Zhao Y, Hu H, Li Y, Wang K, Zou Y. Comparison of various kinds of bone marrow stem cells for the repair of infarcted myocardium: single clonally purified non-hematopoietic mesenchymal stem cells serve as a superior source. J Cell Biochem 2006; 99: 1132–1147.
140. Min JJ, Ahn Y, Moon S, Kim YS, Park JE, Kim SM, Le UN, Wu JC, Joo SY, Hong MH, Yang DH, Jeong MH, Song CH, Jeong YH, Yoo KY, Kang KS, Bom HS. In vivo bioluminescence imaging of cord blood derived mesenchymal stem cell transplantation into rat myocardium. Ann Nucl Med 2006; 20: 165–170.
141. Liu CH, Hwang SM. Cytokine interactions in mesenchymal stem cells from cord blood. Cytokine 2005; 32: 270–279.
142. Lu LL, Liu YJ, Yang SG, Zhao QJ, Wang X, Gong W, Han ZB, Xu ZS, Lu YX, Liu D, Chen ZZ, Han ZC. Isolation and characterization of human umbilical cord mesenchymal stem cells with hematopoiesis-supportive function and other potentials. Haematologica 2006; 91: 1017–1026.
143. Wynn RF, Hart CA, Corradi-Perini C, O'Neill L, Evans CA, Wraith JE, Fairbairn LJ, Bellantuono I. A small proportion of mesenchymal stem cells strongly expresses functionally active CXCR4 receptor capable of promoting migration to bone marrow. Blood 2004; 104: 2643–2645.
144. Bensidhoum M, Chapel A, Francois S, Demarquay C, Mazurier C, Fouillard L, Bouchet S, Bertho JM, Gourmelon P, Aigueperse J, Charbord P, Gorin NC, Thierry D, Lopez M. Homing of in vitro expanded Stro-1- or Stro-1+ human mesenchymal stem cells into the NOD/SCID mouse and their role in supporting human CD34 cell engraftment. Blood 2004; 103: 3313–3319.
145. Son BR, Marquez-Curtis LA, Kucia M, Wysoczynski M, Turner AR, Ratajczak J, Ratajczak MZ, Janowska-Wieczorek A. Migration of bone marrow and cord blood mesenchymal stem cells in vitro is regulated by stromal-derived factor-1-CXCR4 and hepatocyte growth factor-c-met axes and involves matrix metalloproteinases. Stem Cells 2006; 24: 1254–1264.
146. Bierkens JG, Hendry JH, Testa NG. Recovery of the proliferative and functional integrity of mouse bone marrow in long-term cultures established after whole-body irradiation at different doses and dose rates. Exp Hematol 1991; 19: 81–86.
147. Stute N, Fehse B, Schroder J, Arps S, Adamietz P, Held KR, Zander AR. Human mesenchymal stem cells are not of donor origin in patients with severe aplastic anemia who underwent sex-mismatched allogeneic bone marrow transplant. J Hematother Stem Cell Res 2002; 11: 977–984.
148. Pozzi S, Lisini D, Podesta M, Bernardo ME, Sessarego N, Piaggio G, Cometa A, Giorgiani G, Mina T, Buldini B, Maccario R, Frassoni F, Locatelli F. Donor multipotent mesenchymal stromal cells may engraft in pediatric patients given either cord blood or bone marrow transplantation. Exp Hematol 2006; 34: 934–942.
149. Koc ON, Gerson SL, Cooper BW, Dyhouse SM, Haynesworth SE, Caplan AI, Lazarus HM. Rapid hematopoietic recovery after coinfusion of autologous-blood stem cells and culture-expanded marrow mesenchymal stem cells in advanced breast cancer patients receiving high-dose chemotherapy. J Clin Oncol 2000; 18: 307–316.

150. Lazarus HM, Koc ON, Devine SM, Curtin P, Maziarz RT, Holland HK, Shpall EJ, McCarthy P, Atkinson K, Cooper BW, Gerson SL, Laughlin MJ, Loberiza FR, Jr., Moseley AB, Bacigalupo A. Cotransplantation of HLA-identical sibling culture-expanded mesenchymal stem cells and hematopoietic stem cells in hematologic malignancy patients. Biol Blood Marrow Transplant 2005; 11: 389–398.
151. Ball LM, Bernardo ME, Roelofs H, Lankester A, Cometa A, Egeler RM, Locatelli F, Fibbe WE. Co-transplantation of ex vivo expanded mesenchymal stem cells accelerates lymphocyte recovery and may reduce the risk of graft failure in haploidentical hematopoietic stem cell transplantation. Blood 2007; 110(7): 2764–7.
152. Le Blanc K, Samuelsson H, Gustafsson B, Remberger M, Sundberg B, Arvidson J, Ljungman P, Lonnies H, Nava S, Ringden O. Transplantation of mesenchymal stem cells to enhance engraftment of hematopoietic stem cells. Leukemia 2007; 21: 1733–1738.
153. Chan SL, Choi M, Wnendt S, Kraus M, Teng E, Leong HF, Merchav S. Enhanced in vivo homing of uncultured and selectively amplified cord blood CD34+ cells by cotransplantation with cord blood-derived unrestricted somatic stem cells. Stem Cells 2007; 25: 529–536.
154. Han JY, Goh RY, Seo SY, Hwang TH, Kwon HC, Kim SH, Kim JS, Kim HJ, Lee YH. Cotransplantation of cord blood hematopoietic stem cells and culture-expanded and GM-CSF-/SCF-transfected mesenchymal stem cells in SCID mice. J Korean Med Sci 2007; 22: 242–247.
155. Rasmusson I, Ringden O, Sundberg B, Le Blanc K. Mesenchymal stem cells inhibit the formation of cytotoxic T lymphocytes, but not activated cytotoxic T lymphocytes or natural killer cells. Transplantation 2003; 76: 1208–1213.
156. Le Blanc K, Tammik C, Rosendahl K, Zetterberg E, Ringden O. HLA expression and immunologic properties of differentiated and undifferentiated mesenchymal stem cells. Exp Hematol 2003; 31: 890–896.
157. Le Blanc K, Tammik L, Sundberg B, Haynesworth SE, Ringden O. Mesenchymal stem cells inhibit and stimulate mixed lymphocyte cultures and mitogenic responses independently of the major histocompatibility complex. Scand J Immunol 2003; 57: 11–20.
158. Krampera M, Pasini A, Pizzolo G, Cosmi L, Romagnani S, Annunziato F. Regenerative and immunomodulatory potential of mesenchymal stem cells. Curr Opin Pharmacol 2006; 6: 435–441.
159. Bartholomew A, Sturgeon C, Siatskas M, Ferrer K, McIntosh K, Patil S, Hardy W, Devine S, Ucker D, Deans R, Moseley A, Hoffman R. Mesenchymal stem cells suppress lymphocyte proliferation in vitro and prolong skin graft survival in vivo. Exp Hematol 2002; 30: 42–48.
160. Djouad F, Bony C, Apparailly F, Louis-Plence P, Jorgensen C, Noel D. Earlier onset of syngeneic tumors in the presence of mesenchymal stem cells. Transplantation 2006; 82: 1060–1066.
161. Djouad F, Plence P, Bony C, Tropel P, Apparailly F, Sany J, Noel D, Jorgensen C. Immunosuppressive effect of mesenchymal stem cells favors tumor growth in allogeneic animals. Blood 2003; 102: 3837–3844.
162. Gotherstrom C, Ringden O, Westgren M, Tammik C, Le Blanc K. Immunomodulatory effects of human foetal liver-derived mesenchymal stem cells. Bone Marrow Transplant 2003; 32: 265–272.
163. Nauta AJ, Westerhuis G, Kruisselbrink AB, Lurvink EG, Willemze R, Fibbe WE. Donor-derived mesenchymal stem cells are immunogenic in an allogeneic host and stimulate donor graft rejection in a nonmyeloablative setting. Blood 2006; 108: 2114–2120.
164. Poncelet AJ, Vercruysse J, Saliez A, Gianello P. Although pig allogeneic mesenchymal stem cells are not immunogenic in vitro, intracardiac injection elicits an immune response in vivo. Transplantation 2007; 83: 783–790.
165. Lee ST, Jang JH, Cheong JW, Kim JS, Maemg HY, Hahn JS, Ko YW, Min YH. Treatment of high-risk acute myelogenous leukaemia by myeloablative chemoradiotherapy followed by co-infusion of T cell-depleted haematopoietic stem cells and culture-expanded marrow

mesenchymal stem cells from a related donor with one fully mismatched human leucocyte antigen haplotype. Br J Haematol 2002; 118: 1128–1131.
166. Van Damme A, Vanden Driessche T, Collen D, Chuah MK. Bone marrow stromal cells as targets for gene therapy. Curr Gene Ther 2002; 2: 195–209.
167. Peterson B, Zhang J, Iglesias R, Kabo M, Hedrick M, Benhaim P, Lieberman JR. Healing of critically sized femoral defects, using genetically modified mesenchymal stem cells from human adipose tissue. Tissue Eng 2005; 11: 120–129.
168. Ye M, Wang XJ, Zhang YH, Lu GQ, Liang L, Xu JY, Chen SD. Transplantation of bone marrow stromal cells containing the neurturin gene in rat model of Parkinson's disease. Brain Res 2007; 1142: 206–216.
169. Bartholomew A, Patil S, Mackay A, Nelson M, Buyaner D, Hardy W, Mosca J, Sturgeon C, Siatskas M, Mahmud N, Ferrer K, Deans R, Moseley A, Hoffman R, Devine SM. Baboon mesenchymal stem cells can be genetically modified to secrete human erythropoietin in vivo. Hum Gene Ther 2001; 12: 1527–1541.
170. Abdallah BM, Haack-Sorensen M, Burns JS, Elsnab B, Jakob F, Hokland P, Kassem M. Maintenance of differentiation potential of human bone marrow mesenchymal stem cells immortalized by human telomerase reverse transcriptase gene despite [corrected] extensive proliferation. Biochem Biophys Res Commun 2005; 326: 527–538.
171. Mangi AA, Noiseux N, Kong D, He H, Rezvani M, Ingwall JS, Dzau VJ. Mesenchymal stem cells modified with Akt prevent remodeling and restore performance of infarcted hearts. Nat Med 2003; 9: 1195–1201.
172. Studeny M, Marini FC, Champlin RE, Zompetta C, Fidler IJ, Andreeff M. Bone marrow-derived mesenchymal stem cells as vehicles for interferon-beta delivery into tumors. Cancer Res 2002; 62: 3603–3608.
173. Lu FZ, Fujino M, Kitazawa Y, Uyama T, Hara Y, Funeshima N, Jiang JY, Umezawa A, Li XK. Characterization and gene transfer in mesenchymal stem cells derived from human umbilical-cord blood. J Lab Clin Med 2005; 146: 271–278.
174. Chan J, O'Donoghue K, de la FJ, Roberts IA, Kumar S, Morgan JE, Fisk NM. Human fetal mesenchymal stem cells as vehicles for gene delivery. Stem Cells 2005; 23: 93–102.
175. Kobune M, Kawano Y, Ito Y, Chiba H, Nakamura K, Tsuda H, Sasaki K, Dehari H, Uchida H, Honmou O, Takahashi S, Bizen A, Takimoto R, Matsunaga T, Kato J, Kato K, Houkin K, Niitsu Y, Hamada H. Telomerized human multipotent mesenchymal cells can differentiate into hematopoietic and cobblestone area-supporting cells. Exp Hematol 2003; 31: 715–722.
176. Ho YC, Chung YC, Hwang SM, Wang KC, Hu YC. Transgene expression and differentiation of baculovirus-transduced human mesenchymal stem cells. J Gene Med 2005; 7: 860–868.
177. Devine SM, Bartholomew AM, Mahmud N, Nelson M, Patil S, Hardy W, Sturgeon C, Hewett T, Chung T, Stock W, Sher D, Weissman S, Ferrer K, Mosca J, Deans R, Moseley A, Hoffman R. Mesenchymal stem cells are capable of homing to the bone marrow of non-human primates following systemic infusion. Exp Hematol 2001; 29: 244–255.
178. Friedenstein AJ, Deriglasova UF, Kulagina NN, Panasuk AF, Rudakowa SF, Luria EA, Ruadkow IA. Precursors for fibroblasts in different populations of hematopoietic cells as detected by the in vitro colony assay method. Exp Hematol 1974; 2: 83–92.
179. Spees JL, Gregory CA, Singh H, Tucker HA, Peister A, Lynch PJ, Hsu SC, Smith J, Prockop DJ. Internalized antigens must be removed to prepare hypoimmunogenic mesenchymal stem cells for cell and gene therapy. Mol Ther 2004; 9: 747–756.
180. Schuurman R, van Steenis B, van Strien A, van der NJ, Sol C. Frequent detection of bovine polyomavirus in commercial batches of calf serum by using the polymerase chain reaction. J Gen Virol 1991; 72 (Pt 11): 2739–2745.
181. Sundin M, Ringden O, Sundberg B, Nava S, Gotherstromm C, Le Blanc K. No alloantibodies against mesenchymal stromal cells, but presence of anti-fetal calf serum antibodies, after transplantation in allogeneic hematopoietic stem cell recipients. Haematologica 2007; 92(9): 1208–15.

182. Mannello F, Tonti GA. Concise review: no breakthroughs for human mesenchymal and embryonic stem cell culture: conditioned medium, feeder layer, or feeder-free; medium with fetal calf serum, human serum, or enriched plasma; serum-free, serum replacement nonconditioned medium, or ad hoc formula? All that glitters is not gold! Stem Cells 2007; 25: 1603–1609.
183. Kocaoemer A, Kern S, Kluter H, Bieback K. Human AB serum and thrombin-activated platelet-rich plasma are suitable alternatives to fetal calf serum for the expansion of mesenchymal stem cells from adipose tissue. Stem Cells 2007; 25: 1270–1278.
184. Beck L Jr, D'Amore PA. Vascular development: cellular and molecular regulation. FASEB J 1997; 11: 365–373.
185. Asahara T, Murohara T, Sullivan A, Silver M, van der ZR, Li T, Witzenbichler B, Schatteman G, Isner JM. Isolation of putative progenitor endothelial cells for angiogenesis. Science 1997; 275: 964–967.
186. Takahashi T, Kalka C, Masuda H, Chen D, Silver M, Kearney M, Magner M, Isner JM, Asahara T. Ischemia- and cytokine-induced mobilization of bone marrow-derived endothelial progenitor cells for neovascularization. Nat Med 1999; 5: 434–438.
187. Shintani S, Murohara T, Ikeda H, Ueno T, Sasaki K, Duan J, Imaizumi T. Augmentation of postnatal neovascularization with autologous bone marrow transplantation. Circulation 2001; 103: 897–903.
188. Hunting CB, Noort WA, Zwaginga JJ. Circulating endothelial (progenitor) cells reflect the state of the endothelium: vascular injury, repair and neovascularization. Vox Sang 2005; 88: 1–9.
189. Rafii S, Lyden D. Therapeutic stem and progenitor cell transplantation for organ vascularization and regeneration. Nat Med 2003; 9: 702–712.
190. Urbich C, Dimmeler S. Endothelial progenitor cells: characterization and role in vascular biology. Circ Res 2004; 95: 343–353.
191. Hristov M, Erl W, Weber PC. Endothelial progenitor cells: mobilization, differentiation, and homing. Arterioscler Thromb Vasc Biol 2003; 23: 1185–1189.
192. Hirschi KK, Goodell MA. Hematopoietic, vascular and cardiac fates of bone marrow-derived stem cells. Gene Ther 2002; 9: 648–652.
193. Dimmeler S, Zeiher AM. Vascular repair by circulating endothelial progenitor cells: the missing link in atherosclerosis? J Mol Med 2004; 82: 671–677.
194. Hristov M, Weber C. Endothelial progenitor cells: characterization, pathophysiology, and possible clinical relevance. J Cell Mol Med 2004; 8: 498–508.
195. Goon PK, Lip GY, Boos CJ, Stonelake PS, Blann AD. Circulating endothelial cells, endothelial progenitor cells, and endothelial microparticles in cancer. Neoplasia 2006; 8: 79–88.
196. Dimmeler S, Aicher A, Vasa M, Mildner-Rihm C, Adler K, Tiemann M, Rutten H, Fichtlscherer S, Martin H, Zeiher AM. HMG-CoA reductase inhibitors (statins) increase endothelial progenitor cells via the PI 3-kinase/Akt pathway. J Clin Invest 2001; 108: 391–397.
197. Ingram DA, Mead LE, Tanaka H, Meade V, Fenoglio A, Mortell K, Pollok K, Ferkowicz MJ, Gilley D, Yoder MC. Identification of a novel hierarchy of endothelial progenitor cells using human peripheral and umbilical cord blood. Blood 2004; 104: 2752–2760.
198. Hill JM, Zalos G, Halcox JP, Schenke WH, Waclawiw MA, Quyyumi AA, Finkel T. Circulating endothelial progenitor cells, vascular function, and cardiovascular risk. N Engl J Med 2003; 348: 593–600.
199. Gulati R, Jevremovic D, Peterson TE, Chatterjee S, Shah V, Vile RG, Simari RD. Diverse origin and function of cells with endothelial phenotype obtained from adult human blood. Circ Res 2003; 93: 1023–1025.
200. Bompais H, Chagraoui J, Canron X, Crisan M, Liu XH, Anjo A, Tolla-Le Port C, Leboeuf M, Charbord P, Bikfalvi A, Uzan G. Human endothelial cells derived from circulating progenitors display specific functional properties compared with mature vessel wall endothelial cells. Blood 2004; 103: 2577–2584.

201. Prater DN, Case J, Ingram DA, Yoder MC. Working hypothesis to redefine endothelial progenitor cells. Leukemia 2007; 21: 1141–1149.
202. Ingram DA, Mead LE, Moore DB, Woodard W, Fenoglio A, Yoder MC. Vessel wall-derived endothelial cells rapidly proliferate because they contain a complete hierarchy of endothelial progenitor cells. Blood 2005; 105: 2783–2786.
203. Urbich C, Heeschen C, Aicher A, Dernbach E, Zeiher AM, Dimmeler S. Relevance of monocytic features for neovascularization capacity of circulating endothelial progenitor cells. Circulation 2003; 108: 2511–2516.
204. Ziegler BL, Valtieri M, Porada GA, De Maria R, Muller R, Masella B, Gabbianelli M, Casella I, Pelosi E, Bock T, Zanjani ED, Peschle C. KDR receptor: a key marker defining hematopoietic stem cells. Science 1999; 285: 1553–1558.
205. Peichev M, Naiyer AJ, Pereira D, Zhu Z, Lane WJ, Williams M, Oz MC, Hicklin DJ, Witte L, Moore MA, Rafii S. Expression of VEGFR-2 and AC133 by circulating human CD34(+) cells identifies a population of functional endothelial precursors. Blood 2000; 95: 952–958.
206. Gehling UM, Ergun S, Schumacher U, Wagener C, Pantel K, Otte M, Schuch G, Schafhausen P, Mende T, Kilic N, Kluge K, Schafer B, Hossfeld DK, Fiedler W. In vitro differentiation of endothelial cells from AC133-positive progenitor cells. Blood 2000; 95: 3106–3112.
207. Kim SY, Park SY, Kim JM, Kim JW, Kim MY, Yang JH, Kim JO, Choi KH, Kim SB, Ryu HM. Differentiation of endothelial cells from human umbilical cord blood AC133-CD14+ cells. Ann Hematol 2005; 84: 417–422.
208. Murga M, Yao L, Tosato G. Derivation of endothelial cells from. Stem Cells 2004; 22: 385–395.
209. Chung YS, Zhang WJ, Arentson E, Kingsley PD, Palis J, Choi K. Lineage analysis of the hemangioblast as defined by FLK1 and SCL expression. Development 2002; 129: 5511–5520.
210. Shalaby F, Ho J, Stanford WL, Fischer KD, Schuh AC, Schwartz L, Bernstein A, Rossant J. A requirement for Flk1 in primitive and definitive hematopoiesis and vasculogenesis. Cell 1997; 89: 981–990.
211. Case J, Mead LE, Bessler WK, Prater D, White HA, Saadatzadeh MR, Bhavsar JR, Yoder MC, Haneline LS, Ingram DA. Human CD34+AC133+VEGFR-2+ cells are not endothelial progenitor cells but distinct, primitive hematopoietic progenitors. Exp Hematol 2007; 35: 1109–1118.
212. Gennaro G, Menard C, Michaud SE, Rivard A. Age-dependent impairment of reendothelialization after arterial injury: role of vascular endothelial growth factor. Circulation 2003; 107: 230–233.
213. Rivard A, Fabre JE, Silver M, Chen D, Murohara T, Kearney M, Magner M, Asahara T, Isner JM. Age-dependent impairment of angiogenesis. Circulation 1999; 99: 111–120.
214. Murohara T. Therapeutic vasculogenesis using human cord blood-derived endothelial progenitors. Trends Cardiovasc Med 2001; 11: 303–307.
215. Emanueli C, Lako M, Stojkovic M, Madeddu P. In search of the best candidate for regeneration of ischemic tissues: are embryonic/fetal stem cells more advantageous than adult counterparts? Thromb Haemost 2005; 94: 738–749.
216. Liu C, Sun Z, Du X, Chen X, Feng J, Jia B. Implantation of endothelial progenitor cells into laser-induced channels in rat ischemia hindlimb augments neovascularization. Ann Vasc Surg 2005; 19: 241–247.
217. Nagano M, Yamashita T, Hamada H, Ohneda K, Kimura K, Nakagawa T, Shibuya M, Yoshikawa H, Ohneda O. Identification of functional endothelial progenitor cells suitable for the treatment of ischemic tissue using human umbilical cord blood. Blood 2007; 110: 151–160.
218. Duan HX, Cheng LM, Wang J, Hu LS, Lu GX. Angiogenic potential difference between two types of endothelial progenitor cells from human umbilical cord blood. Cell Biol Int 2006; 30: 1018–1027.

219. Yamaguchi J, Kusano KF, Masuo O, Kawamoto A, Silver M, Murasawa S, Bosch-Marce M, Masuda H, Losordo DW, Isner JM, Asahara T. Stromal cell-derived factor-1 effects on ex vivo expanded endothelial progenitor cell recruitment for ischemic neovascularization. Circulation 2003; 107: 1322–1328.
220. Ma N, Ladilov Y, Moebius JM, Ong L, Piechaczek C, David A, Kaminski A, Choi YH, Li W, Egger D, Stamm C, Steinhoff G. Intramyocardial delivery of human CD133+ cells in a SCID mouse cryoinjury model: bone marrow vs. cord blood-derived cells. Cardiovasc Res 2006; 71: 158–169.
221. Grunewald M, Avraham I, Dor Y, Bachar-Lustig E, Itin A, Jung S, Chimenti S, Landsman L, Abramovitch R, Keshet E. VEGF-induced adult neovascularization: recruitment, retention, and role of accessory cells. Cell 2006; 124: 175–189.
222. Pesce M, Orlandi A, Iachininoto MG, Straino S, Torella AR, Rizzuti V, Pompilio G, Bonanno G, Scambia G, Capogrossi MC. Myoendothelial differentiation of human umbilical cord blood-derived stem cells in ischemic limb tissues. Circ Res 2003; 93: e51–e62.
223. Schmidt D, Mol A, Breymann C, Achermann J, Odermatt B, Gossi M, Neuenschwander S, Pretre R, Genoni M, Zund G, Hoerstrup SP. Living autologous heart valves engineered from human prenatally harvested progenitors. Circulation 2006; 114: I125–I131.
224. Kalka C, Tehrani H, Laudenberg B, Vale PR, Isner JM, Asahara T, Symes JF. VEGF gene transfer mobilizes endothelial progenitor cells in patients with inoperable coronary disease. Ann Thorac Surg 2000; 70: 829–834.
225. Hiasa K, Egashira K, Kitamoto S, Ishibashi M, Inoue S, Ni W, Zhao Q, Nagata S, Katoh M, Sata M, Takeshita A. Bone marrow mononuclear cell therapy limits myocardial infarct size through vascular endothelial growth factor. Basic Res Cardiol 2004; 99: 165–172.
226. Walter DH, Rittig K, Bahlmann FH, Kirchmair R, Silver M, Murayama T, Nishimura H, Losordo DW, Asahara T, Isner JM. Statin therapy accelerates reendothelialization: a novel effect involving mobilization and incorporation of bone marrow-derived endothelial progenitor cells. Circulation 2002; 105: 3017–3024.
227. Qiu HY, Fujimori Y, Nishioka K, Yamaguchi N, Hashimoto-Tamaoki T, Sugihara A, Terada N, Nagaya N, Kanda M, Kobayashi N, Tanaka N, Westerman KA, Leboulch P, Hara H. Postnatal neovascularization by endothelial progenitor cells immortalized with the simian virus 40T antigen gene. Int J Oncol 2006; 28: 815–821.
228. Ikeda Y, Fukuda N, Wada M, Matsumoto T, Satomi A, Yokoyama S, Saito S, Matsumoto K, Kanmatsuse K, Mugishima H. Development of angiogenic cell and gene therapy by transplantation of umbilical cord blood with vascular endothelial growth factor gene. Hypertens Res 2004; 27: 119–128.
229. Yi C, Xia W, Zheng Y, Zhang L, Shu M, Liang J, Han Y, Guo S. Transplantation of endothelial progenitor cells transferred by vascular endothelial growth factor gene for vascular regeneration of ischemic flaps. J Surg Res 2006; 135: 100–106.
230. Herder C, Tonn T, Oostendorp R, Becker S, Keller U, Peschel C, Grez M, Seifried E. Sustained expansion and transgene expression of coagulation factor VIII-transduced cord blood-derived endothelial progenitor cells. Arterioscler Thromb Vasc Biol 2003; 23: 2266–2272.
231. Bazan-Peregrino M, Seymour LW, Harris AL. Gene therapy targeting to tumor endothelium. Cancer Gene Ther 2007; 14: 117–127.
232. Seftor RE, Seftor EA, Koshikawa N, Meltzer PS, Gardner LM, Bilban M, Stetler-Stevenson WG, Quaranta V, Hendrix MJ. Cooperative interactions of laminin 5 gamma2 chain, matrix metalloproteinase-2, and membrane type-1-matrix/metalloproteinase are required for mimicry of embryonic vasculogenesis by aggressive melanoma. Cancer Res 2001; 61: 6322–6327.
233. Baudino TA, McKay C, Pendeville-Samain H, Nilsson JA, Maclean KH, White EL, Davis AC, Ihle JN, Cleveland JL. c-Myc is essential for vasculogenesis and angiogenesis during development and tumor progression. Genes Dev 2002; 16: 2530–2543.

234. Stessels F, Van den EG, Van dA, I, Salgado R, Van den HE, Harris AL, Jackson DG, Colpaert CG, van Marck EA, Dirix LY, Vermeulen PB. Breast adenocarcinoma liver metastases, in contrast to colorectal cancer liver metastases, display a non-angiogenic growth pattern that preserves the stroma and lacks hypoxia. Br J Cancer 2004; 90: 1429–1436.
235. Passalidou E, Stewart M, Trivella M, Steers G, Pillai G, Dogan A, Leigh I, Hatton C, Harris A, Gatter K, Pezzella F. Vascular patterns in reactive lymphoid tissue and in non-Hodgkin's lymphoma. Br J Cancer 2003; 88: 553–559.
236. Passalidou E, Trivella M, Singh N, Ferguson M, Hu J, Cesario A, Granone P, Nicholson AG, Goldstraw P, Ratcliffe C, Tetlow M, Leigh I, Harris AL, Gatter KC, Pezzella F. Vascular phenotype in angiogenic and non-angiogenic lung non-small cell carcinomas. Br J Cancer 2002; 86: 244–249.
237. Gothert JR, Gustin SE, van Eekelen JA, Schmidt U, Hall MA, Jane SM, Green AR, Gottgens B, Izon DJ, Begley CG. Genetically tagging endothelial cells in vivo: bone marrow-derived cells do not contribute to tumor endothelium. Blood 2004; 104: 1769–1777.
238. Larrivee B, Niessen K, Pollet I, Corbel SY, Long M, Rossi FM, Olive PL, Karsan A. Minimal contribution of marrow-derived endothelial precursors to tumor vasculature. J Immunol 2005; 175: 2890–2899.
239. Machein MR, Renninger S, Lima-Hahn E, Plate KH. Minor contribution of bone marrow-derived endothelial progenitors to the vascularization of murine gliomas. Brain Pathol 2003; 13: 582–597.
240. Lyden D, Hattori K, Dias S, Costa C, Blaikie P, Butros L, Chadburn A, Heissig B, Marks W, Witte L, Wu Y, Hicklin D, Zhu Z, Hackett NR, Crystal RG, Moore MA, Hajjar KA, Manova K, Benezra R, Rafii S. Impaired recruitment of bone-marrow-derived endothelial and hematopoietic precursor cells blocks tumor angiogenesis and growth. Nat Med 2001; 7: 1194–1201.
241. Arbab AS, Pandit SD, Anderson SA, Yocum GT, Bur M, Frenkel V, Khuu HM, Read EJ, Frank JA. Magnetic resonance imaging and confocal microscopy studies of magnetically labeled endothelial progenitor cells trafficking to sites of tumor angiogenesis. Stem Cells 2006; 24: 671–678.
242. Asahara T, Masuda H, Takahashi T, Kalka C, Pastore C, Silver M, Kearne M, Magner M, Isner JM. Bone marrow origin of endothelial progenitor cells responsible for postnatal vasculogenesis in physiological and pathological neovascularization. Circ Res 1999; 85: 221–228.
243. Moore XL, Lu J, Sun L, Zhu CJ, Tan P, Wong MC. Endothelial progenitor cells' "homing" specificity to brain tumors. Gene Ther 2004; 11: 811–818.
244. Ricousse-Roussanne S, Barateau V, Contreres JO, Boval B, Kraus-Berthier L, Tobelem G. Ex vivo differentiated endothelial and smooth muscle cells from human cord blood progenitors home to the angiogenic tumor vasculature. Cardiovasc Res 2004; 62: 176–184.
245. Oh HK, Ha JM, O E, Lee BH, Lee SK, Shim BS, Hong YK, Joe YA. Tumor angiogenesis promoted by ex vivo differentiated endothelial progenitor cells is effectively inhibited by an angiogenesis inhibitor, TK1-2. Cancer Res 2007; 67: 4851–4859.
246. Vajkoczy P, Blum S, Lamparter M, Mailhammer R, Erber R, Engelhardt B, Vestweber D, Hatzopoulos AK. Multistep nature of microvascular recruitment of ex vivo-expanded embryonic endothelial progenitor cells during tumor angiogenesis. J Exp Med 2003; 197: 1755–1765.
247. Ribatti D. The involvement of endothelial progenitor cells in tumor angiogenesis. J Cell Mol Med 2004; 8: 294–300.
248. Kopp HG, Ramos CA, Rafii S. Contribution of endothelial progenitors and proangiogenic hematopoietic cells to vascularization of tumor and ischemic tissue. Curr Opin Hematol 2006; 13: 175–181.
249. Duda DG, Cohen KS, Kozin SV, Perentes JY, Fukumura D, Scadden DT, Jain RK. Evidence for incorporation of bone marrow-derived endothelial cells into perfused blood vessels in tumors. Blood 2006; 107: 2774–2776.

250. De Palma M, Venneri MA, Naldini L. In vivo targeting of tumor endothelial cells by systemic delivery of lentiviral vectors. Hum Gene Ther 2003; 14: 1193–1206.
251. Wei J, Blum S, Unger M, Jarmy G, Lamparter M, Geishauser A, Vlastos GA, Chan G, Fischer KD, Rattat D, Debatin KM, Hatzopoulos AK, Beltinger C. Embryonic endothelial progenitor cells armed with a suicide gene target hypoxic lung metastases after intravenous delivery. Cancer Cell 2004; 5: 477–488.
252. De Palma M, Venneri MA, Roca C, Naldini L. Targeting exogenous genes to tumor angiogenesis by transplantation of genetically modified hematopoietic stem cells. Nat Med 2003; 9: 789–795.
253. Jiang Y, Jahagirdar BN, Reinhardt RL, Schwartz RE, Keene CD, Ortiz-Gonzalez XR, Reyes M, Lenvik T, Lund T, Blackstad M, Du J, Aldrich S, Lisberg A, Low WC, Largaespada DA, Verfaillie CM. Pluripotency of mesenchymal stem cells derived from adult marrow. Nature 2002; 418: 41–49.
254. Verfaillie CM, Schwartz R, Reyes M, Jiang Y. Unexpected potential of adult stem cells. Ann N Y Acad Sci 2003; 996: 231–234.
255. Kogler G, Sensken S, Wernet P. Comparative generation and characterization of pluripotent unrestricted somatic stem cells with mesenchymal stem cells from human cord blood. Exp Hematol 2006; 34: 1589–1595.
256. Coenen M, Kogler G, Wernet P, Brustle O. Transplantation of human umbilical cord blood-derived adherent progenitors into the developing rodent brain. J Neuropathol Exp Neurol 2005; 64: 681–688.
257. Kim BO, Tian H, Prasongsukarn K, Wu J, Angoulvant D, Wnendt S, Muhs A, Spitkovsky D, Li RK. Cell transplantation improves ventricular function after a myocardial infarction: a preclinical study of human unrestricted somatic stem cells in a porcine model. Circulation 2005; 112: I96–104.
258. Kogler G, Radke TF, Lefort A, Sensken S, Fischer J, Sorg RV, Wernet P. Cytokine production and hematopoiesis supporting activity of cord blood-derived unrestricted somatic stem cells. Exp Hematol 2005; 33: 573–583.
259. McGuckin CP, Forraz N, Baradez MO, Navran S, Zhao J, Urban R, Tilton R, Denner L. Production of stem cells with embryonic characteristics from human umbilical cord blood. Cell Prolif 2005; 38: 245–255.
260. Forraz N, Pettengell R, McGuckin CP. Characterization of a lineage-negative stem-progenitor cell population optimized for ex vivo expansion and enriched for LTC-IC. Stem Cells 2004; 22: 100–108.
261. Kucia M, Halasa M, Wysoczynski M, Baskiewicz-Masiuk M, Moldenhawer S, Zuba-Surma E, Czajka R, Wojakowski W, Machalinski B, Ratajczak MZ. Morphological and molecular characterization of novel population of CXCR4+ SSEA-4+ Oct-4+ very small embryonic-like cells purified from human cord blood: preliminary report. Leukemia 2007; 21: 297–303.
262. Kucia M, Reca R, Campbell FR, Zuba-Surma E, Majka M, Ratajczak J, Ratajczak MZ. A population of very small embryonic-like (VSEL) CXCR4(+)SSEA-1(+)Oct-4+ stem cells identified in adult bone marrow. Leukemia 2006; 20: 857–869.
263. Jay KE, Rouleau A, Underhill TM, Bhatia M. Identification of a novel population of human cord blood cells with hema-topoietic and chondrocytic potential. Cell Res. 2004; 14: 268–282.
264. Zhao Y, Wang H, Mazzone T. Identification of stem cells from human umbilical cord blood with embryonic and hematopoietic characteristics. Exp Cell Res 2006; 312: 2454–2464.
265. Net Cord. https://www.netcord.org. 2007.
266. Fisk NM, Roberts IA, Markwald R, Mironov V. Can routine commercial cord blood banking be scientifically and ethically justified? PLoS Med 2005; 2: e44.

Section II
Umbilical Cord Blood Stem Cell Transplantation

Chapter 7
Cord Blood Transplantation for Pediatric Non-Malignant Conditions

Tatjana Kilo and Peter J. Shaw

Introduction and Description of the Evolution of the Field

Although the majority of hematopoietic stem cell transplantations (HSCT) are done for patients with malignant diseases, it should be remembered that a high proportion of pediatric transplants are done for non-malignant disease, and this is particularly true for unrelated transplants. HSCT is a curative option for many inherited and acquired non-malignant diseases that show abnormalities of the blood or bone marrow (BM)-derived cells. Most patients who could benefit from HSCT lack a suitable related donor and either may not have a suitable or unrelated BM donor identified or the patient cannot wait for the delay of a search of the unrelated marrow donor registries. Cord blood (CB) transplantation (CBT) has been shown to be a viable alternative for these patients. There may also be a theoretical benefit, especially for patients with inborn metabolic errors, if CB cells have greater capacity of de-differentiate into non-hematopoietic tissues [1].

Despite the rarity of non-malignant disease as an indication for HSCT when compared with the total transplant numbers, in particular for adults with malignancy, they have made a fundamental contribution to the field of HSCT. The first related BM transplant (BMT) was performed for severe combined immunodeficiency (SCID) in 1968 [2]; the first unrelated transplant for severe aplastic anemia in 1973 [3], and the first haploidentical transplants, for a mucopolysaccharidosis (MPS) without T-cell depletion (TCD) and SCID with TCD in 1980 [4, 5]. Transplants for non-malignant diseases have also contributed to the field of CBT: the first allogeneic CBT was successfully performed for non-malignant disease in 1988, when a patient with Fanconi anemia (FA) was successfully transplanted from his human leukocyte antigen (HLA)-identical sibling [6]. The first CBT performed from an HLA-identical sibling, born after in vitro fertilization (IVF) and pre-implantation genetic diagnosis (PGD), was also for FA [7, 8]. The first unrelated CBT were

P.J. Shaw (✉)
Head, BMT Service, Senior Staff Oncologist, Oncology Unit, Clinical Associate Professor, Discipline of Paediatrics & Child Health, Children's Hospital at Westmead, Sydney, NSW 2145, Australia

N. Bhattacharya, P. Stubblefield (eds.), *Frontiers of Cord Blood Science*,
DOI 10.1007/978-1-84800-167-1_7,

Table 7.1 Unrelated transplants for non-malignant diseases registered with the CIBMTR: patients transplanted between 1988 and 2006

Year of report	BM/PBSC	Cord blood
1992–1994	325	5
1995–1997	379	119
1998–2000	496	199
2001–2003	577	332
2004–2006*	529	343
Total (1988–2006)	2483	999

*05/06 data incomplete.

performed in 1993 by the Duke group for a group of patients with malignant and non-malignant diseases [9].

Since then related and unrelated CBT have been carried out for an increasing number of patients with an increasing variety of non-malignant diseases over the past years [9, 10]. The vast majority of CBT for non-malignant (and malignant) disease are unrelated, and the numbers of unrelated CBT for non-malignant disease are starting to approach the number of transplants performed using BM or peripheral blood stem cells (PBSC) (see Table 7.1).

The top eight diagnoses for unrelated cord blood transplant for non-malignant disease are as follows:

Disease	Number
FA	120
SCID, all types	109
Hurler MPS I	90
Severe aplastic anemia	80
Wiskott–Aldrich syndrome (WAS)	75
Krabbe's disease	48
Adrenoleukodystrophy (ALD)	48
Osteopetrosis	45

The data presented here are preliminary and were obtained from the Statistical Center of the Center for International Blood and Marrow Transplant Research (CIBMTR). The analysis has not been reviewed or approved by the Advisory or Scientific Committee of the CIBMTR.

Reasons Why One Should Use Cord Blood in These Diseases

Lack of Donor

One major limitation to proceed to allogeneic BMT is the lack of a suitable HLA-matched related or unrelated donor. Although the number of unrelated CB units (224,343) available on the international registries is a small proportion of the total number of unrelated donors (10,733,542, as reported to BMDW [11]), CB can be used successfully for HSCT across HLA disparities that would not be tolerated with an unrelated adult marrow donor. With less stringent criteria for HLA, it is possible to find a suitable cord unit for a patient where a matched unrelated donor would not be found (or not found quickly enough – see next) and this is the type of patient who would either not proceed to transplant at all, or would have had a haploidentical BMT, in the past. Such haploidentical procedures were previously done under restricted circumstances, but now with the ability to harvest large numbers of CD34 positive cells from peripheral blood, the range of diseases and weight of patients that can be transplanted is widening. Many of the diseases that are transplanted are recessive, and it is not unusual that these diseases are associated with ethnic groups that are under-represented on the BM donor registries. With the ability to readily tolerate a one- or two-antigen mismatch, it is possible to find donors for patients who have one of these rare HLA-antigens, as they can be mismatched at this locus.

Finding a donor for an uncommon haplotype

- Patient MC inherited his mother's haplotype HLA A 34 B 65 DR 03 - ranked > 6000th in frequency with the NMDP.
- Over 30 family donors were typed, and none had a suitable type.
- There was no suitable unrelated adult donor
- A cord blood unit was identified that matched the paternal haplotype and also matched DRB1; leaving a 2/6 mismatch at the HLA A 34 B 65.

Lack of Time

One of the main reasons that haploidentical HSCT was applied so early in transplants for diseases such as SCID was the urgency of proceeding to BMT; many groups recommend BMT as soon as possible or within 3 months of diagnosis; for many years this was impossible with an unrelated donor. Cord blood stem cells are cryopreserved and readily available for transplant centers, which is a major advantage if stem cells are needed quickly. As time goes on, more and more cord units can be searched on with known low-resolution A and B types and known high-resolution DRB1 typing. It may be possible to find suitable units almost immediately; currently over 90% of cord units on the registries have Class II molecular typing available, compared to about 60% of BM donors (see Table 7.6). Further samples are immediately available for confirmatory testing. This avoids one of several delays that can occur when assessing a BM donor. These include waiting for the potential donor to be contacted and called back in for further testing, donor evaluation, work up, and harvest and even potential deferral or becoming unavailable to donate. This can be critically important for many progressive neurodegenerative disorders, when the time to transplant affects survival and (mostly neurological) outcome (e.g. Krabbe's disease).

There are several diseases where BMT has been tried and was unsuccessful in the past, and one of the reasons may be the delay due to the long search time for an unrelated BM donor. So although these diseases are listed with BMT not being recommended, for example for Hunter's disease (Type II MPS), now that a CB unit could be available in less than 2 weeks, the potential application of HSCT using CBT in these diseases may have to be re-evaluated.

In some disorders when time is less pressing, it might be possible to wait for a new matched sibling to be born. In the past, this was with a random 1:4 chance, or could be known for diseases where antenatal diagnosis is carried out and HLA typing could confirm the mother was carrying an unaffected fetus, who may also match the affected child. More recently, PGD to select an embryo produced by IVF that was both unaffected by the disease and HLA identical to the patient has been performed. This is of particular relevance to the haemoglobinopathies and other diseases where there is more time available before HSCT is necessary. CB may be collected and used if it is necessary to proceed to transplant before the sibling is old enough to safely donate BM.

Although such an option is attractive, it will not always be possible, because:

1. The family size may be complete and they may not want another child
2. The procedure of IVF and PGD is expensive and may not be available
3. Even where available, the procedure is draining and may not work, or the family may abandon it [7]
4. The collected cord unit may have insufficient cells, but one may then be able to wait for the donor to be old enough to donate safely
5. There are many technical, ethical and legal concerns [12, 13, 14]

The use of such technology to produce a savior sibling is also advantageous in that the donor benefits from being known to be free of the disease affecting their sibling. It is also acceptable in cultures where the concept of antenatal diagnosis followed by therapeutic termination of an affected pregnancy is unacceptable. Although there may be perceived ethical dilemmas facing families in this situation, in practice thinking about having another child to help when these illnesses are diagnosed is usually the second question parents ask [15].

If a donor is needed urgently, there is the alternative option to use one of the parents for a haplo-identical BMT. This has been feasible since 1980, with the combination of a small baby, for example with SCID, and the harvesting of large volumes of BM from a parent that were aggressively T-cell depleted with sheep red-blood cell rosetting or similar techniques; techniques which are inadmissible in the days of vJCD. Such procedures were successful without conditioning the patients, because they were already immunodeficient. However, immune recovery was often limited. Larger patients with diseases characterized by greater immune competence have been successfully transplanted with unmanipulated BM (UBM) [5], or more recently with PBSC harvest and CD34 selection [16].

A haploidentical transplant from a parental donor does carry a potential disadvantage for patients with autosomal recessive metabolic disorders, particularly enzyme deficiencies. Even if the parent is phenotypically healthy, his or her stem cells might not be capable of curing the underlying disorder, e.g. for MPS type I (Hurler), a high activity of enzyme is crucial for neurological outcome [17]. A heterozygous carrier might be unaffected, but still have a reduced activity. CB units can be tested for enzyme activity and, where possible, a unit with a high activity can be chosen [18]. However, the importance of enzyme activity in the graft has not yet been evaluated in comparative studies or extended to other metabolic disorders. This topic is discussed below in the section "Mucopolysaccharidoses." This potential disadvantage, however, might be less important in other non-malignant diseases, e.g. in BM failure (BMF) syndromes.

In patients not immunocompromised by their underlying disease, a haploidentical transplant also carries a significant risk of graft-versus-host disease (GVHD), even if TCD is used [17, 19].

Lack of GVHD

A third advantage of CBT for non-malignant diseases is the lower risk of acute and chronic GVHD [20]. In several studies, CBT has shown to cause less GVHD than BM or PBSC, even in the setting of substantial HLA incompatibility [9, 10].

Unlike patient with leukemia, who might benefit from increased graft-versus-leukemia (GVL) effect with GVHD, GVHD is of no possible benefit in the non-malignant patient group; therefore, CBT might be beneficial. However, because GVHD is of no benefit in such patients, there has been a long history in using T-cell-depleted grafts for such diseases and they carry a lower incidence of GVHD. Rocha et al. compared the rate of acute and chronic GVHD between unrelated transplants using UBM, T-cell-depleted BM (T-BM), and CBT. There was a significantly higher cumulative incidence by day 100 in the UBM group: acute GVHD grade II–IV 56% and grade III–IV 30% as opposed to T-BM (19% and 8%) and CBT (33% and 22%) [21]. This illustrates that the advantages of less GVHD with CBT are particularly true in the setting of unmanipulated grafts, but less prominent if TCD is used. T-cell-depleted grafts, however, are associated with a higher risk of rejection and delayed T-cell reconstitution. Many non-malignant diseases are known to have a higher risk of graft rejection anyway [10], which might be a disadvantage of this donor choice. Delayed T-cell reconstitution is a particular concern in T-immunodeficiencies.

The risk of rejection after a T-cell-depleted graft can mean that if rejection ensues and a second transplant is being undertaken, a CBT may be preferable to a second unrelated procedure but without TCD [22, 23].

It is the general opinion in the CBT community that a higher cell dose is advantageous and usually there is no upper limit to such a dose. However, the patients we are discussing here are often quite young and so light and it is not unusual for these patients to receive very high cell doses, often over 10×10^7 nucleated cells/kg. A recent study showed that lower weight and higher CD3 count were associated with a higher incidence in GVHD, probably due to the early onset engraftment syndrome or erythroderma which is often seen in patients receiving high cell doses of CB (Fig. 7.1) [24].

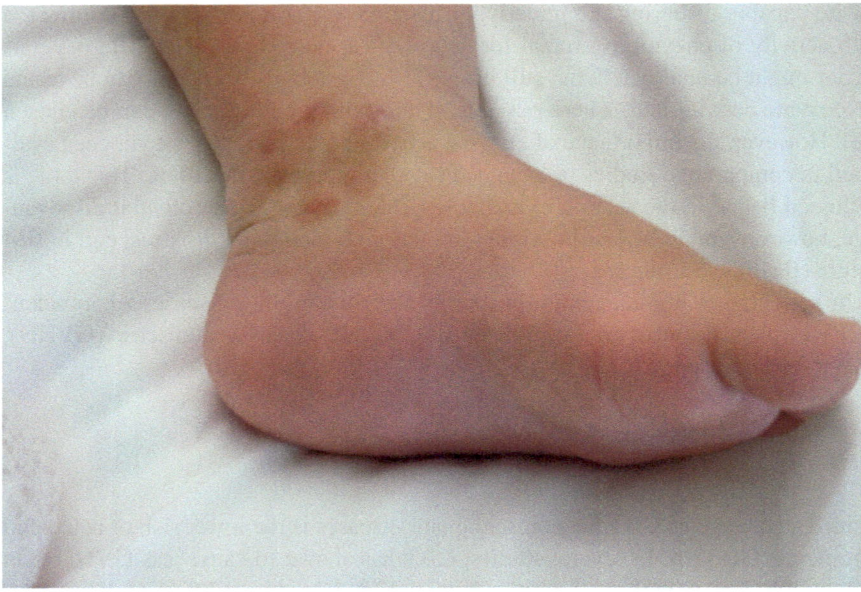

Fig. 7.1 Photograph of biopsy-proved skin GvHD after unrelated cord blood transplant for Wiskott–Aldrich syndrome (cell dose 9×10^7/kg). Skin rash appeared on day +10, when the WBC was 0.2×10/l; and photograph is taken on day +14 after 3 days of steroids, when neutrophil recovery was just starting

Potential Disadvantages of Using Cord Blood

Transmission of Other Diseases

It is true that a CB unit is likely to have a lower risk of carrying cytomegalovirus (CMV), which remains as one of the major infective problems post-BMT. But the risk of the unwitting transmission of a congenital defect with a CBT must be higher than that with an adult BM donor. It is theoretically possible to test a CB unit for specific genetic disorders, but this is time-consuming and routine testing for common diseases at time of collection is not usually performed [25]. In extremely rare diseases, family history as well as follow-up on mother and donor might not reveal a disorder. Even though this risk seems to be extremely low, it is necessary to inform parents about this risk. This is because the families we are discussing here have already been confronted with the diagnosis of an extremely rare disease, so telling them that the chance of acquisition of some other disease is also extremely rare is of little comfort to them. Two recent reports, of a CB recipient subsequently developing donor-derived leukemia or myelodysplastic syndrome with monosomy 7, highlight the potential for acquiring diseases from the donor [26, 27].

Non-Engraftment

One of the known disadvantages of CBT is delayed engraftment [28, 29] and immune reconstitution [30, 31, 32] compared to unrelated UBM grafts.

The Rocha study quoted earlier showed that the probability of neutrophil recovery by day 60 was highest in the UBM group (96%) as compared to 90% in the T-BM and 80% in CBT, with mean days to recovery being 18, 16, and 32 days, respectively. The platelet recovery by day 180 was similar with 85%, 85%, and 90%, but the time to recovery was significantly faster in the UBM and T-BM (mean 29 days for both) than in the CBT group (mean 81 days) [28].

Non-engraftment or graft failure is more common among patients who have not received chemotherapy or experienced alloimmunization with multiple transfusions. Many non-malignant diseases, particularly BMF syndromes and haemoglobinopathies, carry a higher risk of non-engraftment. In CBT, non-malignant disease has been shown to be a risk factor for graft failure [10, 33] and amongst those, BMF syndromes and haemoglobinopathies had the highest risk [33].

A high number of graft failures in non-malignant disease was also reported by Bradley et al. Of the 21 children (seven with non-malignant disorders) given, a reduced intensity conditioning prior to with reduced intensity CBT, six patients experienced primary graft failure with autologous reconstitution, four of them with non-malignant diseases. All the four were successfully re-transplanted with CB. The combination of non-malignant disease, with little prior therapy, CB as a source of stem cells and reduced intensity conditioning will challenge our ability to achieve donor engraftment with minimal toxicity [34].

Graft failure and delayed immune reconstitution account for much of the higher risk of morbidity and mortality from infection, which is a special concern in patients with pre-existing infections, e.g. immunodeficiency syndromes.

Current Issues for Specific Diseases

We describe here various aspects relevant to specific diseases. As well as individual series or case reports, these diseases are often included in larger series of patients. We include reference to these at the end of each section.

Haemoglobinopathies

Thalassemia

Beta thalassemia major is one of the most prevalent haemoglobinopathies throughout the world, resulting from absent or reduced production of β-chains in hemoglobin synthesis leading to ineffective erythropoiesis and severe hemolytic anemia. Patients are transfusion dependent and at risk of transmitted infections, and complications secondary to iron overload. Stem cell transplantation (SCT) is a curative option for these patients and has been shown to have better results if done early, especially before organ damage occur.

However, even if overall results with transplant are acceptable, patients with thalassemia treated in countries with adequate medical resources are not at immediate risk and increasingly effective supportive care can significantly ameliorate both clinical symptoms and prolong life expectancy.

One of the obstacles to SCT in patients with thalassemia is graft rejection secondary to alloimmunization from transfusion dependency and erythroid hyperplasia of the marrow.

The probability of rejection with a standard myeloablative regimen and BM or PBSC transplant in thalassemia is reported as 4–12%, depending on the patient's risk class of risk (Pesaro criteria) prior to SCT [35, 36, 37]. Apart from the risk of graft rejection, transplant-related mortality (TRM) and GVHD are the major complications in these patients, with an 8–15% risk of TRM, even in matched sibling transplants in early stages of disease [35, 38] and a probability of chronic GVHD of 27% [39]. Any HSCT procedure is likely to be a cost-effective option as compared to the high lifetime cost of transfusion and chelation – the estimated lifetime cost of therapy for β-thalassemia major in the United Kingdom was reported in 1999 to exceed 800,000 Great British Pounds [40].

In countries such as Thailand, therapy with hypertransfusion and desferal is expensive and has limited availability. If one does not have adequate medical resources, then the option of taking CB at birth from matched siblings and performing a matched CBT early in the course of disease gives the best chance of success of the transplant and also makes good economic sense. Issaragrisil et al. [41] describe the use of matched sibling CBT, with no GVHD and a high probability of cure in a Lucarelli class I patient. Under these constraints, they recommend that patients should undergo transplant early in the course of the disease to have a high chance of cure [42, 43]. In a small group of patients transplanted with CB from related donors, Miniero et al. report engraftment in six out of 10 patients [44]. Walters et al. showed in a group of 14 patients sustained engraftment in 11 patients; however, some of those received combined CB and BM/PBSC transplants [45].

Locatelli et al. describe a series of 44 patients who underwent related CBT for thalassemia ($n = 33$) and sickle cell disease (SCD; n = 11) [46]. The overall survival (OS) in their study was 100%, with a 79% event-free survival (EFS) for thalassemia and 90% for SCD (difference not significant). Patients with thalassemia had a higher risk of graft failure (7/33 = 21%) than SCD (1/11 = 9%). The probabilities of acute and limited chronic GVHD in engrafted patients were 11% and 6% respectively, confirming the low rate of GVHD in related CBT recipients.

Amongst the thalassemia patients, there was an advantage in EFS depending on the type of preparative regimen used [busulphan (Bu), thiotepa, cyclophosphamide (Cy) or Bu, thiotepa, fludarabine EFS 94% vs. Bu/Cy alone 62%] suggesting an advantage of a third drug added to the preparative regimen. The use of methotrexate (MTX) as part of GVHD prophylaxis was associated with higher treatment failure (EFS in patients receiving MTX was 55% as opposed to 90% in those who did not receive MTX). This has been reported previously in a series of acute leukemia patients undergoing CBT [47]. Whether the cytotoxicity of MTX is detrimental to cell replication with low cells doses is uncertain. However, in a report of Thomson et al. this was not observed [31].

Until recently, unrelated HSCT was considered unacceptable for disease such as thalassemia, because of the increased TRM in a disease that is associated with prolonged survival with supportive therapy.

Krishnamurti et al. analyzed donor availability in patients with haemoglobinopathies. Less than 30% of these patients have a matched sibling donor. Patients with haemoglobinopathies often come from ethnic backgrounds underrepresented in BMT registries, decreasing the chance of finding a suitable matched donor. This report showed that it is possible to find at least a 5/6 HLA-matched CB unit for all patients and a potential 6/6 CB unit for 60% of sickle cell patients and 80% of thalassaemic patients [48].

In several single case reports of unrelated CBT for thalassemia, prompt engraftment was observed [49, 50, 51, 52]. Jaing et al. report successful engraftment and complete donor chimerism in a group of 5 patients after unrelated CBT in Taiwan. All of these patients survived, but experienced grade II–III GVHD, however none of them developed extensive chronic GVHD [51]. Jaing et al. extended their experience to double CBT in five thalassaemics. Although all engrafted, one developed late graft failure with autologous recovery (6/6 match, but lowest cell dose). The four remaining patients showed 100% single donor chimerism and became transfusion independent. Four patients experienced acute GVHD grade I–III. No extensive chronic GVHD was observed, but all four patients had limited chronic GVHD involving the skin. One patient later developed Evans syndrome and died of hemorrhage [53]. Whether double CBT will be associated with a higher rate of GvHD than single cord is of particular importance for non-malignant indications for BMT, where GVHD is of no protective benefit.

Except for the report by Hall et al. all of the cases are from countries where access to supportive therapy is limited and costly. Considering the risk of TRM and morbidity with unrelated SCT, the indication should be questioned in countries with adequate supportive therapy.

Thalassemia is a classic example where one might consider “waiting” for a matched sibling to be born. The techniques of IVF and PGD may in some cases lead the parents to the choice of initiating a pregnancy with the near certainty that the baby will be free of thalassemia, that compatible stem cells can be collected at birth, may be sufficient for CBT, or will have an HLA-identical donor available for later BMT.

Other cases of CBT for thalassemia are included in Rocha 1998 [54], Wagner 1995 [10], Styczynski 2004 [55], Rocha 2000 [56], and Gluckman 1997 [33].

Sickle Cell Disease

SCD is an inherited blood disorder with an abnormal type of hemoglobin (HbS) that results in sickle cell-shaped red blood cells causing obstructions of vessels with end organ damage causing substantial morbidity and mortality. Patients need frequent red cell transfusions to maintain HbS levels low to prevent recurrent cerebrovascular complications, hence leading to secondary complications of iron overload and alloimmunization against red cell antigens or HLA antigens. It has been known that SCD is curable by HSCT for many years, depending on severity of pre-existing symptoms the TRM is reported as 6–10% [57, 58] and chronic GVHD occurring in about 12% [59]. Previous publications with BM or PBSC from matched siblings demonstrated an OS of 90% and an EFS of 80% with rejection (8–15%) being the major cause of treatment failure [60, 61].

In the previously mentioned study of Locatelli, the EFS for SCD patients after related umbilical CBT was 90% [46] with a lower rate of graft failure than in the thalassaemic patient group, low probability of acute or chronic GVHD, and an OS of 100%.

Adamkiewicz et al. present three children with SCD and cerebrovascular accidents undergoing unrelated 4/6 mismatched CBT [62]. One patient had graft failure, two patients engrafted. All patients developed moderate to severe acute GVHD with one patient experiencing extensive chronic GVHD.

Other cases of CBT for SCD are included in Rocha 1998 [54], Wagner 1995 [10], Rocha 2000 [56] and Gluckman 1997 [33].

For both thalassemia and SCD, persistent mixed chimerism or partial engraftment has been previously reported, and unlike in aplastic anemia [63], was not always associated with graft failure. Even with a low percentage of donor cells, the amount of mature red blood cells might be sufficient enough for the patient to become clinically asymptomatic and thus transfusion independent [58, 64].

Given that we are dealing with diseases which are non-malignant, and that the aim is merely to correct the underlying problem, and the observation that mixed chimerism can correct the disease phenotype, it is logical to attempt to use non-myeloablative conditioning in such diseases; the original cohort of patients reported by Slavin's group included thalassemia, Gaucher's disease, Blackfan-Diamond anemia, and FA [65]. However, the observation that in some cases, stable mixed chimerism can correct the disease is not easy to achieve intentionally, and such attempts have not led to sustained engraftment even with BM or PBSC from matched siblings once immunosuppression is withdrawn [66].

Bone Marrow Failure (BMF) Syndromes

BMF syndromes in children comprise several entities that can be hereditary or acquired. For many of these diseases, HSCT is a curative treatment option, and the source of stem cells is not critical. The final decision of what source of stem cells to use may depend more on timing and donor availability rather than whether this is a matched or mismatched family donor, or unrelated marrow or CB. We have listed many of the diseases where CBT has been performed in Table 7.2 and restricted our comments to the more common disorders or where there are particular advantages (or disadvantages) related to the use of CB as a stem cell source.

Table 7.2 Application of cord blood transplant in various disease characterized by bone marrow failure (BMF)

Disorder	Natural history and alternative therapy	Use of cord blood for transplant
Amegakaryocytic thrombocytopenia	Bleeding complications, development of aplastic anemia and leukemia	MacMillan 1998 [86]; Rocha 2000 [56]
Aplastic anemia	Complications secondary to pancytopenia, risk of malignant transformation; Immunosuppressive therapy	Gluckman 1997 [33]; Rocha 2000 [56]; Rocha 1998 [54]; Wagner 1995 [10]; Rubinstein 1998 [85]; Styczynski 2004 [55]; Ohga 2006 [87]
Diamond-Blackfan anemia	Steroid therapy. Cyclosporin; Refractory patients become transfusion dependent and are at risk of iron overload; Increased risk of aplastic anemia, leukaemia and other cancers	Dianzani, 2000 [88]; Gluckman 1997 [33]; Wagner 1995 [10]; Rubinstein 1998 [85]; Wagner 1996 [20]; Wagner 2002 [84]; Bonno 1997 [89]; Rocha 2000 [56]
Dyskeratosis congenita	Death in second decade of complications from BMF, infections, pulmonary complications and malignancy; Growth factors, steroids and antibiotics	Nobili 2002 [90]; Gluckman 1997 [33]; Rocha 1998 [54]
Osteopetrosis	Complications from BMF; Infantile form leading to early death in first 10 years; Vitamin D, growth factors, interferon; Steroid therapy controversial; Surgical care	Wagner 1995 [10]; Wagner 1996 [20]; Gluckman 1997 [33]; Rubinstein 1998 [85]; Wagner 2002 [84]; Rocha 1998 [54]; Rocha 2000 [56]
Paroxysmal nocturnal hemoglobinuria	Survival about 10 years, hemolysis, BMF, risk of thrombosis (often cause of death); Supportive therapy, anticoagulation, studies with anti-complement agents; ATG for aplastic anemia	Shaw 1999 [67]
Severe congenital neutropenia	Early death due to neutropenia and infections, risk of transformation to myelodysplastic syndrome and leukaemia; Majority of patients responding to G-CSF therapy with significant improved survival rate unless developing MDS/leukaemia	Mino 2004 [91]; Nakazawa 2004 [92]; Kurtzberg 1996 [9]; Rocha 2000 [56]
Shwachman Diamond syndrome	Recurrent infections, development of aplastic anemia, complications due to pancytopenia; Long-term survival variable, shortened if aplastic anemia; Death from infection or malignant transformation; Supportive therapy, growth factors, pancreatic enzymes	Vibhakar 2005 [93]

Shaw et al. report a cohort of 13 patients with BMF syndromes, three of them transplanted with unrelated CB and 10 with sibling BM. They observed a faster engraftment, less GVHD and a lower overall mortality rate with BM, the mortality rate by day 100 being 20% in the matched sibling patients, and 66% in the CB group (overall mortality rates being 40% and 66%, respectively) [67].

Fanconi Anemia (FA)

More patients have undergone unrelated CBT for FA than any other condition. This rare autosomal recessive disease is characterized by congenital abnormalities, chromosomal fragility, and cancer susceptibility and is the archetypal BMF syndrome. Early mortality is often associated with complications of BMF or secondary malignancies, AML being the most frequent. Currently, HSCT can restore normal hematopoiesis, but has been associated with a high treatment-related morbidity and mortality secondary to graft rejection or GVHD, as a result of severe tissue damage and absence of sufficient repair mechanisms. Other risk factors identified as carrying a higher chance of success were [62, 68, 69]:

- Matched sibling BMT
- Younger age
- Higher pre-transplant platelet counts
- Absence of previous treatment with androgens
- Normal liver functions tests

Transplants performed after a long period of aplasia, especially after leukemic transformation, carry poor results.

It should be obvious that all of these risk factors can be minimized if HSCT is performed earlier in the course of disease and now, with the availability of IVF and PGD, even the presence of a matched sibling is a factor which can be manipulated in some cases. FA is the disease where PGD to select an embryo produced by IVF that was both unaffected by FA and HLA identical to the patient was first performed [7]. Subsequent cases have been reported for different conditions [8, 70, 71].

Satisfactory results with an OS of around 60–75% depending on age, risk factors, and conditioning regimens have been achieved transplanting FA patients from matched sibling donors [68, 72, 73]; however, the results are less promising when alternative donors were used, successful outcome being reported in the range of around 30–45% [68, 69, 73, 74, 75]. Avoiding radiotherapy in these susceptible patient group and replacing it with fludarabine showed good OS results of around 70–80% also in unrelated BMT [75, 76].

The Eurocord experience summarized CBT in 44 children (seven matched siblings, 37 unrelated) for FA with a survival of 36% 2 years after transplant [77]. These results are similar to those reported by Guardiola [69] where SCT was performed from BM donors [78, 79].

The Minnesota group has considerable experience in FA and use of CBT. They have shown that fludarabine is an important factor in achieving engraftment in this difficult disease, and the hope and expectation is that this will translate into long-term improvements in EFS, with early results in matched family donors being encouraging (including three sibling cords) [80]. Fludarabine-containing conditioning regimens have been reported by others to show early survival with limited toxicity and mild GVHD in the presence of full engraftment, but only with small numbers to date [23, 81, 82, 83].

It may well be that the improvement in results with CBT in thalassemia and SCD also related to the use of fludarabine and this may become an important part of the HSCT conditioning.

Other cases of CBT for FA are included in Rocha 1998 [54], Wagner 1995 [10], Wagner 2002 [84], Kurtzberg 1996 [9], Wagner 1996 [20], Styczynski 2004 [55], Gluckman 1997 [33], and Rubinstein 1998 [85].

Primary Immuno deficiencies

Congenital immune deficiency syndromes are a rare but important cause of morbidity and mortality in early childhood. In severe cases, HSCT is the treatment of choice. The SCID are a group of various genetic disorders with impairment of T-cell differentiation with or without B-cell disorder. Most prevalent are X-linked SCID and ADA-deficiency with a frequency of 50–60% and 20%, respectively. Reticular dysgenesis, T-B-SCID, T-B+-SCID other than X-linked SCID are rare disorders [94]. Because SCID invariably leads to an early death due to infections, usually within the first year, the treatment of choice has been an urgent allogeneic HSCT for more than 30 years [2, 79]. The non-SCID immune deficiencies also have a poor long-term outlook and this is why this group of diseases have been at the forefront of clinical BMT, as mentioned in the introduction. The established standard transplant type for children with SCID is either HLA-identical or T-cell-depleted haploidentical marrow, usually from a parental donor. The OS rate for all SCID patients with SCT is around 78% [78] varying with type of transplant, age, need for a preparative regimen, and underlying infections. A recent study of Myers et al. showed that transplant results are much better (survival rate 95%) when carried out shortly after birth [95].

Related donor transplant leads to good outcomes, especially as GVHD is rare and preparative regimens often not necessary. Survival rates with matched related donors can be as high as 80–90% [78, 96]. About 77% of haploidentical graft recipients survive [78], whereas the survival in matched unrelated donor transplant is around 50–70% [97].

The main factors contributing to transplant-related morbidity and TRM are opportunistic infections and malnutrition. These problems can be especially troublesome if the patient is infected before the transplant; hence rapid recovery of both myeloid and lymphoid function is important [98].

Time until immune reconstitution is crucial in these frequently infected patients already lacking sufficient immune function for weeks or months prior to transplant. In the unmanipulated graft containing mature T cells, T-cell engraftment can be observed as early as 2 weeks, whereas in T-cell-depleted grafts normal T-cell function is observed only after 3–4 months [78, 79, 99]. Many patients lacking HLA-identical donors are treated successfully with haplo-identical stem cells. Although a TCD haploidentical BMT has been successful at reconstituting the T-cell immune system [4], there are problems associated with this source of stem cells. The lack of conditioning and HLA mismatch is associated with a long period of time for T-cell engraftment to occur, failure of B-cell engraftment and function (split chimerism, patients still requiring long-term immunoglobulin replacement [78]) as well as increased resistance to engraftment, in particular with the non-SCID immune deficiencies.

In these diseases, CB is a potentially excellent source of stem cells, as the benefits include reliable recovery of immune function when a high cell dose is infused, a low risk of GVHD, and low viral transmission rate. This is in part because it is often possible to source a cord unit for these small patients who firstly has an excellent cell dose and secondly is available quickly. Disadvantages include lack of viral-specific cytotoxic T-cells and slower engraftment when small stem cell doses per body weight used. There is no potential for a booster transplant from the same donor, but boosters with a second CB unit have been described [100]. However, the slow immune reconstitution remains a potential risk, which is definitely slower than in UBM [97], but similar or even faster than in TCD marrow [100, 101].

SCT performed from different stem cell sources performed in a group of 89 SCID patients was described by Buckley et al. [78], with 12 HLA identical related and 77 TCD haploidentical donors. Amongst the haplo-identical patients, 20 patients required booster transplants to overcome poor B and T-cell function. In three cases, the boost was with unrelated CB. In the children receiving a CBT as boost, T-cells were detectable shortly after transplant, but their function remained suppressed, mainly due to anti-GVHD therapy. Two of these patients survived.

Bhattacharya et al. describe unrelated CBT in 14 patients, eight with SCID and six with other immunodeficiencies; 12 received unrelated and 2 received sibling CBT at a median age of 3.5 months [100]. The two patients with sibling CBT underwent transplant without conditioning, all others received preparative regimens. After receiving a median cell dose of 8×10^7/kg, all patients engrafted, with a median of 22 days to neutrophil and 51 days to platelet engraftment. Median time to T-cell engraftment was 61 days, ranging from 10 to 222 days. Eleven of 12 surviving patients developed full donor T-cell chimerism, but only six had full donor B-cell chimerism. All 12 surviving patients achieved sufficient T-cell immune reconstitution, even the patient with mixed T-cell chimerism, but five are still receiving immunoglobulin replacement. One patient had grade II–IV GVHD, one grade II. Both received matched grafts (10/10 and 6/6, respectively), but the patient with severe GVHD had significant materno-fetal engraftment. Despite significant HLA mismatches in the other patients, they did not get GVHD. The combination of GVHD and pre-existing infections contributed to a poorer outcome. Two patients died of multi-organ failure related to infectious complications, one experiencing infection and severe GVHD, one died early prior to engraftment. This report compares favorably with similar studies with TCD haploidentical BM from the same group [102] with an OS of 63% and an engraftment 49%.

Knutsen et al. report their 2-year experience with CBT in severe T-cell immunodeficiency in eight cases with SCID, reticular dysgenesis, combined immunodeficiency, and WAS [103]. Seven of eight patients survived, six of them being well. One patient with reticular dysgenesis failed to engraft, but did so after a second CBT. All patients had hematopoietic full donor chimerism with neutrophil engraftment between 11 and 16 days. T-cell development was observed relatively early, between day 60 and 100 resulting in stable long-term T-cell engraftment with normal lymphoproliferative responses. In this series, engraftment of B cell was observed early, in contrast to previous experience in TCD grafts, where half of the patients retained host B-cells. All the patients in this series received conditioning. All patients developed acute GVHD, but the majority (seven patients) develop only grade I in the presence of GVHD prophylaxis with cyclosporine and corticosteroids. One patient with combined immunodeficiency, who received a two-antigen mismatch graft (serological HLA-DR mismatch), developed acute GVHD grade IV, and eventually died of infection after responding to second line therapy.

Tsuji et al. published their experience in HSCT for 30 patients with primary immunodeficiency diseases over the past 30 years; the survival rate being better in patients transplanted since 1996. The group included seven patients receiving unrelated CBT [104]. Of these seven, six showed neutrophil engraftment between days 9 and 23. Twenty-seven of the 30 patients had pre-existing infections. Amongst CBT recipients, five had SCID and three had WAS. All cases received preparative regimens and GVHD prophylaxis. TCD haploidentical donor stem cells were used for nine transplants in eight patients, matched related BM in eight and matched unrelated BM in seven patients. Primary graft failure occurred in two of nine TCD haploidentical transplant patients, seven engrafted, one after a second procedure (78%). All but one of the engrafted patients had mixed chimerism and poor T-cell function. All patients whose T-cell number did not reach 1×10^9/l within 6 months of transplant died within 5 years.

In patients whose grafts were not TCD, sustained engraftment was achieved in 21 of 22 patients (95%), with most of them being fully donor on chimerism. OS in the patients receiving T-cell replete grafts was 80.4% at 5 years.

Thirty-three percent of the evaluable patients had grade II–IV GVHD with three patients dying. The incidence of chronic GVHD was six out of 24 evaluable patients (25%), five of them being extensive, but resolved in all but one. Amongst the CBT recipients two had acute GVHD, one being grade II, one grade IV. The patient (WAS, 1 locus mismatch) with GVHD grade IV died on day 216 of thrombotic microangiopathy in the context of extensive chronic GVHD. Two developed extensive GVHD. Of the CBT recipients, one other patient with SCID died of veno-occlusive disease on day 5. All others are alive.

Ziegner et al. performed unrelated 5/6 matched CBT in three patients with X-linked immunodeficiencies: X-linked lymphoproliferative syndrome and X-linked Hyper-IgM. All patients had grade I GVHD, survived and showed normal numbers and function of T and B cells 3 years after transplant [105].

Goebel et al. describe a serial transplantation in two brothers with SCID. The first brother received a 4/6 unrelated CBT leading to severe acute GVHD, limited chronic GVHD, and complete donor chimerism. His brother received UBM from the first with no GVHD but mixed chimerism [106].

Fagioli et al. describe two children with different type of SCID undergoing successful unrelated CBT after conditioning with Bu/Cy and anti-thymocyte globulin (ATG). Both patients developed GVHD, grade I in one and grade III in the other with no chronic GVHD. Both are alive, one with full engraftment, the other with mixed chimerism [107].

Other cases of CBT for SCID are reported in Wagner 1995 [10], Rocha 2000 [56], Gluckman 1997 [33], and Rubinstein 1998 [85].

Wiskott–Aldrich-Syndrome (WAS)

WAS is a X-chromosomal recessive genetic disorder characterized by cellular and humoral immunodeficiency, thrombocytopenia, platelet abnormalities, and eczema. It is associated with an increased risk of autoimmune diseases and hematologic malignancy.

Although the median survival has improved over the past decades, WAS is still associated with a significant morbidity and mortality rate. Infections and bleeding are the major causes of death, but a significant number of patients also developed malignancies, primarily lymphoreticular tumors, and leukemia. If HSCT is successful, hematological and immunological defects are corrected and eczema resolves. The 5-year probability of survival is reported as around 70% with best result for matched sibling marrow transplants (87%), 71% for matched unrelated donors and only 52% with other related donors. Age is a major risk factor, with much better outcomes reported for unrelated HSCT if the patient is less than 5 years of age at the time of transplant with the results of a matched unrelated transplant approaching those of a matched sibling in this age group [108]. TCD haploidentical transplants also have been successfully performed [109].

When a matched sibling donor is unavailable, CBT has been used as an alternative source. WAS is less immediately life-threatening as compared to other immunodeficiencies. This means HSCT can usually be done as a semi-elective procedure in stable patients. Like FA, in this scenario, CBT from a planned matched sibling might be an option.

Knutsen et al. report three children with WAS transplanted with umbilical CB (4/6 in two, 5/6 in one patient). Acute GVHD grade I–II occurred in two of these children; none had chronic GVHD. Immunological reconstitution was demonstrated in all patients resulting in T-, B-, and NK-cell development as well as functional B-cell antibody response in two patients [110].

Kaneko et al. report a 14-month-old boy with WAS and recurrent CMV pneumonia, who underwent successful unrelated CBT. The patient showed sufficient engraftment even in the presence of long-term ganciclovir therapy [111].

Other cases of CBT for WAS are included in Wagner 1995 [10], Thomson 2000 [31], Styczynski 2004 [55], Rocha 2000 [56], and Rubinstein, 1998 [85] (Table 7.3).

Table 7.3 Application of cord blood transplant in various other primary immunodeficiencies

Disorder	Natural History and alternative therapy	Role of CBT
ADA	SCID group: supportive therapy, anti-infective medication; Enzyme replacement; Gene therapy	Bhattacharya 2005 [100]
Bare lymphocyte syndrome	SCID-like	Rocha 2000 [56]; Gluckman 1997 [33]
Chediak-Higashi syndrome	Death secondary to infection and hemorrhage in first decade.	Rocha 2000 [56]
Chronic granulomatous disease	Variable. Early death; Supportive therapy; Studies with INF-y	Bhattacharya 2003 [112]; Rocha 2000 [56]
Combined immunodeficiency (CID)	Infections	Broom 2006 [113]; Slatter 2006 [114]; Knutsen 2000 [103]
Common variable immunodeficiency (CVID)	Infections	Kurtzberg 1996 [9]
Leukocyte adhesion deficiency	Early death due to infection in infancy	Rocha 2000 [56]; Gluckman 1997 [33]
Di-George Syndrome CHARGE association	Infections 2nd cause of mortality after cardiac deaths; Thymic transplant; Supportive therapy; BMT: controversial, selected cases only	Ohtsuka 2004 [115]; Bhattacharya 2005 [100]
IPEX	Immune dysregulation, endocrinopathy and enteropathy	Bhattacharya 2005 [100]
MCH II deficiency	SCID-like	Bhattacharya 2005 [100]
Omenn syndrome	SCID group	Bhattacharya 2005 [100]
Purine-nucleoside phosphorylase deficiency	SCID group, delayed onset	Myers 2004 [116]
Reticular dysgenesis	SCID group, plus myeloid lineage affected	Bhattacharya 2005 [100]; Knutsen 2000 [103]; Rocha 2000 [56]
Thymic dysplasia (Nezelof syndrome)		Knutsen 2000 [103]
X-linked agamma-globulinaemia	Immunoglobulin replacement. Life expectancy up to four decades	Howard 2003 [118]
X-linked hyper-IgM syndrome	Chronic liver disease 3rd decade, intermittent neutropenia. Immunoglobuline replacement, G-CSF	Ziegner 2001 [105]
X-linked lympho-proliferative disease	Fatal EBV infections, half develop liver failure, lymphoma development. Immunosuppression, chemotherapy	Vowels 1993 [119]; Ziegner 2001 [105]; Wagner 1995 [10]; Rocha 2000 [56]
X-linked anhidrotic ectodermal dysplasia with immunodeficiency	Recurrent severe infections and dysmorphia. Hypogammaglobulinaemia, low NK-cells. Immunoglobuline replacement	Tono 2007 [117]

Inherited Metabolic Diseases – General

Inborn metabolic diseases are a complex heterogenous group of rare inherited diseases. For some of these diseases, some of their symptoms can be ameliorated with HSCT. These disorders show enzyme deficiencies resulting in accumulation of toxic metabolites in various tissues. There are only limited alternative options for the management of these conditions, many characterized by severe progressive neurological deterioration and eventually death in the first or second decade of life. Allogeneic SCT can prevent progression of some deficiencies, but has considerable risks of morbidity and mortality from infection, organ toxicity, and GVHD. Donor stem cells are capable of delivering sufficient enzyme inside and outside the blood compartment. This can arrest or slow the progression of the disease, improving OS and quality of life. Unfortunately many children who might benefit from transplantation lack an appropriately matched donor or are diagnosed at an advanced stage of disease. In most progressive diseases, HSCT can only provide maximal benefit if performed early in life. In many cases, HSCT is only reasonable if done when only mild symptoms are present or even before clinical symptoms occur. Even if HSCT is successful, the underlying enzyme deficiency is only corrected after several months, so the disease may progress for some time after transplant. The decision when and whether to proceed to transplant depends on the natural history of the underlying disorder.

Enzymes penetrate the blood–brain barrier poorly. If the central nervous system (CNS) is involved, the success is thought to be dependent on donor monocyte/macrophage cells carrying enzyme and replacement of microglial cells by cells of donor origin. Since this process is very slow, there is a delay between transplant and possible disease stabilization [120], which might be acceptable in a slowly progressive disease (e.g. ALD), but does not improve the outcome for rapid progressive diseases (e.g. Krabbe's disease).

SCT has been performed in more than 20 rare metabolic disorders [121], but many are reported as single cases only so far. In most of these diseases, CBT has also been used as a source of stem cells, at least in more recent cases. Since several of these metabolic disorders are slowly progressive, it is important to evaluate the long-term outcome of HSCT. Experience regarding long-term outcome is limited and general transplant recommendations cannot be given. As a general principle, performing BMT earlier produces better outcomes. For Hurler's syndrome, X-linked ALD and osteopetrosis, HSCT has been performed for several years and detailed studies are available with promising results given the natural history of the disease. SCT is therefore generally recommended. Most other inherited metabolic diseases lack larger studies and long-term follow-up, and in some disorders SCT is contraindicated. Peters et al. summarize the indications for SCT as recommended by the Inborn Errors Group of the European Group For Blood and Marrow Transplantation (EBMT) [122]. Although SCT is considered to be contraindicated in some disorders, use of CBT in more recent publications, for example MPS type II [24], underlines the need to re-evaluate the indications in this rapidly changing field.

Probably because patients with metabolic diseases have a normal, intact immune, and hematopoietic system, primary graft failure and late rejection is quite common in this group (see section on MPS I next).

Immature CB stem cells have shown to cause less frequent and less GVHD than BM-derived stem cells. Unlike malignancies, GVHD has no beneficial effect, so CBT can be a good alternative source of stem cells, especially when no matched sibling is available. Similarly, this might be achieved with a heavily T-cell-depleted BM or PBSC graft if a matched unrelated donor is available.

There is the theoretical advantage of cord blood stem cells differentiating into non-hematological cells, but this needs to be proved in the future [1].

The biggest group of metabolic disorders where HSCT has been performed are the lysosomal storage diseases, in particular the MPS and leukodystrophies. In MPS, glycosaminoglycans accumulate resulting in organ damage mainly in brain, heart, liver, cornea, and bones/cartilage. Leukodystrophies (sphingolipidoses) show demyelination in the central and peripheral nervous system caused by accumulation of sphingolipids.

The largest series of CBT for such metabolic diseases comes from the Cord Blood Transplantation Study (COBLT) group and was recently published [24]. They report 69 children with lysosomal and peroxisomal storage diseases (MPS types I to III, mucolipidosis type II, ALD, metachromatic leukodystrophy, globoid cell leukodystrophy, and Tay-Sachs disease). The conditioning regimen for all patients consisted of Bu/Cy and ATG.

OS at 6 months was 80% and 72% at 1 year, with long-term survival of 68% with a median follow-up of 24.5 months (range: 1.9–58.5 months). In this study group, the total amount of infused nucleated cells was higher (median cell dose 8.7×10^7/kg) than most CBT series. Together with an overall small sized patient, this resulted in a high rate of engraftment (probability of engraftment was 78% by day 42 and 84% by day 100).

However, a lower weight and higher CD3 count was also associated with GVHD, but the cumulative incidence of grade III and IV acute GVHD was 9%, as compared to a II–IV rate of 36%, probably due to the early onset engraftment syndrome or erythroderma which is often seen in these patients receiving high cell doses of CB. Given that chronic GVHD is of no benefit to these patients either, the number developing chronic GVHD will need to be monitored, currently reported at 11 with limited and two with extensive chronic GVHD.

Of concern was that severe CNS toxicity was reported in 10%, and these patients are often being transplanted for diseases where the main purpose is to avoid CNS toxicity. The long-term outcome on neuro-cognitive function was, however, not addressed in this study.

In comparison to a parallel COBLT study for patients with leukaemia [123], the metabolic disease group had faster neutrophil recovery, more acute GVHD on day 100 and more chronic GVHD.

The rate of non-engraftment in the non-malignant group was low, with primary graft failure in three patients (4%) with no secondary graft failure. Thus, the high rate of non-engraftment frequently seen in children not exposed to previous chemotherapy was not observed in this study, results were similar to leukemic patients receiving Bu, melphalan, and ATG as a preparative regimen.

In this group, the degree of HLA mismatch did not influence engraftment, GVHD or OS, whereas in the leukaemia group a better match was associated with better

OS [120]. This may reflect these patients having had no prior therapy, and so being better able to tolerate complications related to the HLA-mismatch.

Mucopolysaccharidoses

According to current recommendations for SCT in metabolic storage diseases, SCT is not recommended in MPS type II, III, and IV and its role for Hurler/Scheie and Scheie syndrome is less clear [122], but some authors recently reported transplants mainly from CB in these conditions (see Table 7.4).

Hurler's Syndrome

Hurler's syndrome is the most severe for of MPS type I, an autosomal recessive metabolic storage disease caused by α-L-iduronidase deficiency, resulting in accumulation of glycosaminoglycans in various organs. Patients present with severe, progressive neurological deterioration, cardiomyopathy, skeletal abnormalities, corneal clouding, hepatomegaly, and finally death in childhood.

Allogeneic SCT before the age of 2 years has proved to prevent further disease progression. Most experience and long-term follow-up exists for patients trans-

Table 7.4 Application of cord blood transplant in various inborn metabolic disorders

Disorder	Natural history and alternative therapy	Role of CBT
MPS II, Hunter		Martin 2006 [24]; Wagner 1995 [10]; Rocha 2000 [56]
MPS III, Sanfillipo		Martin 2006 [24]; Rocha 2000 [56]
MPS IV Morquio		Rocha 2000 [56]
MPS VI, Maroteaux-Lamy	Usually fatal by early adulthood, most deaths secondary to cardiopulmonary complications; Normal neurological development	Lee 2000 [135]; Rocha 2000 [56]
Batten disease (NCL)	Severe progressive neurological deterioration and death in first decade; SCT tried in few cases; Potential gene therapy	Gluckman 1997 [33]
Metachromatic leukodystrophy	Potential gene therapy	Martin 2006 [24]; Rocha 2000 [56]
I-cell disease	Limited therapy	Martin 2006 [24]
Niemann-Pick disease	Early death in infancy type A, pulmonary complications in type B, others variable	Rocha 2000 [56]
Gaucher's disease	Enzyme replacement, but not a life-long cure	Rocha 2000 [56]
Tay Sachs	Fatal	Martin 2006 [24]
Lesch-Nyhan syndrome		Kurtzberg 1996 [9]

planted for Hurler's syndrome. Since 1980, more than 200 patients with Hurler's syndrome have undergone allogeneic SCT, mostly from BM donors [124, 125, 126]. Since more than half the children lack a suitable marrow donor and time from diagnosis to transplant is crucial, an alternative source of stem cells is needed to perform transplant in a timely fashion. There is general consensus in the metabolic community that the diagnosis of MPS I should lead to an early HSCT. Delays will allow further neurological progression to occur and so CBT is potentially a good, fast option. This is supported by the fact that MPS I is the third commonest indication for unrelated CBT reported to the CIBMTR, after FA and SCID (see Table 7.1).

Staba et al. report 20 children with MPS-1, also conditioned with Bu/Cy/ATG [18]. One advantage of CB is shown in that the median age at transplant in this series was 16 months, as opposed to previous studies using BM: Peters et al. report two groups of patients undergoing BMT for MPS I, the first 54 with a median age of 1.8 years at time of related (matched sibling and haplo-identical related) transplant [17] and a second group with 40 children undergoing unrelated SCT at a median age of 1.7 years [124]. This age difference is crucial in a disease where outcome is related to the age of transplantation, especially when the cut off for successful SCT is considered around 2 years of age. In the Peters papers, for the matched siblings, 85% engrafted, with complete donor chimerism in 58% and 27% mixed chimerism. The rate of acute GVHD II-IV by day 100 was 32%. In the haploidentical subgroup, only 65% engrafted (62% full donor, 3% mixed chimerism) and 55% developed acute GVHD II–IV by day 100. In the unrelated group, they observed a survival rate of 50% (20 patients), with a probability of acute GVHD grade II–IV of 30%, and 18% for extensive chronic GVHD [124]. Out of these, only 13 have complete donor chimerism, two have mixed chimerism, and five have autologous recovery.

The OS of the whole group was 54%; with a 5-year survival of 75% for matched siblings and 53% for haploidentical recipients. This paper also reports that GVHD was adversely associated with neurological outcome. However, since the patient group receiving a haplo-identical transplant had a higher incidence of GVHD as well as a potential of receiving a graft from a potentially heterozygous carrier with lower enzyme activity, the impact of GVHD on neurological outcome remains unclear.

In the Staba series, potential CB units were tested for leukocyte α-L-iduronidase activity and those with high-normal activity were selected. The EFS was 85%, with 17 of the 20 children alive with complete donor chimerism and normal enzyme activity.

Boelens et al. analyzed the outcome of HSCT in 146 patients with Hurler's syndrome with a focus on risk factor analysis for graft failure. There was a higher risk for graft failure when TCD grafts or reduced intensity conditioning was used. Although the chance of being alive with engraftment did not vary by cell source, CBT resulted in full-donor chimerism and all recipients had normal enzyme levels [127]. Considering that the success of SCT in Hurler's syndrome depends on the enzyme level provided by the graft, the amount of donor chimerism achieved is crucial. CB could become the preferred stem cell source for metabolic conditions requiring normal enzyme levels. This is supported by Church et al. who studied activity of donor enzyme 1 year after the SCT in 39 patients with Hurler's syndrome. No mixed chimerism was seen in CBT recipients. Patients with full donor chimerism had lower enzyme levels post-transplant when transplanted from a heterozygous carrier as compared to an unaffected donor ($p < 0.0001$) [128]. The long-term clinical outcome related to enzyme activity needs to be assessed in the future, but these two studies may influence a clinician toward unrelated CB as opposed to a heterozygous family member if there is no unaffected matched sibling available.

Other cases of CBT for Hurler's syndrome are included in Wagner 1995 [10], Rocha 2000 [56], Gluckman 1997 [33], and Rubinstein 1998 [85].

Globoid-Cell Leukodystrophy (Krabbe's Disease)

Globoid-cell leukodystrophy is an autosomal recessive disorder, caused by deficiency of lysosomal galactocerebrosidase, leading to accumulation of galactolipids. This results in inflammation and demyelination of the developing brain resulting in rapid progressive neurological deterioration and death. Depending on the clinical phenotype infantile, late infantile, juvenile, and adult forms exist. Like other leukodystrophies, HSCT can improve neurological outcome as well as OS in the juvenile form of the disease when performed early in the course of the disease. However, in the infantile form, symptoms appear before the age of 6 months and death usually occurs before 2 years of age. Previous HSCT have been performed after clinical symptoms occurred and have not been successful.

Patients with Krabbe's disease face two major obstacles, lack of a suitable donor and time. With CBT, the chance of finding a suitable donor is very high and can significantly shorten time to transplant. But even if a donor is readily available, by the time the diagnosis is established by clinical symptoms, it is too late for successful transplant.

A recent study of Escolar et al. compares the outcome of unrelated CBT in children with infantile Krabbe's disease transplanted at the time of clinical diagnosis with those transplanted in the neonatal period. In the latter group, the diagnosis was made pre-natally or at time of birth in an asymptomatic child because of family history [129]. A major finding was that use of HSCT from unrelated CB donors in asymptomatic newborns favorably altered the natural history of the disease, whereas infants transplanted after symptoms occurred hardly showed any neurological improvement. This study shows that unrelated CBT performed in the neonatal period results in substantially improved neurological and overall outcome when compared with no therapy or SCT performed after the symptoms development.

Under these circumstances, it is almost impossible to recruit a suitable BM donor in the time frame required, so CB enables patients to undergo SCT as soon as possible. Diagnosis was made in the newborn group pre-natally or shortly after birth, and their age range at time of transplant was 12–44 days (median 28 days). In the group of symptomatic infants diagnosis was made between 4 and 9 months of age with transplant performed at age range 142–352 days. The conditioning regimen consisted again of Bu/Cy with or without ATG. In the newborn group, 100% survived, with engraftment. One patient who did not receive ATG survived with mixed chimerism and presents with normal enzyme level. Similarly, all of the infants survived the early transplant period, but the subsequent survival rate was only 43% because of disease progression.

Both groups showed rapid engraftment, related to the high dose of nucleated cells per kg. This is faster than that reported previously in older, heavier patients [85].

There was a marked difference in neurological outcome between the two groups. Whereas the infant group hardly experienced any benefit from SCT, the neonates showed significant development with only some degree of gross motor function impairment.

However, since this a very recently performed study, the long-term outcome of these patients can only be determined with further follow-up. A staging system to predict outcome after unrelated CBT for infantile Krabbe's disease was recently published [130].

This promising early outcome in what was previously a uniformly fatal disease raises issues about the appropriateness of neonatal screening for a wider range of such metabolic disorders. It also means that previous attempts for other diseases with early onset that have been tried and failed may have to be revisited, ideally in the context of well-controlled trials.

Other cases of CBT for globoid cell leukodystrophy are included in Wagner 1996 [20], Rocha et al. 2000 [56].

X-Linked Adrenoleukodystrophy

X-linked ALD is a condition resulting from deficient degradation of very-long-chain fatty acids in the peroxisomes. The childhood form presents at median around 7 years of age with adrenal insufficiency and cerebral demyelination progressing to severe disability and death, usually within 2–5 years of onset. If performed at early stage, HSCT has proved to be effective. Currently, it is the only long-term treatment for boys affected with ALD [131, 132]. The major series report of Peters et al. describes outcome of 126 patients, 12 of which had CB donors [133]. As in other diseases, the speed with which BMT can be performed is important. When an asymptomatic sibling of an affected child is diagnosed, there may well be ample time to find a well-matched unrelated BM donor. But if a patient is diagnosed at an early stage of neurological involvement, rapid identification of a CB unit may give a vital advantage in proceeding to BMT quickly.

Beam et al. reported the outcome of unrelated CBT in 12 patients with ALD. Median age at time of transplant was 7 years (ranging from neonate to 9.75 years). All umbilical cord had normal levels of very long fatty chain acids, provided a median of 6.98×10^7 nucleated cells per kilogram and were matching at least four of six HLA loci. This series demonstrated similar outcome to that seen with HLA-matched BM donors. Patients transplanted earlier continue to develop at a normal level, supporting the importance of this rapidly available source of HSC [134].

Other cases of CBT for ALD are included in Wagner 1996 [20], Rocha 2000 [56], Gluckman 1997 [33], and Rubinstein 1998 [85].

Other Non-Malignant Disorders

A condition where CBT has been used on some occasions is severe multisystem Langerhans cell histiocytosis (LCH), which usually has a poor prognosis if unresponsive to chemotherapy. Meyer-Wentrup et al. report the successful unrelated one antigen mismatch CBT in a 15-month-old boy. Engraftment was delayed, requiring prolonged G-CSF administration. Despite full donor chimerism, transfusion independency was achieved only by day +220. Further complications were grade III acute GVHD, limited chronic GVHD, renal impairment, and recurrent sepsis, but LCH did not recur [136]. Two more case reports describe successful unrelated CBT in patients with refractory LCH [137, 138]. Other patients have been described in Gluckman 1997 [33] and Rocha 2000 [56].

Another case report describes a successful unrelated CBT in a patient with Evans syndrome, an acquired disorder consisting of autoimmune hemolytic anemia and thrombocytopenia. After failing intensive conservative treatment and two autologous SCTs this patient received a 7/10 matched CBT resulting in prompt and sustained engraftment (Table 7.5) [139].

Table 7.5 Application of cord blood transplant in other rare non-malignant disorders

Disorder	Natural history and alternative therapy	Role of CBT
Hemophagocytic lymphohistiocytosis	Early death without SCT	Mizumoto 2006 [140]; Styczynski 2004 [55]; Rocha 2000 [56]; Gluckman 1997 [33]
Chronic active EBV infection		Iguchi 2006 [141]; Ishimura 2005 [142]
EBV associated lymphoproliferative disease		Toubo 2004 [143]
Duchenne muscular dystrophy	Progressive disease with death in second decade	Zhang 2005 [144]; Zhang 2005 [145]; No long-term evaluation
Hemophilia	Factor substitution	Andolina 2004 – unsuccessful CBT for this disease [146]

Table 7.6 Advantages and disadvantages of different stem cell sources

	MUD	MUD TCD	Haplo-identical (family, parental)	CBT
Time to donor identification	Usually at least 3 months or more	Usually at least 3 months or more	Rapid	<1 month
Donor not available	Often	Often	Rarely	No
Risk for donor	Yes	Yes	Yes	None
Rearranging date SCT	Difficult	Difficult	Relatively easy	Easy
Molecular typing available A+B+DRB1	60%	60%	Not needed	90%
Mismatch transplant possible with satisfactory results	No	No	Yes	Yes
Rare haplotype reduces chance of finding donor	Yes	Yes	No	Slightly
Factors contributing to engraftment	HLA match	HLA match	Cell dose	Cell dose
Second HSC graft, booster or donor lymphocyte infusion possible	Yes	Yes	Yes	No
Risk of viral infection with graft	Yes	Yes	Yes	Low
Risk of transmitting congenital diseases	No	No	No	Yes
Risk of developing GVHD	High	Lower	Lower	Lower

How Do We Balance the Place of Cord Blood Against Other Sources of Stem Cells?

Available stem cell sources for various types of diseases are BM, peripheral blood, T-BM or PBSC, haplo-identical transplant, and CBT from related or unrelated donors (Table 7.6).

How Can We Improve?

In many areas of clinical practice, HSCT is regarded as a treatment of last resort. Even in Oncology, there are strong proponents of chemotherapy alone approaches who are reluctant to consider BMT for some or all of their patients. When you are dealing with a non-malignant disease and often with a child who may be quite well at the time of presentation or diagnosis, one needs clear evidence to present to the family so they can trust the BMT team's recommendation to proceed to what is a high-risk procedure, with a real and immediate risk of death. Unless such evidence is compelling, families may not be able to contemplate HSCT until the disease is too far advanced for the procedure to be of any benefit. For many of these diseases, an early transplant-related death may be the lesser of two evils. But if we replace the morbidity or mortality of the underlying disease with complications of transplant, then we have not benefited these families.

These patients are usually young, and so light, and an adequate cell dose is rarely a problem – for a recent patient of our own, we had a choice of four cord units, all of which were a 5/6 match; all had a cell dose $>10 \times 10^7$/kg and all were in Australia. Our adult colleagues would love to have the advantage we pediatric BMT physicians have with small patients! Double cord transplants are being explored, and are an obvious benefit for adult patients, but if these do carry a greater risk of GVHD, then again they are not necessarily the best option for patients with non-malignant disease. The COBLT study is the first to suggest that perhaps one can have too big a cell dose, and so matching may well become more important.

Given the fact that GVHD lacks benefit and is often detrimental in patients with non-malignant disease, TCD as a method of GVHD prophylaxis has been used widely for BMT. As CB banks increase, then the hope is that we may be able to find better-matched donors for our patients. In the COBLT studies, there was an advantage in having a better-matched cord unit in the patients with malignancy, but this trend was not confirmed in the patients with non-malignant disease, perhaps because these previously untreated patients can tolerate an HLA-mismatch better. Whether this remains true or not when we can analyze larger numbers of patients remains to be seen.

As mentioned above for the haemoglobinopathies, non-myeloablative conditioning may appear a better option particularly for patients with thalassemia. A high rate of rejection has already been seen, the rate of GVHD is not less than with a standard myeloablative graft and use of a CB unit is even more likely to be associated with rejection. For the time being, families who are rearranging their lives to attempt to cure their child's illness may not be prepared to risk an experimental conditioning regimen which carries a high likelihood of needing to be repeated. For many of the diseases here, a failed first transplant and need for a second also takes too long if the disease has progressive neurological involvement.

Summary

In conclusion, for patients who need allogeneic HSCT for non-malignant conditions, related or unrelated CBT is a good option. Current experience shows that unrelated CBT is a feasible procedure for children with BMF and inborn errors; however, the number of patients and the follow-up time in these disease categories is limited to date suggesting that additional experience is needed to determine the benefits of these alternative therapies. In immunodeficiencies, CBT is an effective option with results as good as other sources of stem cells. CB directed banking is recommended in families with patients of haemoglobinopathies if a transplant might be indicated in the future. For several inborn metabolic disorders, CBT is a curative alternative for patients lacking an appropriate BM donor. If the condition requires urgent transplant, a search for an unrelated CBT donor should be made simultaneously as a BM donor search. If both types of donors are available, the decision for BM versus CB depends upon the clinical situation.

References

1. Kurtzberg J, Cord blood transplantation in genetic disorders. Biol Blood Marrow Transplant 2004; 10(10):735–736.
2. Gatti RA, Meuwissen HJ, Allen HD et al., Immunological reconstitution of sex-linked lymphopenic immunological deficiency. Lancet 1968; 2(7583):1366–1369.
3. Speck B, Zwaan FE, van Rood JJ et al., Allogeneic bone marrow transplantation in a patient with aplastic anemia using a phenotypically HLA-identical unrelated donor. Transplantation 1973; 16(1):24–28.
4. Reisner Y, Kapoor N, Kirkpatrick D et al., Transplantation for severe combined immunodeficiency with HLA-A,B,D,DR incompatible parental marrow cells fractionated by soybean agglutinin and sheep red blood cells. Blood 1983; 61(2):341–348.
5. Hobbs JR, Hugh-Jones K, Barrett AJ et al., Reversal of clinical features of Hurler's disease and biochemical improvement after treatment by bone-marrow transplantation. Lancet 1981; 2(8249):709–712.
6. Gluckman E, Broxmeyer HA, Auerbach AD et al., Hematopoietic reconstitution in a patient with Fanconi's anemia by means of umbilical-cord blood from an HLA-identical sibling. N Engl J Med 1989; 321(17):1174–1178.
7. Grewal SS, Kahn JP, Macmillan ML et al., Successful hematopoietic stem cell transplantation for Fanconi anemia from an unaffected HLA-genotype-identical sibling selected using preimplantation genetic diagnosis. Blood 2004; 103(3):1147–1151.
8. Bielorai B, Hughes MR, Auerbach AD et al., Successful umbilical cord blood transplantation for Fanconi anemia using preimplantation genetic diagnosis for HLA-matched donor. Am J Hematol 2004; 77(4):397–399.
9. Kurtzberg J, Laughlin M, Graham ML et al., Placental blood as a source of hematopoietic stem cells for transplantation into unrelated recipients. N Engl J Med 1996; 335(3):157–166.
10. Wagner JE, Kernan NA, Steinbuch M et al., Allogeneic sibling umbilical-cord-blood transplantation in children with malignant and non-malignant disease. Lancet 1995; 346(8969):214–219.
11. http://www.BMDW.org.(accessed 9/9/2006).
12. Wagner JE, Kahn JP, Wolf SM et al., Preimplantation testing to produce an HLA-matched donor infant. JAMA 2004; 292(7):803–804.
13. Wolf SM, Kahn JP, Wagner JE, Using preimplantation genetic diagnosis to create a stem cell donor: issues, guidelines & limits. J Law Med Ethics 2003; 31(3):327–339.
14. Spriggs M, Savulescu J, "Saviour siblings". J Med Ethics 2002; 28(5):289.
15. Pennings G, Schots R, Liebaers I, Ethical considerations on preimplantation genetic diagnosis for HLA typing to match a future child as a donor of haematopoietic stem cells to a sibling. Hum Reprod 2002; 17(3):534–538.
16. Gaipa G, Dassi M, Perseghin P et al., Allogeneic bone marrow stem cell transplantation following CD34+ immunomagnetic enrichment in patients with inherited metabolic storage diseases. Bone Marrow Transplant 2003; 31(10):857–860.

17. Peters C, Shapiro EG, Anderson J et al., Hurler syndrome: II. Outcome of HLA-genotypically identical sibling and HLA-haploidentical related donor bone marrow transplantation in fifty-four children. The Storage Disease Collaborative Study Group. Blood 1998; 91(7):2601–2608.
18. Staba SL, Escolar ML, Poe M et al., Cord-blood transplants from unrelated donors in patients with Hurler's syndrome. N Engl J Med 2004; 350(19):1960–1969.
19. Yabe H, Inoue H, Matsumoto M et al., Unmanipulated HLA-haploidentical bone marrow transplantation for the treatment of fatal, nonmalignant diseases in children and adolescents. Int J Hematol 2004; 80(1):78–82.
20. Wagner JE, Rosenthal J, Sweetman R et al., Successful transplantation of HLA-matched and HLA-mismatched umbilical cord blood from unrelated donors: analysis of engraftment and acute graft-versus-host disease. Blood 1996; 88(3):795–802.
21. Rocha V, Cornish J, Sievers EL et al., Comparison of outcomes of unrelated bone marrow and umbilical cord blood transplants in children with acute leukemia. Blood 2001; 97(10):2962–2971.
22. Shaw PJ, Bleakley M, Lau L, Unrelated cord blood transplant as salvage following non-engraftment of unrelated marrow transplant? Bone Marrow Transplant 2004; 34(3): 275–276.
23. Motwani J, Lawson SE, Darbyshire PJ, Successful HSCT using nonradiotherapy-based conditioning regimens and alternative donors in patients with Fanconi anaemia – experience in a single UK centre. Bone Marrow Transplant 2005; 36(5):405–410.
24. Martin PL, Carter SL, Kernan NA et al., Results of the cord blood transplantation study (COBLT): outcomes of unrelated donor umbilical cord blood transplantation in pediatric patients with lysosomal and peroxisomal storage diseases. Biol Blood Marrow Transplant 2006; 12(2):184–194.
25. Gluckman E, Rocha V, Chastang C, Cord blood banking and transplant in Europe. Eurocord. Bone Marrow Transplant 1998; 22 Suppl 1:S68–S74.
26. Fraser CJ, Hirsch BA, Dayton V et al., First report of donor cell-derived acute leukemia as a complication of umbilical cord blood transplantation. Blood 2005; 106(13):4377–4380.
27. Sevilla J, Querol S, Molines A et al., Transient donor cell-derived myelodysplastic syndrome with monosomy 7 after unrelated cord blood transplantation. Eur J Haematol 2006; 77(3): 259–263.
28. Gluckman E, Rocha V, Chevret S, Results of unrelated umbilical cord blood hematopoietic stem cell transplant. Transfus Clin Biol 2001; 8(3):146–154.
29. Frassoni F, Podesta M, Maccario R et al., Cord blood transplantation provides better reconstitution of hematopoietic reservoir compared with bone marrow transplantation. Blood 2003; 102(3):1138–1141.
30. Locatelli F, Maccario R, Comoli P et al., Hematopoietic and immune recovery after transplantation of cord blood progenitor cells in children. Bone Marrow Transplant 1996; 18(6): 1095–1101.
31. Thomson BG, Robertson KA, Gowan D et al., Analysis of engraftment, graft-versus-host disease, and immune recovery following unrelated donor cord blood transplantation. Blood 2000; 96(8):2703–2711.
32. Abu-Ghosh A, Goldman S, Slone V et al., Immunological reconstitution and correlation of circulating serum inflammatory mediators/cytokines with the incidence of acute graft-versus-host disease during the first 100 days following unrelated umbilical cord blood transplantation. Bone Marrow Transplant 1999; 24(5):535–544.
33. Gluckman E, Rocha V, Boyer-Chammard A et al., Outcome of cord-blood transplantation from related and unrelated donors. Eurocord Transplant Group and the European Blood and Marrow Transplantation Group. N Engl J Med 1997; 337(6):373–381.
34. Bradley MB, Satwani P, Baldinger L et al., Reduced intensity allogeneic umbilical cord blood transplantation in children and adolescent recipients with malignant and non-malignant diseases. Bone Marrow Transplant 2007; 40(7): 621–631.

35. Lucarelli G, Galimberti M, Polchi P et al., Bone marrow transplantation in patients with thalassemia. N Engl J Med 1990; 322(7):417–421.
36. Lucarelli G, Clift RA, Galimberti M et al., Marrow transplantation for patients with thalassemia: results in class 3 patients. Blood 1996; 87(5):2082–2088.
37. Storb RF, Lucarelli G, McSweeney PA et al., Hematopoietic cell transplantation for benign hematological disorders and solid tumors. Hematol Am Soc Hematol Educ Program 2003;372–397.
38. Lucarelli G, Galimberti M, Polchi P et al., Marrow transplantation in patients with thalassemia responsive to iron chelation therapy. N Engl J Med 1993; 329(12):840–844.
39. Gaziev D, Polchi P, Galimberti M et al., Graft-versus-host disease after bone marrow transplantation for thalassemia: an analysis of incidence and risk factors. Transplantation 1997; 63(6):854–860.
40. Karnon J, Zeuner D, Brown J et al., Lifetime treatment costs of beta-thalassemia major. Clin Lab Haematol 1999; 21(6):377–385.
41. Issaragrisil S, Visuthisakchai S, Suvatte V et al., Brief report: transplantation of cord-blood stem cells into a patient with severe thalassemia. N Engl J Med 1995; 332(6):367–369.
42. Issaragrisil S, Umbilical cord blood transplantation for thalassemia. Curr Hematol Rep 2005; 4(6):415–416.
43. Issaragrisil S, Cord blood transplantation in thalassemia. Blood Cells 1994; 20(2–3): 259–262.
44. Miniero R, Rocha V, Saracco P et al., Cord blood transplantation (CBT) in haemoglobinopathies. Eurocord. Bone Marrow Transplant 1998; 22 Suppl 1:S78–S79.
45. Walters MC, Quirolo L, Trachtenberg ET et al., Sibling donor cord blood transplantation for thalassemia major: Experience of the Sibling Donor Cord Blood Program. Ann N Y Acad Sci 2005; 1054:206–213.
46. Locatelli F, Rocha V, Reed W et al., Related umbilical cord blood transplantation in patients with thalassemia and sickle cell disease. Blood 2003; 101(6):2137–2143.
47. Locatelli F, Rocha V, Chastang C et al., Factors associated with outcome after cord blood transplantation in children with acute leukemia. Eurocord-Cord Blood Transplant Group. Blood 1999; 93(11):3662–3671.
48. Krishnamurti L, Abel S, Maiers M et al., Availability of unrelated donors for hematopoietic stem cell transplantation for haemoglobinopathies. Bone Marrow Transplant 2003; 31(7):547–550.
49. Hall JG, Martin PL, Wood S et al., Unrelated umbilical cord blood transplantation for an infant with beta-thalassemia major. J Pediatr Hematol Oncol 2004; 26(6):382–385.
50. Tan PH, Hwang WY, Goh YT et al., Unrelated peripheral blood and cord blood hematopoietic stem cell transplants for thalassemia major. Am J Hematol 2004; 75(4):209–212.
51. Jaing TH, Hung IJ, Yang CP et al., Successful unrelated cord blood transplantation in a child with beta-thalassemia major. J Trop Pediatr 2005; 51(2):122–124.
52. Fang J, Huang S, Chen C et al., Unrelated umbilical cord blood transplant for beta-thalassemia major. J Trop Pediatr 2003; 49(2):71–73.
53. Jaing TH, Yang CP, Hung IJ et al., Transplantation of unrelated donor umbilical cord blood utilizing double-unit grafts for five teenagers with transfusion-dependent thalassemia. Bone Marrow Transplant 2007;40(4):307–311.
54. Rocha V, Chastang C, Souillet G et al., Related cord blood transplants: the Eurocord experience from 78 transplants. Eurocord Transplant group. Bone Marrow Transplant 1998; 21 Suppl 3:S59-S62.
55. Styczynski J, Cheung YK, Garvin J et al., Outcomes of unrelated cord blood transplantation in pediatric recipients. Bone Marrow Transplant 2004; 34(2):129–136.
56. Rocha V, Wagner JE Jr, Sobocinski KA et al., Graft-versus-host disease in children who have received a cord-blood or bone marrow transplant from an HLA-identical sibling. Eurocord and International Bone Marrow Transplant Registry Working Committee on Alternative Donor and Stem Cell Sources. N Engl J Med 2000; 342(25):1846–1854.

57. Johnson FL, Look AT, Gockerman J et al., Bone-marrow transplantation in a patient with sickle-cell anemia. N Engl J Med 1984; 311(12):780–783.
58. Walters MC, Patience M, Leisenring W et al., Bone marrow transplantation for sickle cell disease. N Engl J Med 1996; 335(6):369–376.
59. Sullivan KM, Parkman R, Walters MC, Bone marrow transplantation for non-malignant disease. Hematology (Am Soc Hematol Educ Program) Volume 2000; 319–338.
60. Vermylen C, Cornu G, Ferster A et al., Bone marrow transplantation in sickle cell disease: the Belgian experience. Bone Marrow Transplant 1993; 12 Suppl 1:116–117.
61. Walters MC, Storb R, Patience M et al., Impact of bone marrow transplantation for symptomatic sickle cell disease: an interim report. Multicenter investigation of bone marrow transplantation for sickle cell disease. Blood 2000; 95(6):1918–1924.
62. Adamkiewicz TV, Mehta PS, Boyer MW et al., Transplantation of unrelated placental blood cells in children with high-risk sickle cell disease. Bone Marrow Transplant 2004; 34(5):405–411.
63. Hill RS, Petersen FB, Storb R et al., Mixed hematologic chimerism after allogeneic marrow transplantation for severe aplastic anemia is associated with a higher risk of graft rejection and a lessened incidence of acute graft-versus-host disease. Blood 1986; 67(3):811–816.
64. Andreani M, Manna M, Lucarelli G et al., Persistence of mixed chimerism in patients transplanted for the treatment of thalassemia. Blood 1996; 87(8):3494–3499.
65. Slavin S, Nagler A, Naparstek E et al., Nonmyeloablative stem cell transplantation and cell therapy as an alternative to conventional bone marrow transplantation with lethal cytoreduction for the treatment of malignant and nonmalignant hematologic diseases. Blood 1998; 91(3):756–763.
66. Iannone R, Casella JF, Fuchs EJ et al., Results of minimally toxic nonmyeloablative transplantation in patients with sickle cell anemia and beta-thalassemia. Biol Blood Marrow Transplant 2003; 9(8):519–528.
67. Shaw PH, Haut PR, Olszewski M et al., Hematopoietic stem-cell transplantation using unrelated cord-blood versus matched sibling marrow in pediatric bone marrow failure syndrome: one center's experience. Pediatr Transplant 1999; 3(4):315–321.
68. Guardiola P, Socie G, Pasquini R et al., Allogeneic stem cell transplantation for Fanconi anaemia. Severe Aplastic Anaemia Working Party of the EBMT and EUFAR. European Group for Blood and Marrow Transplantation. Bone Marrow Transplant 1998; 21 Suppl 2:S24–S27.
69. Guardiola P, Pasquini R, Dokal I et al., Outcome of 69 allogeneic stem cell transplantations for Fanconi anemia using HLA-matched unrelated donors: a study on behalf of the European Group for Blood and Marrow Transplantation. Blood 2000; 95(2):422–429.
70. Kuliev A, Rechitsky S, Tur-Kaspa I et al., Preimplantation genetics: Improving access to stem cell therapy. Ann N Y Acad Sci 2005; 1054:223–227.
71. Kuliev A, Rechitsky S, Verlinsky O et al., Preimplantation diagnosis and HLA typing for haemoglobin disorders. Reprod Biomed Online 2005; 11(3):362–370.
72. Gluckman E, Bone marrow transplantation in Fanconi's anemia. Stem Cells 1993; 11 Suppl 2:180–183.
73. Gluckman E, Auerbach AD, Horowitz MM et al., Bone marrow transplantation for Fanconi anemia. Blood 1995; 86(7):2856–2862.
74. Barker JN, Davies SM, Defor T et al., Survival after transplantation of unrelated donor umbilical cord blood is comparable to that of human leukocyte antigen-matched unrelated donor bone marrow: results of a matched-pair analysis. Blood 2001; 97(10):2957–2961.
75. de la Fuente J., Reiss S, McCloy M et al., Non-TBI stem cell transplantation protocol for Fanconi anaemia using HLA-compatible sibling and unrelated donors. Bone Marrow Transplant 2003; 32(7):653–656.
76. Tischkowitz M, Dokal I, Fanconi anaemia and leukaemia – clinical and molecular aspects. Br J Haematol 2004; 126(2):176–191.
77. Gluckman E, Results of unrelated cord blood transplant in patients with bone marrow failure syndromes. Biol Blood Marrow Transplant 2004; 10(10):736–737. Ref Type: Abstract.

78. Buckley RH, Schiff SE, Schiff RI et al., Hematopoietic stem-cell transplantation for the treatment of severe combined immunodeficiency. N Engl J Med 1999; 340(7):508–516.
79. Buckley RH, Schiff SE, Sampson HA et al., Development of immunity in human severe primary T cell deficiency following haploidentical bone marrow stem cell transplantation. J Immunol 1986; 136(7):2398–2407.
80. Tan PL, Wagner JE, Auerbach AD et al., Successful engraftment without radiation after fludarabine-based regimen in Fanconi anemia patients undergoing genotypically identical donor hematopoietic cell transplantation. Pediatr Blood Cancer 2006; 46(5):630–636.
81. de Medeiros CR, Silva LM, Pasquini R, Unrelated cord blood transplantation in a Fanconi anemia patient using fludarabine-based conditioning. Bone Marrow Transplant 2001; 28(1):110–112.
82. Aker M, Varadi G, Slavin S et al., Fludarabine-based protocol for human umbilical cord blood transplantation in children with Fanconi anemia. J Pediatr Hematol Oncol 1999; 21(3):237–239.
83. Yoshimasu T, Tanaka R, Suenobu S et al., Prompt and durable hematopoietic reconstitution by unrelated cord blood transplantation in a child with Fanconi anemia. Bone Marrow Transplant 2001; 27(7):767–769.
84. Wagner JE, Barker JN, Defor TE et al., Transplantation of unrelated donor umbilical cord blood in 102 patients with malignant and nonmalignant diseases: influence of CD34 cell dose and HLA disparity on treatment-related mortality and survival. Blood 2002; 100(5): 1611–1618.
85. Rubinstein P, Carrier C, Scaradavou A et al., Outcomes among 562 recipients of placental-blood transplants from unrelated donors. N Engl J Med 1998; 339(22):1565–1577.
86. Macmillan ML, Davies SM, Wagner JE et al., Engraftment of unrelated donor stem cells in children with familial amegakaryocytic thrombocytopenia. Bone Marrow Transplant 1998; 21(7):735–737.
87. Ohga S, Ichino K, Goto K et al., Unrelated donor cord blood transplantation for childhood severe aplastic anemia after a modified conditioning. Pediatr Transplant 2006; 10(4): 497–500.
88. Dianzani I, Garelli E, Ramenghi U, Diamond-Blackfan Anaemia: an overview. Paediatr Drugs 2000; 2(5):345–355.
89. Bonno M, Azuma E, Nakano T et al., Successful hematopoietic reconstitution by transplantation of umbilical cord blood cells in a transfusion-dependent child with Diamond-Blackfan anemia. Bone Marrow Transplant 1997; 19(1):83–85.
90. Nobili B, Rossi G, De SP et al., Successful umbilical cord blood transplantation in a child with dyskeratosis congenita after a fludarabine-based reduced-intensity conditioning regimen. Br J Haematol 2002; 119(2):573–574.
91. Mino E, Kobayashi R, Yoshida M et al., Umbilical cord blood stem cell transplantation from unrelated HLA-matched donor in an infant with severe congenital neutropenia. Bone Marrow Transplant 2004; 33(9):969–971.
92. Nakazawa Y, Sakashita K, Kinoshita M et al., Successful unrelated cord blood transplantation using a reduced-intensity conditioning regimen in a 6-month-old infant with congenital neutropenia complicated by severe pneumonia. Int J Hematol 2004; 80(3):287–290.
93. Vibhakar R, Radhi M, Rumelhart S et al., Successful unrelated umbilical cord blood transplantation in children with Shwachman-Diamond syndrome. Bone Marrow Transplant 2005; 36(10):855–861.
94. Fischer A, Severe combined immunodeficiencies (SCID). Clin Exp Immunol 2000; 122(2):143–149.
95. Myers LA, Patel DD, Puck JM et al., Hematopoietic stem cell transplantation for severe combined immunodeficiency in the neonatal period leads to superior thymic output and improved survival. Blood 2002; 99(3):872–878.
96. Antoine C, Muller S, Cant A et al., Long-term survival and transplantation of haemopoietic stem cells for immunodeficiencies: report of the European experience 1968-99. Lancet 2003; 361(9357):553–560.

97. Dalal I, Reid B, Doyle J et al., Matched unrelated bone marrow transplantation for combined immunodeficiency. Bone Marrow Transplant 2000; 25(6):613–621.
98. Knutsen AP, Wall DA, Kinetics of T-cell development of umbilical cord blood transplantation in severe T-cell immunodeficiency disorders. J Allergy Clin Immunol 1999; 103(5 Pt 1): 823–832.
99. Fischer A, Landais P, Friedrich W et al., European experience of bone-marrow transplantation for severe combined immunodeficiency. Lancet 1990; 336(8719):850–854.
100. Bhattacharya A, Slatter MA, Chapman CE et al., Single centre experience of umbilical cord stem cell transplantation for primary immunodeficiency. Bone Marrow Transplant 2005; 36(4):295–299.
101. Muller SM, Kohn T, Schulz AS et al., Similar pattern of thymic-dependent T-cell reconstitution in infants with severe combined immunodeficiency after human leukocyte antigen (HLA)-identical and HLA-nonidentical stem cell transplantation. Blood 2000; 96(13): 4344–4349.
102. Gennery AR, Dickinson AM, Brigham K et al., CAMPATH-1 M T-cell depleted BMT for SCID: long-term follow-up of 19 children treated 1987-98 in a single center. Cytotherapy 2001; 3(3):221–232.
103. Knutsen AP, Wall DA, Umbilical cord blood transplantation in severe T-cell immunodeficiency disorders: two-year experience. J Clin Immunol 2000; 20(6):466–476.
104. Tsuji Y, Imai K, Kajiwara M et al., Hematopoietic stem cell transplantation for 30 patients with primary immunodeficiency diseases: 20 years experience of a single team. Bone Marrow Transplant 2006; 37(5):469–477.
105. Ziegner UH, Ochs HD, Schanen C et al., Unrelated umbilical cord stem cell transplantation for X-linked immunodeficiencies. J Pediatr 2001; 138(4):570–573.
106. Goebel WS, Nelson RP, Jr., Brahmi Z et al., Serial transplantation resulting in tolerance to an unrelated cord blood graft. Transplantation 2006; 81(11):1596–1599.
107. Fagioli F, Biasin E, Berger M et al., Successful unrelated cord blood transplantation in two children with severe combined immunodeficiency syndrome. Bone Marrow Transplant 2003; 31(2):133–136.
108. Filipovich AH, Stone JV, Tomany SC et al., Impact of donor type on outcome of bone marrow transplantation for Wiskott-Aldrich syndrome: collaborative study of the International Bone Marrow Transplant Registry and the National Marrow Donor Program. Blood 2001; 97(6):1598–1603.
109. Rumelhart SL, Trigg ME, Horowitz SD et al., Monoclonal antibody T-cell-depleted HLA-haploidentical bone marrow transplantation for Wiskott-Aldrich syndrome. Blood 1990; 75(4):1031–1035.
110. Knutsen AP, Steffen M, Wassmer K et al., Umbilical cord blood transplantation in Wiskott Aldrich syndrome. J Pediatr 2003; 142(5):519–523.
111. Kaneko M, Watanabe T, Watanabe H et al., Successful unrelated cord blood transplantation in an infant with Wiskott-Aldrich syndrome following recurrent cytomegalovirus disease. Int J Hematol 2003; 78(5):457–460.
112. Bhattacharya A, Slatter M, Curtis A et al., Successful umbilical cord blood stem cell transplantation for chronic granulomatous disease. Bone Marrow Transplant 2003; 31(5): 403–405.
113. Broom MA, Wang LL, Otta SK et al., Successful umbilical cord blood stem cell transplantation in a patient with Rothmund-Thomson syndrome and combined immunodeficiency. Clin Genet 2006; 69(4):337–343.
114. Slatter MA, Bhattacharya A, Flood TJ et al., Use of two unrelated umbilical cord stem cell units in stem cell transplantation for Wiskott-Aldrich syndrome. Pediatr Blood Cancer 2006; 47(3):332–334.
115. Ohtsuka Y, Shimizu T, Nishizawa K et al., Successful engraftment and decrease of cytomegalovirus load after cord blood stem cell transplantation in a patient with DiGeorge syndrome. Eur J Pediatr 2004; 163(12):747–748.

116. Myers LA, Hershfield MS, Neale WT et al., Purine nucleoside phosphorylase deficiency (PNP-def) presenting with lymphopenia and developmental delay: successful correction with umbilical cord blood transplantation. J Pediatr 2004; 145(5):710–712.
117. Tono C, Takahashi Y, Terui K et al., Correction of immunodeficiency associated with NEMO mutation by umbilical cord blood transplantation using a reduced-intensity conditioning regimen. Bone Marrow Transplant 2007;39(12):801–804.
118. Howard V, Myers LA, Williams DA et al., Stem cell transplants for patients with X-linked agammaglobulinemia. Clin Immunol 2003; 107(2):98–102.
119. Vowels MR, Tang RL, Berdoukas V et al., Brief report: correction of X-linked lymphoproliferative disease by transplantation of cord-blood stem cells. N Engl J Med 1993; 329(22):1623–1625.
120. Krivit W, Sung JH, Shapiro EG et al., Microglia: the effector cell for reconstitution of the central nervous system following bone marrow transplantation for lysosomal and peroxisomal storage diseases. Cell Transplant 1995; 4(4):385–392.
121. Boelens JJ, Trends in haematopoietic cell transplantation for inborn errors of metabolism. J Inherit Metab Dis 2006; 29(2–3):413–420.
122. Peters C, Steward CG, Hematopoietic cell transplantation for inherited metabolic diseases: an overview of outcomes and practice guidelines. Bone Marrow Transplant 2003; 31(4): 229–239.
123. Wall DA, Carter SL, Kernan NA et al., Busulfan/melphalan/antithymocyte globulin followed by unrelated donor cord blood transplantation for treatment of infant leukemia and leukemia in young children: the Cord Blood Transplantation study (COBLT) experience. Biology of Blood and Marrow Transplantation 2005; 11(8):637–646.
124. Peters C, Balthazor M, Shapiro EG et al., Outcome of unrelated donor bone marrow transplantation in 40 children with Hurler syndrome. Blood 1996; 87(11):4894–4902.
125. Krivit W, Aubourg P, Shapiro E et al., Bone marrow transplantation for globoid cell leukodystrophy, adrenoleukodystrophy, metachromatic leukodystrophy, and Hurler syndrome. Curr Opin Hematol 1999; 6(6):377–382.
126. Krivit W, Peters C, Shapiro EG, Bone marrow transplantation as effective treatment of central nervous system disease in globoid cell leukodystrophy, metachromatic leukodystrophy, adrenoleukodystrophy, mannosidosis, fucosidosis, aspartylglucosaminuria, Hurler, Maroteaux-Lamy, and Sly syndromes, and Gaucher disease type III. Curr Opin Neurol 1999; 12(2):167–176.
127. Boelens JJ, Wynn RF, O'Meara A et al., Outcomes of hematopoietic stem cell transplantation for Hurler's syndrome in Europe: a risk factor analysis for graft failure. Bone Marrow Transplant 2007; 40(3):225–233.
128. Church H, Tylee K, Copper A et al., Biochemical monitoring after haematopoietic stem cell transplant for Hurler syndrome (MPSIH): implications for functional outcome after transplant in metabolic disease. Bone Marrow Transplant 2007; 39(4) :207–210.
129. Escolar ML, Poe MD, Provenzale JM et al., Transplantation of umbilical-cord blood in babies with infantile Krabbe's disease. N Engl J Med 2005; 352(20):2069–2081.
130. Escolar ML, Poe MD, Martin HR et al., A staging system for infantile Krabbe disease to predict outcome after unrelated umbilical cord blood transplantation. Pediatrics 2006; 118(3):e879–e889.
131. Shapiro E, Krivit W, Lockman L et al., Long-term effect of bone-marrow transplantation for childhood-onset cerebral X-linked adrenoleukodystrophy. Lancet 2000; 356(9231): 713–718.
132. Shapiro EG, Lockman LA, Balthazor M et al., Neuropsychological outcomes of several storage diseases with and without bone marrow transplantation. J Inherit Metab Dis 1995; 18(4):413–429.
133. Peters C, Charnas LR, Tan Y et al., Cerebral X-linked adrenoleukodystrophy: the international hematopoietic cell transplantation experience from 1982 to 1999. Blood 2004; 104(3):881–888.

134. Beam D, Poe M, Provenzale J et al., Outcomes of Unrelated Umbilical Cord Blood Transplantation for X-Linked Adrenoleukodystrophy. Biol Blood Marrow Transplant 2007; 13(6):665–674.
135. Lee V, Li CK, Shing MM et al., Umbilical cord blood transplantation for Maroteaux-Lamy syndrome (mucopolysaccharidosis type VI). Bone Marrow Transplant 2000; 26(4):455–458.
136. Meyer-Wentrup F, Foell J, Wawer A et al., Unrelated cord blood transplantation in an infant with severe multisystem Langerhans cell histiocytosis: clinical outcome, engraftment and culture of monocyte-derived dendritic cells. Bone Marrow Transplant 2004; 33(8):875–876.
137. Suminoe A, Matsuzaki A, Hattori H et al., Unrelated cord blood transplantation for an infant with chemotherapy-resistant progressive Langerhans cell histiocytosis. J Pediatr Hematol Oncol 2001; 23(9):633–636.
138. Nagarajan R, Neglia J, Ramsay N et al., Successful treatment of refractory Langerhans cell histiocytosis with unrelated cord blood transplantation. J Pediatr Hematol Oncol 2001; 23(9):629–632.
139. Urban C, Lackner H, Sovinz P et al., Successful unrelated cord blood transplantation in a 7-year-old boy with Evans syndrome refractory to immunosuppression and double autologous stem cell transplantation. Eur J Haematol 2006; 76(6):526–530.
140. Mizumoto H, Hata D, Yamamoto K et al., Familial hemophagocytic lymphohistiocytosis with the MUNC13-4 mutation: a case report. Eur J Pediatr 2006; 165(6):384–388.
141. Iguchi A, Kobayashi R, Sato TZ et al., Successful report of reduced-intensity stem cell transplantation from unrelated umbilical cord blood in a girl with chronic active Epstein-Barr virus infection. J Pediatr Hematol Oncol 2006; 28(4):254–256.
142. Ishimura M, Ohga S, Nomura A et al., Successful umbilical cord blood transplantation for severe chronic active Epstein-Barr virus infection after the double failure of hematopoietic stem cell transplantation. Am J Hematol 2005; 80(3):207–212.
143. Toubo T, Suga N, Ohga S et al., Successful unrelated cord blood transplantation for Epstein-Barr virus-associated lymphoproliferative disease with hemophagocytic syndrome. Int J Hematol 2004; 80(5):458–462.
144. Zhang C, Feng HY, Huang SL et al., Therapy of Duchenne muscular dystrophy with umbilical cord blood stem cell transplantation. Zhonghua Yi Xue Yi Chuan Xue Za Zhi 2005; 22(4):399–405.
145. Zhang C, Chen W, Xiao LL et al., Allogeneic umbilical cord blood stem cell transplantation in Duchenne muscular dystrophy. Zhonghua Yi Xue Za Zhi 2005; 85(8):522–525.
146. Andolina M, Maximova N, Rabusin M et al., Failure of a sibling umbilical cord blood transplantation to correct hemophilia A. Haematologica 2004; 89(7):ECR22.

Chapter 8
Cord Blood Transplantation for Hematologic Malignancies

Karen Quillen

Since the first cord blood transplant in 1988 for a child with Fanconi's anemia, cord blood transplantation is widely accepted for the treatment of pediatric leukemia in patients without a sibling donor. The outcome of matched or one-antigen mismatched umbilical cord blood transplants is comparable to matched unrelated marrow transplantation. An adequate cell dose is generally around 2.5–3.0 × 10E7 nucleated cells/kg. The issue of an adequate cell dose has limited the use of cord blood grafts in adults with acute leukemia. The outcome of cord blood transplantation in adults appears to vary with institutional experience, which partially relates to the slower neutrophil and immune recovery. New strategies such as double-unit cord blood transplantation will help to shorten the period of cytopenias, elucidate the mechanisms of hematopoietic engraftment, and broaden the applicability of cord blood transplantation to adults with leukemia.

Cord Blood Transplantation in Children with Acute Leukemia

The first human cord blood transplant was performed in 1988 by Dr. Gluckman and colleagues in Paris; a 5-year-old boy with Fanconi's anemia received his HLA-identical sister's cord blood that had been cryopreserved [1]. This patient is disease-free more than 15 years later with complete donor chimerism.

Many children have subsequently received cord blood transplants from related donors (generally a sibling), for a variety of conditions such as marrow failure syndromes, congenital immunodeficiencies, metabolic disorders, hemoglobinopathies, hematologic malignancies, and solid tumors. Cord blood transplants have two main advantages over marrow or peripheral blood stem cell grafts in the related donor setting: first, cord blood collection is risk-free for the donor, avoiding the need for general anesthesia (in the case of marrow harvest) or growth factor mobilization

K. Quillen (✉)
Department of Laboratory Medicine, Boston University Medical Center, 88 East Newton St., H-3600, Boston, MA 02118, USA
e-mail: kq@bu.edu

N. Bhattacharya, P. Stubblefield (eds.), *Frontiers of Cord Blood Science*,
DOI 10.1007/978-1-84800-167-1_8,

and leukapheresis (in the case of peripheral blood stem cell harvest); second, a cord blood transplant is generally considered to have a lower risk of graft-versus-host disease (GVHD) than a conventional (unmanipulated) marrow graft.

A retrospective comparison of 113 cord blood transplants and 2,052 marrow transplants in children (15 years of age or younger) for the period 1990–1997, all from HLA-identical sibling donors, was performed through the International Bone Marrow Transplant Registry and Eurocord [2]. Over half of the patients were transplanted for malignancy, most commonly acute leukemia. Recipients of cord blood were younger (median age of 5 years vs. 8 years) and smaller (median weight of 17 kg vs. 26 kg) than recipients of bone marrow. The median cell dose was 4.7 × 10E7 cells/kg for cord blood compared to 3.5 × 10E8 cells/kg for marrow. Despite less intense GVHD prophylaxis (with the omission of methotrexate in 72% of cord blood recipients), cord blood transplants had a lower risk of acute GVHD (14% vs. 24%) and chronic GVHD (5% vs. 14%). Hematopoietic recovery in terms of neutrophil (26 days vs. 18 days) and platelet (44 days vs. 24 days) engraftment was significantly slower for cord blood transplantation compared to marrow. Three-year survival in patients transplanted for malignancy was similar in the two groups (46% for cord blood recipients, 55% for marrow recipients).

Only 30% of patients have an HLA-identical sibling donor. Some of the patients who do not have an HLA-matched related donor may find a matched unrelated marrow donor. For those who do not find an acceptably matched unrelated marrow donor, a mismatched unrelated cord blood transplant is a viable option. The search and procurement process for an unrelated cord blood graft through a cord blood bank is generally much faster (under 1 month) than the comparable process for an unrelated marrow donor (3–4 months) since the cord blood graft is already collected [3].

The New York Blood Center operates the oldest public cord blood bank in the United States and reported on its experience providing unrelated cord blood grafts for 562 patients in the United States and abroad for the period 1992–1998 [4]. HLA-A and -B antigens were determined serologically. HLA-DRB1 alleles were determined by high-resolution (HR) DNA typing. Eighty-six percent of cord blood grafts were one or two-antigen mismatches with the transplant recipient. Two-thirds of patients were under 12 years of age or weighed less than 40 kg. Over 80% of patients were under 18 years of age or weighed less than 60 kg. Three-quarters of patients had hematologic malignancies, mainly acute leukemia in an intermediate or advanced stage of the disease, or acquired bone marrow disorders such as myelodysplastic syndrome or aplastic anemia. The remaining one-quarter of patients had genetic diseases such as Fanconi's anemia or severe combined immunodeficiency.

Myeloid engraftment post-transplantation (absolute neutrophil count $\geq 500/mm^3$) occurred at a median of 28 days. Successful myeloid engraftment (by day 42) was significantly associated with a higher cell dose (>2.4 × 10E7 nucleated cells/kg) and the absence of HLA mismatching in a multivariate analysis. Platelet engraftment post-transplantation (platelet count $\geq 50{,}000/mm^3$) occurred at a median of 90 days. In multivariate analysis, age, infection after transplantation, and GVHD were significant factors affecting platelet engraftment.

The incidence of acute GVHD was almost 70%; about one-third of GVHD cases were grade III or grade IV. In multivariate analysis, age and HLA mismatch were independently associated with acute GVHD. Mortality at day 100 was 39%; the deaths were attributed to infection, respiratory failure, multiorgan failure or GVHD. This figure was felt to compare favorably with bone marrow transplantation from unrelated donors, especially considering that two-antigen mismatches are generally not accepted in unrelated marrow transplantation. The conclusion of this report was that umbilical cord blood is a useful source of allogeneic hematopoietic stem cells for bone marrow reconstitution.

Eurocord is an international registry operating on behalf of the European Group for Blood and Marrow Transplantation (EBMT); it includes more than 180 transplant centers worldwide in 35 countries, all performing cord blood transplants. A retrospective analysis comparing the outcome of unrelated cord blood transplants (UCBT) to unrelated bone marrow transplants (UBMT) in children with acute leukemia for the period 1994–1998 was reported by Eurocord and EBMT [5]. There were 99 UCBT, 262 unmanipulated UBMT, and 180 T-cell-depleted unrelated bone marrow transplants (T-UBMT). The UCBT patients were younger (median age of 6 years) and contained a higher proportion of patients with acute myeloid leukemia (AML, 30%). Fourteen percent of UCBT patients had undergone prior transplants for relapse (12 autologous, 2 allogeneic transplants). The median nucleated cell dose for UCBT was 3.8 × 10E7/kg (range of 2.4–36 × 10E7 cells/kg), one log less than that for UBMT or T-UBMT. HLA-A and -B antigens were determined serologically; HLA-DRB1 alleles were determined by HR DNA typing. Most UBMTs were 6/6 matches (81%); most T-UBMTs were 6/6 matches (54%) or one-antigen mismatched (34%). Most UCBTs were one-antigen mismatched (43%) or two-antigen mismatched (41%).

Myeloid engraftment post-transplantation (absolute neutrophil count ≥500/mm^3) occurred at a median of 32 days for UCBT compared to 18 days for UBMT and 16 days for T-UBMT. Platelet engraftment post-transplantation (platelet count ≥20,000/mm^3) occurred at a median of 81 days for UCBT compared to 29 days for both UBMT and T-UBMT. Treatment-related mortality at day 100 was significantly higher in the UCBT group (39%) compared with the other two groups (19% for UBMT and 14% for T-UBMT). The incidence of acute GVHD and the incidence of grades III/IV GVHD at day 100 was 35%/22% for UCBT, 58%/30% for UBMT, and 20%/8% for T-UBMT. The incidence of chronic GVHD was 25% for UCBT compared to 46% for UBMT and 12% for T-UBMT. A lower incidence of GVHD raises the theoretical concern that a diminished graft-versus-leukemia effect might lead to a higher relapse rate. In this study, relapse at 2 years was the same (38%) for both UCBT and UBMT, but 47% for T-UBMT. Survival at 2 years was 35% for UCBT compared to 49% for UBMT and 41% for T-UBMT. The conclusion of this report is that for children with acute leukemia who lack a matched sibling donor, a simultaneous search of bone marrow donor registries and cord blood banks should be done. The final choice for stem cell source balances donor–recipient histocompatibility with the urgency of the transplant, and the cell dose of the cord blood unit.

A subsequent Eurocord analysis focused exclusively on the role of cord blood transplantation (UCBT) in the treatment of relapsed or high-risk AML in children [6]. Many children with relapsed AML who will potentially benefit from bone marrow transplantation do not have an HLA-matched sibling donor or unrelated donor, or the search for an unrelated donor takes too long. UCBT can be performed safely with up to two-antigen mismatches, and the search process is much faster. This study identified 95 children with AML who underwent UCBT between 1994 and 2002 in 17 countries. The median age at transplantation was 6 years. Ten percent of patients had secondary AML (excluding patients with Fanconi's anemia). Half the patients were in second complete remission (CR2), 29% of patients were at high-risk by virtue of being in relapse or an advanced CR (beyond CR2), and 21% were in first complete remission (CR1). Most of this latter group had unfavorable cytogenetic abnormalities such as monosomy 5 or 7 or 11q23 abnormalities, or had secondary leukemia. Twenty-two patients had undergone prior hematopoietic stem cell transplants (18 autologous transplants in relapse, 4 unrelated marrow transplants with engraftment failure). HLA-A and -B antigens were determined serologically; HLA-DRB1 alleles were determined by HR DNA typing. Eighty percent of grafts were mismatched for one or two antigens; 11% were mismatched for three or more loci. The median collected cell dose was $5.2 \times 10E7$ cells/kg. Significantly, reflecting more recent UCBT practice, half of the patients received a hematopoietic growth factor in the early post-transplantation period.

Myeloid engraftment occurred at a median time of 26 days; six patients did not have neutrophil recovery by day +60. In multivariate analysis, the factors associated with neutrophil recovery were status of disease at transplantation (CR1 or CR2 were favorable) and prophylactic use of hematopoietic growth factor. Platelet engraftment occurred at a median time of 52 days (platelet count $\geq$20,000/mm^3); five patients did not have platelet recovery by day +180. The only significant factor associated with platelet recovery was disease status at the time of transplantation. The incidence of acute GVHD and the incidence of grades III/IV GVHD by day 100 were 35% and 20%, respectively. The incidence of chronic GVHD at 2 years was 15%. Treatment-related mortality (TRM, defined as all causes of non-leukemic deaths occurring after transplantation) was 20%; most of these deaths were caused by infection. In multivariate analysis, TRM was associated with a low collected nucleated cell dose (less than $5.2 \times 10E7$ cells/kg). Overall relapse incidence at 2 years was 29%. Not surprisingly, advanced disease at the time of transplantation (CR3 or higher or no CR) was associated with relapse: the relapse rate was 61% for patients who were not in remission at the time of UCBT. Overall survival and leukemia-free survival (LFS) at 2 years were 49% and 42%, respectively. Both these outcomes were significantly associated in multivariate analysis with disease status at the time of UCBT, and interestingly, by major ABO incompatibility. UCBT occurring after 1997 was significantly associated with LFS in univariate analysis.

The conclusions of this study were threefold. First, LFS after UCBT for childhood AML is associated with disease status at the time of transplantation; relapse incidences for the different stages of disease are felt to be comparable to those reported after unrelated bone marrow transplantation. Second, the outcome of

UCBT is not influenced by three traditional prognostic factors of childhood AML: unfavorable cytogenetics such as monosomy 5 or 7, secondary AML from prior chemoradiation or bone marrow stem cell disorder (such as myelodysplastic syndrome), and the duration of first CR for patients transplanted in CR2. This seems to support a potent graft-versus-leukemia effect for these subsets of traditionally poor-risk factors. Finally, treatment-related mortality (TRM) is significantly influenced by an adequate nucleated cell dose: above the median collected cell dose of 5.2 × 10E7 cells/kg, TRM was 9%, much lower than the overall TRM of 20%. Other studies have suggested that the impact of cell dose is even more significant with increasing HLA disparity (see later section). The effect of cell dose is correlated with infection as the major contributor to non-relapse mortality; this has implications for the prophylaxis and diagnosis of infection in UCBT.

A recent Eurocord update of 323 pediatric patients with acute lymphoblastic leukemia (ALL), who underwent UCBT for the period 1994–2004 was reported [7]. The median age was 6.5 years at UCBT; median cell dose infused was 4.1 × 10E7 cells/kg. Eighty-five percent of cord blood grafts were one- or two-antigen mismatches. Forty-two percent of patients ($n = 136$) were transplanted in second complete remission (CR2); 34% of patients ($n = 111$) were transplanted for advanced disease and 20% of this group had undergone prior autologous transplantation; the remaining were transplanted in first complete remission (CR1), and 89% of this group in CR1 had poor-risk cytogenetics. LFS at 2 years was 36% for the entire cohort. In multivariate analysis, CR1 and CR2 were associated with better LFS (41–42% for these two groups compared to 24% for the patients with advanced disease). The conclusion of this analysis is that UCBT should be offered for children lacking an HLA-identical donor, in an earlier disease state.

Another recent comparison of 503 children with acute leukemia who underwent UCBT and 282 children who underwent UBMT in the United States for the period 1995–2003 was reported on behalf of the New York Blood Center and the IBMTR [8]. All cord blood units were HLA-typed at the antigen level for HLA-A and HLA-B, and at allele level for HLA-DRB1. The majority of UCB grafts were mismatched at one ($n = 201$) or two ($n = 267$) antigens; only 35 were matched. The UBM grafts chosen for comparison had allele-level typing for HLA-A, -B, -C, and -DRB1: 116 were fully matched, 44 one-allele mismatched, and 122 two-allele mismatched. A high cell dose for UCBT was defined as greater than 3 × 10E7 cells/kg. There was no difference in neutrophil and platelet engraftment between the matched marrow recipients and the matched UCBT recipients. Surprisingly, the incidence of acute (grades III/IV) and chronic GVHD was not significantly different for UCBT, matched and mismatched compared to UBMT. Transplant related mortality was significantly higher for two-antigen mismatched UCBT at 46% compared to 21% for matched UBMT. LFS at 5 years was the primary outcome of the study: 60% for matched UCBT; 45% for one-antigen mismatched UCBT with a high cell dose; 38% for matched UBMT, 37% for mismatched UBMT; 36% for one-antigen mismatched UCBT with a low cell dose; and 33% two-antigen mismatched UCBT. These differences in LFS were not statistically significant. The conclusion of this study was that for pediatric patients with acute leukemia who are candidates for hematopoietic stem cell transplantation but do not have a sibling match, a simultaneous search for a suitable cord or marrow graft should be done. A UCB graft with up to two-antigen mismatches is comparable to a UBM graft with up to two-allele mismatches. Japan has successfully developed a network of cord blood banks in recent years. It has reported on 411 cord blood transplants for malignancies for the period 1997–2001, mostly in children [9]. However, unlike the Eurocord or New York Blood Bank/IBMTR data, a much higher proportion (65%) of UCBT was matched or one-antigen mismatched. Disease-free survival at 3-years was 35%; cell dose but not HLA disparity was associated with survival.

In conclusion, sufficient data exist to support comparable efficacy between HLA-matched unrelated marrow and matched or one-antigen mismatched UCB with an adequate cell dose for pediatric patients with acute leukemia. The minimum cell dose is not precisely defined, but should be around 2.5–3.0 × 10E7 nucleated cells/kg. In one study [10] CD34 cell dose (greater than 1.7 × 10E5 cells/kg) was the one factor significantly associated with rate of engraftment, treatment-related mortality, and survival.

Cord Blood Transplantation in Adults

In recent years, the use of UCBT in adults with hematologic malignancies has increased. Eurocord and the European Blood and Marrow Transplant Group performed a retrospective analysis of 682 adult patients with acute leukemia who had undergone UCBT ($n = 98$) or matched UBMT ($n = 584$) with myeloablative conditioning for the period 1998–2002 [11]. The UCBT patients were younger (median age 24.5 years vs. 32 years) and weighed less (median weight 58 kg vs. 68 kg) than the UBMT patients. More UCBT patients had advanced disease (52% beyond CR2 compared to 34%) at the time of transplantation, or had undergone a prior autologous transplant (19% vs. 8%). Ninety percent of UCBT were one- or two-antigen mismatches defined by serologic typing or low-resolution DNA typing for HLA-A and -B, and HR DNA typing for HLA-DRB1. The median cell dose was 2.3 × 10E7 nucleated cells/kg for UCBT recipients compared to 2.9 × 10E8 cells/kg for UBMT recipients. The median number of CD34+ cells in the cord blood grafts was 1.1 × 10E5 cells/kg. Consistent with the Eurocord pediatric series [5], 77% of UCBT recipients received antithymocyte or antilymphocyte globulin as part of their conditioning compared to 37% of UBMT patients. The predominant GVHD prophylaxis regimen was cyclosporine and corticosteroids (70%) in the UCBT patients, and cyclosporine and methotrexate (95%) in the UBMT patients. Data were not given on the use of post-transplant hematopoietic growth factors.

Myeloid engraftment was delayed in UCBT recipients, with the median time to neutrophil recovery occurring at day 26 compared to day 19 for UBMT recipients. The incidence of graft failure was high in this series: 7% in the marrow group and 20% in the cord blood group. The incidence of GVHD (grades II–IV) by day 100 was significantly lower in the UCBT group (26% vs. 39%). The 2-year cumulative incidence of chronic GVHD was 30% for UCBT and 46% for UBMT (not significant). There was no difference in treatment-related mortality (TRM, defined as all causes of non-leukemic deaths occurring after transplantation): 44% for UCBT and 38% for UBMT. However, causes of TRM were predominantly infections or toxicity for UCBT and infections or GVHD for UBMT. Relapse was associated with advanced disease; the rate was 23% for both groups. LFS and overall survival were also similar between the two groups: 33%/36% for UCBT and 38%/42% for UBMT. The conclusion of this study is that mismatched UCBT for acute leukemia in adults is a viable alternative to matched UBMT. Relative to UBMT, UCBT is associated with delayed myeloid recovery, but a lower incidence of acute GVHD despite HLA disparity. Both these outcomes are similar to the pediatric experience. Unlike the pediatric experience reported by the same group, transplant-related mortality was not higher for UCBT compared to UBMT, despite delayed neutrophil recovery which carries a high risk of infection. The fact that this adult series included transplants in a later period (1998–2002) probably points to improved experience managing prolonged neutropenia.

Rocha and colleagues subsequently updated their data to retrospectively compare 139 UCB transplants with 229 haploidentical T-cell-depleted transplants in patients with high-risk ALL ($n = 148$) and AML ($n = 220$) for the same period 1998–2002 [12]. In the AML group, both "alternative" stem cell sources had similar disease-free survival (24–30%) at 2 years. In the ALL group, the UCB patients had superior 2-year DFS compared to the haploidentical patients (36% vs. 13%, $p = 0.01$).

Another recent retrospective analysis of UCBT in adults [13] paints a slightly less promising picture. Data on adult patients who underwent UCBT (one or two HLA mismatches) through the national cord blood program of the New York Blood Center or unrelated marrow transplants (0 or 1 HLA mismatch) through the IBMTR for the period 1996–2001 in the United States were collected. There were 367 recipients of matched bone marrow (UBMT), 83 recipients of one-antigen mismatched bone marrow (UMBMT), and 150 recipients of one or two-antigen mismatched cord blood (UCBT). Patients who had undergone prior transplantation were excluded. UCBT patients were younger (median age around 30 years) and weighed less (median weight 68 kg). Unlike the Eurocord study above, hematologic diagnoses other than acute leukemia were included; specifically, the marrow recipients had a much higher proportion of patients with chronic myelogenous leukemia (CML) compared to the UCBT recipients (40% UBMT, 45% UMBMT, 25% UCBT). Similarly, the UBMT group had a higher proportion of good-risk patients (first complete remission, first chronic phase for CML, and refractory anemia): 40% for the UBMT group, 33% for the UMBMT group, 20% for UCBT. Conversely, the cord blood recipients had a much higher proportion of advanced disease (relapse, primary induction failure, CML blast crisis, or secondary AML from myelodysplastic syndrome): 43% for UCBT, 29% for UBMT, and 25% for UMBMT. The median cell dose was $2.2 \times 10E7$ cells/kg for the UCBT group compared to $2.2–2.4 \times 10E8$ cells/kg for the marrow recipients.

Consistent with prior studies, median times to neutrophil recovery were significantly longer in UCBT patients (27 days UCBT, 20 days UMBMT, and 18 days

UBMT). Median times to platelet recovery (platelet count >20,000/mm^3) were 60 days in UCBT, and 29 days for both marrow groups. The incidence of acute GVHD was the highest in the UMBMT group at 52%, and similar between the UCBT and UBMT groups (41% and 48%, respectively). The incidence of chronic GVHD was the highest in the UCBT group at 51% compared to 40% in the UMBMT group and 35% in the UBMT group although the proportion of patients with extensive chronic GVHD was the lowest in the UCBT group. Treatment-related mortality (all non-relapse causes of death) was the lowest for UBMT at 46% compared to 65% in the UMBMT group and 63% in the UCBT group. Relapse rates were similar in the three groups (17% UCBT, 14% UMBMT, 23% UBMT). LFS at 3 years was significantly higher for UBMT at 33% compared to 23% for UCBT and 19% for UMBMT; as expected, LFS was associated with age and disease status. Overall survival at 3 years was 35% for UBMT patients compared to 26% for UCBT patients and 20% for the UMBMT group. The conclusion of this study is that in the absence of a matched unrelated marrow donor, a one-antigen mismatched marrow graft or cord blood mismatched for one or two antigens are acceptable alternatives and have similar outcomes. The treatment-related mortality in this series appears high, even for the matched marrow recipients whose TRM was 46%, considering that 40% of this group of UBMT patients had good risk disease (CR1, CML first chronic phase, or refractory anemia).

Other recently published series support the notion that the outcome of UCBT in adults varies greatly. The Cord Blood Transplantation study group in the United States [14] reported on the adult subset of a prospective study of UCBT. Enrollment required a minimum of 1 × 10E7 nucleated cells/kg in the cord blood graft, and no more than two HLA mismatches at HLA-A and -B (low- or intermediate-resolution DNA typing) and HLA-DRB1 (high-resolution DNA typing). Thirty-four subjects with a median age of 35 years were entered. Most patients had a two-antigen mismatched graft. Diagnoses were predominantly acute leukemia (28/34 patients); most patients were determined to be at poor risk by National Marrow Donor Program criteria. The primary end point was survival at 180 days; the result was 30%.

In contrast, one single-institution study in Japan is much more promising [15]. This was a retrospective comparative analysis of 45 adults who received matched UBMT and 68 adults who received one or two-antigen mismatched UCBT for the period 1997–2003. Median age of the UCBT group was 36 years and median weight was 55 kg. More patients in the UCBT group had AML (57% vs. 33%); of the AML patients who received UCBT, more than half had advanced disease (beyond CR2). More patients in the UBMT group had CML (40% vs. 7%); 60% of CML patients who underwent UBMT had advanced disease. All UCBT patients received prophylactic G-CSF. Median cell dose was 2.5 × 10E7 cells/kg for the UCBT group, and 3.3 × 10E8 cells/kg for the UBMT group. The UBMT group was HLA-matched (87%) or one-antigen mismatched (13%). Three-quarters of the UCBT group were one- or two-antigen mismatched; one-quarter was three or four-antigen mismatched. Despite slower neutrophil (22 days vs.18 days) and platelet (40 days vs. 25 days) recoveries in UCBT patients, they had lower treatment-related mortality at 1 year (9% vs. 29%), and superior disease-free survival at 2 years (74% vs. 44%) compared with UBMT patients. Of note, relapse or refractory disease was the biggest contributor to UCBT deaths, not infection as in other series.

This same group recently updated their experience comparing 100 adults who received UCBT with 71 adults who received related donor grafts (55 bone marrow, 21 peripheral blood stem cell) for hematologic malignancies during 1997–2005 [16]. All patients received a TBI-containing myeloablative regimen. Most (76%) of the related grafts were fully matched for HLA-A, -B, and -DRB1. Of the cord blood grafts, the majority (54%) were two-antigen mismatches. Most patients received G-CSF post-transplant. Cumulative incidence of severe GVHD (grades III/IV) on day 100 was 7% for UCBT and 19% for the related transplants ($p = 0.04$). The cumulative incidence of extensive chronic GVHD at 3 years was 25% for UCBT and 45% for the related transplants ($p = 0.01$). Disease-free survival at 3 years was 70% for UCBT and 60% for related transplant, a difference that was not statistically significant. These are very encouraging statistics. Japan has developed a national cord blood transplantation program within a relatively short period of time with excellent results. The relative HLA homogeneity in this island country compared to the tremendous HLA diversity in a country such as the United States may play a role in these disparate outcomes.

In summary, UCBT in adult leukemia patients with an adequate cell dose is a viable alternative cell source for hematopoietic stem cell transplantation in the absence of an HLA-matched family or unrelated donor. Advances to overcome the limitation of cell dose, especially in the setting of HLA disparity in the future, will extend this option to a greater number of adult patients with hematologic malignancies or other acquired bone marrow disorders such as myelodysplastic syndrome.

New Strategies in Cord Blood Transplantation

Since an adequate cell dose from a single cord blood unit limits its wide applicability to adults, investigators explored the safety and efficacy of using two cord blood units to augment cell dose in high-risk adults and adolescents with hematologic malignancies [17]. Initially, patients were eligible for double-unit UCBT if no single unit containing at least 2.5 × 10E7 cells/kg was identified. Subsequently, eligibility was broadened to include patients who did not have a single unit containing at least 3.5 × 10E7 cells/kg. The largest available UCB unit (at least 1 × 10E7 cells/kg), which was 4–6 antigen matched to the recipient was selected (UCB #1). Then UCB #2 (at least 0.5 × 10E7 cells/kg) was selected to be 4–6 antigen matched to the recipient and to UCB#1. HLA disparity between each unit and the recipient and between the two units was not necessarily at the same loci. Twenty-three patients were included in this report, with a median age of 24 years and a median weight of 73 kg. All had acute leukemia considered to be at high risk of relapse, except one patient who had CML in chronic phase refractory to standard treatment. The median infused cell dose was 3.5 × 10E7 cells/kg combined from both UCB units. The median CD34+ cell dose was 4.9 × 10E5 cells/kg. Double-unit infusion was well tolerated. All patients received G-CSF post-infusion.

All 21 evaluable patients had sustained neutrophil engraftment at a median of 23 days; no patient had secondary graft failure. Hematopoiesis on day 21 bone marrow analysis showed 100% single-donor chimerism in 16/21 (76%) patients and dual-donor chimerism in the remainder; by day 100, all patients (17/17 alive) had single-donor chimerism. The graft factor predictive of engraftment was not the nucleated cell dose or the CD34+ cell dose, but a higher CD3+ cell dose. Of the 8/21 patients who received two UCB units with different degrees of HLA disparity, the better HLA-matched unit predominated in four patients, while the lesser matched unit predominated in four patients. The incidence of grades II–IV GVHD and grades III–IV GVHD was 65% and 13%, respectively. Cumulative incidence of chronic GVHD was 23%. Transplantation-related mortality at 6 months was 22%. Major causes of death were infection or relapse; no patient died of GVHD. Leukemia-free survival at 1 year was 57%, with the major predictor being disease status at the time of transplantation. The conclusion of this study is that double-unit UCBT produces durable single-donor engraftment without any apparent excess of GVHD. A higher CD3+ cell dose determined which unit predominated, which supports the hypothesis that donor predominance is immune-mediated. This strategy enables many more adult patients to have access to UCB grafts (graft made up one or two units) containing an adequate cell dose.

Another approach toward achieving an adequate cell dose is to use ex vivo expansion of UCB cells [18]. A phase 1 trial showed that one particular device was able to expand nucleated cells in UCB 2.4-fold but expansion of CD34+ cells was less successful. Twenty-eight patients enrolled in the trial, of whom only three were over 60 kg. The expanded cells were infused on day 12 and infusion was well tolerated. However, augmentation of UCB transplants with ex vivo-expanded cells did not alter the time to myeloid or platelet engraftment in 21 evaluable patients. The inability to expand primitive stem cells (CD34+lin-) is of some concern although it is possible that this could be improved with a different combination of early-acting cytokines. It is also not possible with this scheme to detect if the expanded cells are contributing to hematopoiesis since they were derived from the original UCB graft.

Along similar lines, other investigators have used low-dose peripheral blood CD34+ cells from a related HLA-haploidentical donor with a primary unrelated umbilical cord blood graft [19]. Eleven adult patients with poor-risk acute leukemia who did not have an HLA-matched donor (related or unrelated) or UCB unit with more than 4.0 × 10E7 cells/kg were studied. Median age was 23 years and median weight was 66 kg. The cord blood grafts were up to two-antigen mismatched containing a median infused cell dose of 2 × 10E7 cells/kg, and a median CD34+ cell dose (available for 7/11 units) of 1.1 × 10E5 cells/kg. Haploidentical donors were siblings who shared a paternal HLA haplotype with the patient ($n = 6$), the mother ($n = 4$), and one father. The haploidentical CD34+ cells were obtained from the family donor by G-CSF mobilization, apheresis, and positive selection, then cryopreserved; the median CD34+ dose of haploidentical cells was 2.3 × 10E6 cells/kg.

Two patients died before myeloid engraftment: one from grade IV GVHD, one from multiorgan failure; both had received maternal haploidentical cells. The remaining nine patients reached an absolute neutrophil count >0.5 × 10E9/L at a median of 11 days in 7/9 patients, neutrophils and mononuclear cells were initially primarily of haploidentical derivation, with subsequent shift to the cord blood genotype; the remaining two patients, both of whom received maternal haploidentical cells, achieved myeloid engraftment with full chimerism of CB cells on days +20 and +36. Complete chimerism exclusively of cord blood cells developed in eight patients, at a median of 30 days. Platelet engraftment (platelet count >20,000/mm^3) occurred at a median of 43 days. Acute GVHD occurred in 6/11 patients (55%) with one death directly attributable to grade IV GVHD. Disease-free survival at 3 years was 40%. CMV infection caused half the deaths. This study achieved the goal of shortening the period of neutropenia (compared to a single-unit cord blood transplant) with neutrophils derived from the haploidentical CD34+ cells. A haploidentical donor is easily available within the patient's family. There is a suggestion that acute GVHD may be potentially more severe with this approach compared to the double-unit cord blood transplant strategy.

In peripheral blood stem cell transplantation, there has been recent interest in the use of non-myeloablative or "reduced-intensity" preparative regimens to reduce regimen-related toxicity and therefore broaden transplant eligibility to older patients with co-morbid medical conditions that may preclude the use of myeloablative conditioning. The key component of such an approach rests on the graft-versus-malignancy effect, which takes time. Several regimens are widely used with varying degrees of myelotoxicity and immunosuppression. Most protocols are exploring the use of such regimens in diseases that have a slower rate of progression (for example, low-grade lymphoma and not acute leukemia) and for which myeloablative allogeneic stem cell transplantation is not the standard of care [20].

The largest single-institution experience with non-myeloablative chemotherapy regimens in unrelated cord blood transplantation included 95 consecutive adults (median age 50, range 18–69, median weight 78 kg), who received fludarabine/cyclophosphamide/TBI (200 cGy) with anti-thymocyte globulin in less heavily pretreated patients [21]. The median cell dose of 3.6 × 10E7 cells/kg was mostly achieved with double-unit cord blood grafts. Most cord blood units were HLA-mismatched at one or two loci. GVHD prophylaxis consisted of cyclosporine and mycophenolate for most patients. Sustained donor engraftment was achieved in 87% of patients. The incidence of acute severe GVHD at day 100 was 25% and the incidence of chronic GVHD at 1 year was 25%. Disease-free and overall survival at 2 years were 43% and 44%, respectively.

Another recent single-institution series [22] included 21 adults transplanted for hematologic malignancies and aplastic anemia with double cord transplants and fludarabine/melphalan/ATG conditioning. The median cell dose was 4.0 × 10E7 cells/kg. Most cord blood units were HLA-mismatched at one or two loci (molecular typing was used for HLA-A, -B, and -DRB1). GVHD prophylaxis consisted of cyclosporine and mycophenolate. Three patients had graft failure (two early, one late). Only 1/21 patients had severe (grades III/IV) acute GVHD, although 40% of patients had grades II–IV GVHD. Disease-free survival at 1 year was 67%.

High-resolution HLA typing by sequencing for HLA-A, -B, -C, -DR, -DQ has become available recently. To determine the impact of HR HLA typing on outcomes after UCBT, DNA of 122 unrelated cord blood graft/recipient pairs were analyzed for mismatches, and compared to the data from the traditional determination of HLA disparity (HLA-A, -B on low-resolution typing, and HLA-DRB1 on HR typing) [23]. By the traditional approach, 13% were fully matched, 40% were one-antigen mismatched, 36% were two-antigen mismatched, 8% were three-antigen mismatched, and 3% were four antigen-matched. By the HR approach, 4% were fully matched, 10% were one-antigen mismatched, 15% two-antigen mismatched, 22% three-antigen mismatched, 25% four-antigen mismatched, 12% five-antigen mismatched, 6% six-antigen mismatched, 5% seven- or eight-antigen mismatched. Remarkably, there was no significant correlation between the number of HR mismatches on the one hand, and acute GVHD grades II–IV and 2-year survival on the other. However, HLA-A locus mismatches on HR typing analyzed in the host-versus-graft direction was associated with reduced cumulative incidence of engraftment. Killer-cell immunoglobulin-like receptor incompatibility for HLA-C in the host-versus-graft direction was also significantly associated with impaired engraftment. Although the role of HR typing in UCBT remains to be defined, it is unlikely to change current practice until the donor pool of cord blood units enlarges.

Conclusion

Unrelated cord blood transplantation has a well-established role in pediatric patients with hematologic malignancies: matched or one-antigen mismatched grafts are equivalent if not superior to matched unrelated marrow in this setting. Of course, the power of cord blood transplantation is the ability to transplant across greater HLA barriers. Two-antigen mismatched grafts produce very encouraging results for children who are transplanted in an early disease state (but have high-risk factors such as unfavorable cytogenetics).

An adequate cell dose is critical to the outcome of cord blood transplantation. Recent practice includes a nucleated cell dose of $2.5 \times 10E7$ cells/kg, or a CD34+ cell dose of $1.7 \times 10E5$ cells/kg. Cell dose appears to be particularly important in the setting of greater HLA disparity.

More UCBT has been performed in adults in recent years as the availability of larger banked cord blood units has improved. As with all UCBT studies, prospective randomized trials are not possible. Two recent retrospective comparisons of UCBT and unrelated marrow transplantation have somewhat different outcomes, but both support the notion that an UCBT with one or two antigen mismatches and an adequate cell dose is a viable option for adults with hematologic malignancies and no matched marrow donor. One single-institution report from Japan has particularly impressive results but may not be reproducible in another country, given Japan's unique population HLA makeup.

Institutional experience is important because prolonged neutropenia and delayed immune reconstitution are expected for UCBT. One single-institution retrospective analysis showed that overall infection rates were higher in UCB recipients compared to recipients of matched unrelated marrow (or peripheral blood stem cells), particularly before day 50, when gram-positive bacteremias predominated. In a larger Eurocord analysis of 510 UCBTs for the period 1994–2002, the incidences of overall, bacterial, viral, and fungal infections were 69%, 49%, 32%, and 10%, respectively. Shorter time to engraftment and UCBT performed after 1998 decreased the risk of all three types of infection in multivariate analysis. CMV seropositivity and HLA disparity (more than three-antigen mismatches) were associated with viral infection. Older age (>16 years) and presence of grades III/IV GVHD were associated with fungal infections. Prevention and management of infection are clearly very important areas of clinical study [24, 25].

New strategies such as double-unit cord blood transplantation or co-transplantation with haploidentical CD34+ cells or mesenchymal stem cells [26, 27] will help to shorten the period of cytopenias, elucidate the mechanisms of cord blood engraftment and broaden the applicability of UCBT to more patients especially adults. Pathophysiologic mechanisms of a preserved graft-versus-malignancy effect in the face of a low incidence of severe GVHD in cord blood grafting will shed light on this "holy grail" of allogeneic stem cell transplantation [3]. The field of cord blood transplantation holds promise for many patients who have few other options, but its success is critically dependent on a broad donor pool particularly for ethnic minorities that are under-represented in traditional bone marrow registries.

References

1. Gluckman E, Broxmeyer HA, Auerbach AD, et al. (1989) Hematopoietic reconstitution in a patient with Fanconi's anemia by means of umbilical-cord blood from an HLA-identical sibling. N Engl J Med 321:1174–1178.
2. Rocha V, Wagner J, Sobocinski K, et al. (2000) Graft-versus-host disease in children who have received a cord-blood or bone marrow transplant from an HLA-identical sibling. N Engl J Med 342: 1846–1854.
3. Tse W, Laughlin M. (2005) Umbilical cord blood transplantation: a new alternative option. In: Berliner N, Lee S, Linenberger M, Vogelsang G, editors. Hematology 2005. Washington, DC: American Society of Hematology pp. 377–383.
4. Rubinstein P, Carrier C, Scaradavou A, et al. (1998) Outcomes among 562 recipients of placental-blood transplants from unrelated donors. N Engl J Med 339:1565–1577.
5. Rocha V, Cornish J, Sievers E, et al. (2001) Comparison of outcomes of unrelated bone marrow and umbilical cord blood transplants in children with acute leukemia. Blood 97: 2962–2971.
6. Michel G, Rocha V, Chevret S, et al. (2003) Unrelated cord blood transplantation for childhood acute myeloid leukemia: a Eurocord group analysis. Blood 102:4290–4297.
7. Rocha V, Michel G, Kabbara N, et al. (2005) Outcomes after unrelated cord blood transplantation in children with acute lymphoblastic leukemia. A Eurocord-Netcord survey. Blood 106:93a.
8. Eapen M, Rubinstein P, Zhang M, et al. (2007) Outcomes of transplantation of unrelated donor umbilical cord blood and bone marrow in children with acute leukaemia: a comparison study. Lancet 369:1947–1954.
9. Isoyama K, Ohnuma K, Kato K et al. (2003) Cord blood transplantation from unrelated donors: a preliminary report from the Japanese cord blood bank network. Leuk Lymphoma 44:429-438.

10. Wagner J, Barker J, DeFor T, et al. (2002) Transplantation of unrelated donor umbilical cord blood in 102 patients with malignant and nonmalignant diseases: influence of CD34 cell dose and HLA disparity on treatment-related mortality and survival. Blood 100:1611–1618.
11. Rocha V, Labopin M, Sanz G, et al. (2004) Transplants of umbilical cord blood or bone marrow from unrelated donors in adults with acute leukemia. N Engl J Med 351:2276–2285.
12. Rocha V, Aversa F, Labopin M, et al. (2005) Outcomes of unrelated cord blood and haploidentical stem cell transplantation in adults with acute leukaemia. Blood 106:92a.
13. Laughlin M, Eapen M, Rubinstein P, et al. (2004) Outcomes after transplantation of cord blood or bone marrow from unrelated donors in adults with leukemia. N Engl J Med 351:2265–2275.
14. Cornetta K, Laughlin M, Carter S, et al. (2005) Umbilical cord blood transplantation in adults: results of the prospective cord blood transplantation (COBLT). Biol Blood Marrow Transplant 11:149–160.
15. Takahashi S, Iseki T, Ooi J, et al.(2004) Single-institute comparative analysis of unrelated bone marrow transplantation and cord blood transplantation for adult patients with hematologic malignancies. Blood 104:3813–3820.
16. Takahashi S, Ooi J, Tomonari A, et al. (2007) Comparative single-institute analysis of cord blood transplantation from unrelated donors with bone marrow or peripheral blood stem-cell transplants from related donors in adult patients with hematologic malignancies after myeloablative conditioning regimen. Blood 109:1322–1330.
17. Barker J, Weisdorf D, DeFor T, et al. (2005) Transplantation of two partially HLA-matched umbilical cord blood units to enhance engraftment in adults with hematologic malignancy. Blood 105:1343–1347.
18. Jaroscak J, Goltry K, Smith A, et al. (2003) Augmentation of umbilical cord blood (UCB) transplantation with ex vivo-expanded UCB cells: results of a phase 1 trial using the Aastrom-Replicell system. Blood 101:5061–5067.
19. Fernandez M, Regidor C, Cabrera R, et al. (2003) Unrelated umbilical cord blood transplants in adults: early recovery of neutrophils by supportive co-transplantation of a low number of highly purified peripheral blood CD34+ cells from an HLA-haploidentical donor. Exp Hematol 31:535–544.
20. Childs R, Chernoff A, Contentin N et al. (2000) Regression of metastatic renal-cell carcinoma after nonmyeloablative allogeneic peripheral-blood stem-cell transplantation. N Engl J Med 343:750–758.
21. Brunstein CG, Barker JN, Defor TE, et al. (2005) Non-myeloablative umbilical cord blood transplantation: promising disease-free survival in 95 consecutive patients. Blood 106:166a.
22. Ballen K, Spitzer T, Yeap, B et al. (2007) Double unrelated reduced-intensity umbilical cord blood transplantation in adults. Biol Blood Marrow Transplant 13:82–89.
23. Kogler G, Enczmann J, Rocha V, et al. (2005) High-resolution HLA typing by sequencing for HLA-A, B, C,DR, DQ in 122 unrelated cord blood/patient pair transplants hardly improves long-term clinical outcome. Bone Marrow Transplant 36:1033–1041.
24. Hamza H, Lisgaris M, Yadavalli G, et al. (2004) Kinetics of myeloid and lymphocyte recovery and infectious complications after unrelated umbilical cord blood versus HLA-matched unrelated donor allogeneic transplantation in adults. Br J Haematol 124:488–498.
25. Rocha V, Chevret S, Ionescu I, et al. (2004) Incidence and risk factors of early severe infections after unrelated cord blood transplantation. A Eurocord-Netcord analysis. Blood 104:590a.
26. Macmillan M, Ramsay N, Atkinson K, et al. (2002) Ex-vivo culture-expanded parental haploidentical mesenchymal stem cells to promote engraftment in recipients of unrelated donor umbilical cord blood: results of a phase I-II clinical trial. Blood 100:836a.
27. Kim D, Chung Y, Kim T, et al. (2004) Cotransplantation of third-party mesenchymal stromal cells can alleviate single-donor predominance and increase engraftment from double cord transplantation. Blood 103:1941–1948.

Chapter 9
Double Umbilical Cord Blood Transplantation in Adults

Karen K. Ballen

The first successful cord blood transplant was reported in 1989 in a child with Fanconi's anemia. Over the last 18 years, there has been a dramatic growth in the use of cord blood as an alternative stem cell source for patients without matched related or unrelated bone marrow donors. Initially, the majority of transplants were performed in children. Recently, the results in adult cord blood transplantation appear promising. We will address in this chapter outcome data for adult cord blood transplantation, with an emphasis on new techniques using double or sequential cord blood transplantation. New indications for cord blood use outside of hematology/oncology will also be explored.

Pre-Clinical Background

Work in the laboratories of Broxmeyer, Knudtzon, Lansford, Metcalf, and others showed that neonatal and cord blood contained a high number of granulocyte-macrophage progenitor cells [1]. Neonatal mice contained adequate progenitor cells for bone marrow reconstitution in irradiated mice [2]. Human cord blood was then shown to have sufficient progenitor cells to provide consistent hematopoietic engraftment [3]. These studies provided the scientific support for the initial trials with cord blood transplantation.

Further work, after some of the initial clinical studies, revealed the unique immunologic properties of umbilical cord blood. Cord blood CD34+ cells in culture increase in cell number every 7–10 days, several hundred folds greater than the increase in cultures of similar cells from adult bone marrow, thereby allowing a 10-fold lower CD34+ cell dose to be used for successful cord blood transplantation [4]. Cord blood cells have greater proliferative capacity; longer telomere length has been proposed as a possible explanation [5].

K.K. Ballen (✉)
Massachusetts General Hospital, Zero Emerson, Suite 118. Boston, MA 02114, USA
e-mail: kballen@partners.org

N. Bhattacharya, P. Stubblefield (eds.), *Frontiers of Cord Blood Science*,
DOI 10.1007/978-1-84800-167-1_9,

The immunologic properties of cord blood differ from mature bone marrow or peripheral blood stem cells, which may contribute to the decreased graft-versus-host disease (GVHD) following cord blood transplantation, with preservation of a graft-versus-leukemia effect [6, 7]. Cord blood contains a high proportion of "naive" phenotype T cells that are CD45RA+/CD45RO− and CD62L+ [8]. The chemokine receptor CCR5, expressed by TH1 T cells, is less abundant among cord blood T cells than adult T cells [9]. Cord blood T cell receptors when compared with adult blood T-cell receptors, have a less complex repertoire [10]. Cord blood cells express T cells with less clonal diversity than expressed by adult peripheral blood.

Cord Blood Unit Availability

Potential human leucocyte antigen (HLA)-matched cord blood units can be found for patients in computerized registries such as National Marrow Donor Program (NMDP), Netcord, the New York Blood Center, and other international registries. Currently, Bone Marrow Donors Worldwide lists 250,000 available cord blood units from 35 different cord blood banks in 21 countries [11]. Most of the units have molecular typing available for Class II HLA alleles, and about half of the units have Class I molecular typing available. In the United States, the NMDP currently lists 50,000 cord blood units [12]. The search process and determination of match can be quite complex, especially when looking for more than one cord blood donor [13]. Searching for a cord blood donor is generally faster than for a bone marrow donor, as there is no living donor to find, contact, retest, and consent [14].

One of the goals of the cord blood program is to increase the number of donations from non-Caucasian donors, since non-Caucasian patients have a more difficult time locating matched donors through the NMDP and other international registries. In the early years of cord blood banking, we found no increase in cord blood donations from minority donors as compared to donations from minority donors to bone marrow registries in the same United States geographic area [15]. In fact, in three of the areas surveyed – California, Florida, and Massachusetts – the cord blood banks recruited a lower percentage of minorities than the corresponding bone marrow donor centers.

As visibility of the cord banking efforts grew, a more diverse donor population was recruited. The American Red Cross cord blood banks revealed a diverse donor population: 64% Caucasian, 16% African American, 12% Hispanic, 4% Asian, 1% Native American, and 3% others [16]. An unexpected finding was a lower CD34+ count for African American donors in the Midwest, Northwest, and North Carolina collection sites. Since the average unit from black donors has a lower CD34+ count, an important prognostic factor, more units may need to be collected to list those with a suitable cell dose. The Cord Blood Transplantation Study (COBLT) also showed lower CD34+/CD38− population in African American and Asian donors [17].

Clinical Studies in Cord Blood Transplantation

Studies in Children – Related Cord Blood Transplants

The first cord blood transplants were performed in children. Lessons learned from the pediatric experience have allowed us to successfully transplant adults. The experience with adult and pediatric cord blood transplantation has been recently reviewed [18, 19].

Umbilical cord blood has been used successfully in related transplants for both malignant and non-malignant diseases [7]. The Eurocord group reported on 102 children with acute leukemia receiving cord blood transplants; forty-two received a related donor transplant [20]. Twelve of these patients received a mismatched graft; neutrophil engraftment was 84% and two-year event free survival was 41%. A nucleated cell dose $>3.7 \times 10$ (7)/kg correlated with engraftment. For non-malignant diseases, there has been experience in patients with thalassemia and sickle cell disease. In the Eurocord study, the 100-day transplant related mortality was 0; four patients experienced grade 2 acute GVHD [21]. One patient with sickle cell disease and seven patients with thalassemia did not have sustained donor engraftment. The two-year probability of event-free survival was 79% for thalassemia, and 90% for sickle cell anemia. Cord blood, which is a naturally T-cell depleted product, has a low risk of GVHD, and may be well suited to the treatment of non malignant diseases, as there is no advantage to GVHD/graft versus leukemia.

Since randomized studies between cord blood and bone marrow would be difficult to accomplish, Rocha et al. performed a retrospective case control study. One hundred and thirteen related cord blood recipients were compared with 2052 related bone marrow recipients [22]. Transplant related mortality was similar between the two groups, although the incidence of GVHD was lower in the recipients of cord blood transplants.

Studies in Children – Unrelated Cord Blood Transplants

The first 25 unrelated cord blood transplants were reported in 1996 by the Duke Transplant Team [23]. Thirty percent of these patients were non-Caucasian, and had searched for an unrelated marrow donor for at least six months. The cord blood unit and the patient were mismatched at 1–3 HLA loci. Twenty-three of 25 patients engrafted. Two patients had GVHD, and the event-free survival was 48% with a median follow-up of 12 months. These data suggested that engraftment could occur even with cord blood units that were mismatched at two loci and that the risk of severe GVHD was low.

The University of Minnesota reported on 102 children, with malignant and non-malignant diseases, transplanted with unrelated umbilical cord blood [24]. Although the incidence of GVHD was low (severe acute GVHD was seen in 11% of patients and chronic GVHD in 10% of patients), the risk of leukemia relapse was also low,

17% for standard risk patients, and 45% for high-risk patients, supporting a preservation of the graft-versus-leukemia effect. These data support a preservation of the graft-versus-leukemia effect without clinical graft-versus-host disease.

Cord blood transplantation has also been shown to be effective in metabolic storage diseases. Twenty children with Hurler's syndrome received conditioning with busulfan, cyclophosphamide, and anti-thymocyte globulin followed by infusion of unrelated, 1, 2, or 3 antigen-mismatched cord blood [25]. With a median follow-up of 905 days, 17 of 20 children are alive with complete donor chimerism and normal peripheral blood alpha-1-iduronidase activity. The low risk of GVHD with cord blood transplantation suggests a unique role for cord blood transplantation for children with non-malignant diseases.

The pediatric experience has provided guidance in developing a successful adult cord blood transplant program. The pediatric data indicate that engraftment can occur without a high risk of GVHD, even if the patient and cord blood donor are mismatched at two antigens [24]. Therefore, the potential donor pool is considerably increased from unrelated bone marrow or peripheral blood stem cells. The incidence of severe GVHD is low, but a graft-versus-leukemia effect is preserved. The cell dose infused is consistently an important marker for improved engraftment and survival; engraftment, particularly platelet engraftment, is prolonged after cord blood transplantation.

Studies in Adults – Single Cord Blood Transplants – Ablative Regimens

In the last 5 years, there has been increased interest in cord blood transplantation for adult patients. Only 30% of patients have a matched sibling donor, and cord blood offers an alternative stem cell source. The initial cord blood studies were performed using single cord blood units, and are outlined in Table 9.1. Laughlin et al. analyzed a large American experience in 68 adults, median age 31 years, who received cord blood transplants [26]. The incidence of neutrophil engraftment was 90%, but the median time to engraftment was 27 days, longer than in historical controls of unrelated bone marrow. A higher number of CD34+ cells in the cord blood units correlated with improved engraftment and survival. Transplant-related mortality was high in this series; 47% of patients died prior to Day +100, with infection the leading cause of death. With a median follow-up of 22 months, the disease-free survival was 26%.

Results in most other adult cord blood transplant studies using single cord blood units have been poor. In a study by Long and colleagues, 57 adult patients with high-risk disease underwent single cord blood transplantation [27]. The median days to neutrophil and platelet engraftment were 26 and 84 respectively. The transplant related mortality at Day +100 was 50%, with the majority of deaths related to infection. Actuarial projected three-year survival was only 19%.

The Cord Blood Transplantation Study Group (COBLT) reported on results of 34 adult patients with high-risk disease receiving cord blood transplantation [28].

Table 9.1 Adult cord blood transplant: single unit ablative regimen

Investigator	*N*	Diseases	Conditioning regimen	Median follow-up (months)	Disease-free survival (%)
Laughlin	68	CML, AML, CLL, ALL, lymphoma	Cy/TBI or Bu/CY/ATG	22	26
Long	57	CML, AML, CLL, ALL, lymphoma, other	Cy/TBI or Bu/Cy/ATG	56	19
Laughlin	116	CML, AML, MDS, ALL	Multiple	40	23
Rocha	98	AML, ALL	Multiple	27	33
Takahashi	68	AML, ALL, MDS, CML, lymphoma	TBI/Cy or TBI/ARA-C	25	76
Cornetta	34	AML,ALL, MDS, lymphoma	TBI/Cy Busulfan/ Melphalan		30 (at 6 months)

AML: Acute myelogeneous Leukemia; ALL: Acute Lymphoblastic Leukemia; CML: Chronic myelogeneous Leukemia; MDS: Myelodysplasia; TBI: total body radiation; Cy:cyclophosphamide; ARA-C: cytosine arabinoside; ATG: anti-thymocyte globulin

The median nucleated cell dose was low at 1.7×10^7 NC/kg; primary graft failure occurred in 28% of patients and there were only two long-term survivors.

Two reports of retrospective case-control studies comparing unrelated bone marrow transplants to unrelated umbilical cord blood transplants in adults were reported in the New England Journal of Medicine in 2004. The International Bone Marrow Transplant Registry compared survival after unrelated umbilical cord blood transplants to survival after unrelated bone marrow transplants [29]. One hundred and sixteen adults with leukemia receiving unrelated, one or two antigen mismatched cord blood transplants were compared with 367 adults receiving matched unrelated donor bone marrow transplants and 83 patients receiving 1 antigen mismatched bone marrow transplants. Deaths related to infection were highest in the cord blood recipients, but acute GVHD was more common in the mismatched bone marrow cohort. Three-year leukemia-free survival was highest (33%) for patients receiving HLA-matched unrelated bone marrow transplants, but comparable (23% for cord blood and 19% for one antigen mismatched bone marrow) for patients receiving the other two donor sources.

The Eurocord group reported results of a retrospective study comparing outcomes of 98 adults with acute leukemia receiving unrelated one or two antigen mismatched cord blood with 584 adults with acute leukemia receiving unrelated matched bone marrow transplants [30]. Neutrophil recovery was delayed after cord blood transplant (26 days versus 19 days). Graft failure occurred in 20% of the cord blood recipients, and 7% of the bone marrow recipients. Although the incidence of acute GVHD was 26% after cord blood transplant, and 39% after unrelated bone marrow transplant, relapse rates were similar. Therefore, this data suggests that the graft-versus-leukemia effect is preserved in cord blood recipients, even without a high rate of clinical GVHD. The two-year leukemia-free survival was comparable in both groups, 33% for cord blood and 38% for unrelated bone marrow. This study suggests (in contrast to the American study above) that outcomes after cord blood transplant may be similar to outcomes after matched unrelated bone marrow transplant.

The results of the American and European studies indicate a survival of 20–35% after unrelated single cord blood transplantation in adults. In contrast, the Japanese group has reported excellent outcomes after single adult cord blood transplantation. The outcomes of 68 adult unrelated cord blood recipients were compared with 45 adult unrelated bone marrow recipients. The 100-day transplant related mortality was a remarkably low 9% for cord blood recipients and 29% for unrelated bone marrow recipients. The two-year probability of disease free survival was 74% for cord blood and 44% for unrelated bone marrow [31]. These results are superior to those reported in the American and European series, perhaps due to the smaller size and genetic homogeneity of this population. Therefore, in Japan, unrelated cord blood is often selected as the preferred stem cell source, even when a matched unrelated donor is available.

Adult Cord Blood Transplantation – Single Cord Blood – Reduced Intensity Regimen

Non-myeloablative or reduced intensity transplant regimens have been used extensively over the last 5 years, to reduced transplant related mortality in patients who are older or who have comorbid features (Table 9.2) [32,33]. The use of this approach is particularly important given the average age of patients at diagnosis of leukemia and lymphoma is 60 years old. The Japanese group treated 20 patients with refractory lymphoma with a reduced intensity regimen of low dose total body radiation, fludarabine, and melphalan, followed by unrelated cord blood transplantation [34]. Transplant-related mortality continued to be similar to a myeloablative regimen, at 41% in this high-risk group of patients. Estimated progression-free

Table 9.2 Adult cord blood transplantation: single unit reduced intensity regimen

Investigator	*N*	Diseases	Conditioning regimen	Median follow-up (months)	Disease-free survival (%)
Miyakoshi	30	AML, ALL, CML, MDS, lymphoma	Fludarabine, Melphalan, low dose TBI	8	33
Chao	13	AML, ALL, MDS, lymphoma	Fludarabine, Cyclophosphamide, ATG	20	24
Yuji	20	Lymphoma	Fludarabine, Melphalan, low dose TBI	12	50

AML: Acute myelogeneous Leukemia; ALL: Acute Lymphoblastic Leukemia; CML: Chronic myelogeneous Leukemia; MDS: Myelodysplasia; TBI: total body radiation; ATG: anti-thymocyte globulin survival was 50%. Thirty patients with refractory leukemias received a similar approach. The transplanted-related mortality, even with a reduced intensity approach, was high at 27% and 1-year overall survival was 33% [35]. The graft failure rate after reduced intensity cord blood transplantation was estimated to be 7% in one retrospective review of 123 patients [36].

The Duke group used a reduced intensity approach, with a conditioning regimen of fludarabine, cyclophosphamide, and horse anti-thymocyte globulin, in 13 refractory hematologic malignancy patients receiving single cord blood units [37]. There was only one treatment-related death prior to 100 days. The one-year event-free survival was 43%.

These studies show that engraftment is delayed and transplant-related mortality is high in adult patients, receiving single cord blood transplants. Most of the deaths, using either a myeloablative or reduced intensity approach, have been due to infection. The cell dose (either nucleated cell/kg or CD34+ cells/kg) correlated with outcome in most studies. Therefore, strategies to improve outcomes have included increasing the cell dose administered by sequential or double cord blood transplantation. Cord blood expansion is another option to improve engraftment and is discussed elsewhere in this book.

Adult Cord Blood Transplantation – Double Cord Blood Transplantation – Myeloablative Regimen

Sequential or double cord blood transplant describes the transplantation of two or more partially matched cord blood units, given to the same patient several hours apart. Thus, the cord blood units are "pooled" in the patient's body, "in vivo." Although immunologic rejection might be a concern with this approach, an early case report of patients infused with multiple, mismatched units suggested that crossed immunologic rejection would not occur [38].

The University of Minnesota transplant program tested the two cord blood unit approach, in both the ablative and reduced intensity setting, as illustrated in Table 9.3. Barker and colleagues treated 23 adults with hematologic malignancies with an ablative conditioning regimen of cytoxan, total body irradiation, and

Table 9.3 Adult cord blood transplantation: double unit ablative regimen

Investigator	*N*	Diseases	Conditioning	Median follow-up (months)	Disease-free survival (%)
Mao	6	Aplastic Anemia	Cytoxan/ATG	20	67
Barker	23	AML, ALL, CML, lymphoma	Cy/TBI/Fludarabine	10	57

AML: Acute myelogeneous Leukemia; ALL: Acute Lymphoblastic Leukemia; CML: Chronic myelogeneous Leukemia; TBI: total body radiation; ATG: anti-thymocyte globulin fludarabine [39]. Each patient received two cord blood units, 4/6 HLA match or better with each other and with the patient. The combined median nucleated cell dose was 3.5×10^7 NC/kg. All 21 evaluable patients engrafted, with a median days to ANC > 500 of 23. Initial chimerism studies revealed the presence of both cord blood units, with one unit predominating by day +100.

Aplastic anemia has also been successfully treated with cord blood transplantation. In a Chinese study, six patients with severe aplastic anemia were conditioned with cyclophosphamide and anti-lymphocyte globulin [40]. Three patients received one cord blood unit and three patients received two cord blood units. Two patients died of infection; five patients had stable mixed chimerism, and four of six are alive and disease-free with a median follow-up of 20 months.

Adult Double Cord Blood Transplantation – Reduced Intensity Regimen

The results of double cord blood transplantation using a reduced intensity regimen are outlined in Table 9.4. Barker and colleagues transplanted either one or two cord blood units to achieve a minimum cell dose of 3.5 × 10 (7) nucleated cells/kg [41]. Patients whose cord blood unit did not meet this cell dose criteria received the double cord blood transplant. Cord blood units were a 4/6 HLA match or better with the patients and with each other. Twenty-one patients received conditioning with busulfan/fludarabine/low dose TBI and 22 patients (the second cohort) received cyclophosphamide/fludarabine/low dose TBI. Cyclosporine and mycophenolate mofetil (MMF) were used for GVHD prophylaxis. Twenty-four of the 43 patients received two cord blood units. The first regimen with busulfan had an incidence of neutrophil engraftment of 76%, with the median days to an ANC of 500 of 26 days. One-hundred-day transplant-related mortality was 48%. The second regimen with cyclophosphamide had an incidence of neutrophil engraftment of 94% with the median days to an ANC of 500 of 10 days. One-hundred-day

Table 9.4 Adult cord blood transplantation: double unit, reduced intensity regimen

Investigator	*N*	Diseases	Conditioning	Median follow-up (months)	Disease-free survival (%)
Barker	24	AML, ALL, CML, MDS, lymphoma	Busulfan/Fludarabine/ low dose TBI or, Cyclophosphamide/ Fludarabine/low dose TBI		31
Ballen	21	AML, ALL, MDS, lymphoma	Fludarabine, Melphalan, Thymoglobulin	18	55

transplant-related mortality was 28%. Overall survival at 1 year was 39%. Interestingly, for patients receiving a reduced intensity regimen, the day +10 myeloid recovery was autologous, and engraftment of the cord units occurred later after transplant. Extensive chimerism data were not reported with this study.

This group recently updated their data in abstract form, to include 95 patients [42]. Seventy-eight patients received a double cord blood transplant and 17 patients received a single cord blood transplant. The conditioning regimen was cyclophosphamide, fludarabine, and low dose total body radiation. Median cell dose was 3.6×10^7 and 94% of the units were either a 4/6 or 5/6 match with the recipient and with each other. Median time to neutrophil engraftment was 12 days with a 6% rate of primary graft failure. Incidence of grade III–IV acute GVHD and chronic GVHD were both 25%. Overall survival was 52% at 1 year and 44% at 2 years.

The Minnesota group has compared, in a retrospective series, outcomes after double and single cord blood transplantation [43]. This study compared 29 patients with acute leukemia who received double cord blood transplants with 14 patients who received single cord blood transplants. All patients received the conditioning regimen of cyclophosphamide, fludarabine, and total body radiation and immunosuppression with CSA and MMF. The minimal total nucleated cell (TNC) dose was 2.5×10^7. The risk of relapse was less (54% versus 11%) for patients in complete remission (CR) 1 or CR 2 who received double cord blood transplants. There was no difference for patients with more advanced disease (CR 3 or relapse). This study suggests that there could be additional benefit in graft-versus-leukemia effect to the double cord blood approach, but the numbers of patients are small in this series.

An additional study from the same group compared outcomes of double umbilical cord blood transplantation ($n = 9$) or HLA-matched sibling transplantation ($n = 12$) using a reduced intensity regimen in patients with advanced Hodgkin lymphoma [44]. The incidence of acute and chronic GVHD, transplant-related mortality, and progression-free survival were similar between these two groups. The 2-year progression-free survival rates were 25% for cord blood recipients and 20% for patients receiving matched sibling donor grafts.

We have pursued the sequential or double cord blood transplant approach in a Phase I study at the Massachusetts General Hospital and Dana Farber Cancer Institute [45]. Patients received a reduced intensity conditioning regimen of fludarabine, melphalan, and rabbit anti-thymocyte globulin. Two cord blood units were infused on the same day; the cord blood units were an HLA 4/6 (A, B, DR) match with each other and with the patient, and achieved a combined cell dose pre-freeze of $>3.7 \times 10$ (7) NC/kg. Twenty-one patients were treated with this approach. The median days to neutrophil engraftment were 20 days, and the median days to platelet engraftment (platelet count $>20 \times 10^9$/L unsupported were 41 days. There were three deaths prior to day +100, one related to a central nervous system (CNS) bleed, one related to sepsis, and one related to an EBV lymphoproliferative disorder. There were three deaths after Day +100, one related to chronic GVHD and sepsis, one related to fungus infection, and one related to an EBV lymphoproliferative disorder. The one-year overall survival was 71% and the one-year disease free survival was 67%.

Adult Cord Blood Transplantation – Chimerism Analysis

Chimerism refers to the amount each cord blood or the recipient contributes to hematopoiesis. Cord blood, particularly double cord blood transplantation, offers unique challenges in the technical aspects and interpretation of post-transplant chimerism [46]. Chimerism assays are usually performed by DNA methods using amplification of short tandem repeat loci by polymerase chain reaction [47]. The published studies of double cord blood transplantation have shown, that typically one cord blood units predominates and provides the majority of the hematopoiesis.

In the study by Barker et al. using a myeloablative conditioning regimen, 76% of the patients showed hematopoiesis from only a single cord by day 21 [39]. By day +100, one cord unit predominated in all patients. Chimerism results have been analyzed in detail for our study of 21 patients treated with a reduced intensity regimen [46, 48].

Ten of 18 evaluable patients had hematopoiesis from only a single cord by 6 weeks, which persisted out to day 100. By day +100, one cord blood unit predominated in all patients.

We have investigated further the characteristics of the predominant or "winning" cord blood unit. Barker and colleagues found no relation between HLA match or cell dose and cord blood predominance. Interestingly, a higher CD3+ dose was associated with cord blood predominance [39]. In our series, the predominant cord blood was the first cord blood infused in 76% of patients [48]. There was a trend to a higher CD34+ cells dose and nucleated cell count in the predominant cord. These interesting observations will need to be tested in a larger cohort of patients.

The use of double cord blood transplantation has decreased the transplant-related mortality in adults and does not appear to increase GVHD. However, infection and immune reconstitution remain significant problems, even with the infusion of two cord blood units.

Combination Cord Blood and Bone Marrow Transplants

The idea of this approach is to achieve initial engraftment from a mismatched bone marrow transplant, followed by rejection of the bone marrow, and long-term engraftment of the cord blood unit. The Spanish group has pioneered this novel idea. In the initial study, eleven adults received single cord blood units and haploidentical CD34+ selected cells from a family member [49]. Neutrophil engraftment occurred at 12 days (range: 9–36 days). Four patients experienced Grade II or higher acute GVHD. Five of the 11 patients survive disease-free with complete cord blood chimerism at 6–43 months post-transplant.

Murine studies indicate increased engraftment with co-transplantation of mesenchymal stromal cells from an additional donor [50]. Using a NOD-scid mouse model, these investigators have shown improved engraftment when two cord blood units were transplanted with bone marrow mesenchymal cells from a third donor.

These studies suggest that some combination of one or two cord blood units plus bone marrow may be beneficial. Ramirez and colleagues have reported a short period of neutropenia in mice treated with human peripheral blood stem cells and cord blood cells [51].

There are now alternatives to single cord blood transplantation for adult patients, and outcomes for adult patients are improving. The double cord blood results appear promising in terms of neutrophil recovery, and a low risk of GVHD, but are more expensive because of the additional cord blood unit required. This approach should be tested in larger studies with diverse patient populations. Finally, the Spanish approach of combined bone marrow and cord blood unit is exciting, particularly for patients who are unable to locate two appropriately matched cord blood units. Patients who do not have a matched sibling donor should search aggressively for either unrelated bone marrow or unrelated cord blood in all national and international registries. Patients without time to find an unrelated bone marrow donor, or who do not have a 10/10 or 9/10 unrelated adult volunteer donor should be considered for cord blood transplant. In adults, the double cord blood transplant approach should be strongly considered. The goal should be to procure a safe donor source, either bone marrow or cord blood, in a timely fashion so no patients are denied potentially curative transplant therapy.

New Applications of Cord Blood Transplantation

The next 5–10 years should be an exciting time in the cord blood transplantation field. Further investigation is needed to compare cord blood with other donor sources, such as haploidentical transplants, autologous transplants, and mismatched unrelated donor transplants. There might be a future indication for cord blood instead of a matched unrelated donor, for example, in elderly patients with a high risk of GVHD.

An exciting opportunity for cord blood transplantation is in non-malignant disease. A possible application might be in the autoimmune diseases, where there are ongoing trials for autologous transplantation for lupus, systemic sclerosis, and multiple sclerosis [52, 53]. Reports of successful allogeneic transplantation for autoimmune disease have recently been published. A potential advantage of cord blood for these non-malignant diseases is the decreased incidence of GVHD.

Perhaps the most exciting uses of umbilical cord blood might be in cardiac or neurologic disease. Cord blood cells are a more primitive population than adult bone marrow, and have increased capacity for multilineage differentiation [54]. Encouraging preliminary results have been seen in animal models of neurologic and cardiac disease. In a mouse model, cord blood cells injected into the tail vein migrated to infarcted myocardial tissue [55]. Infarct size was smaller in the mice treated with cord blood cells.

Cord blood cells can be expanded in culture and induced to differentiate into cells with neural markers [54]. Recently, cord blood cells have been shown to improve functional recovery in rats that have been subjected to strokes, by middle cerebral artery occlusion [56]. Infarct volume was reduced and behavioral performance increased when a higher dose of cord blood cells was infused.

Conclusion

Umbilical cord blood, traditionally a discarded waste product after delivery, has now become an alternative stem cell source for patients without matched related donors. Transplant outcomes in children are similar to the results seen with unrelated donor transplants. Traditionally, adult transplant has been limited by cell dose and an increased risk of infection. However, new techniques, such as double cord blood transplantation, may help to improve engraftment and immune reconstitution. Particularly intriguing is the interest in cord blood for the treatment of nonmalignant disease. We anticipate continued growth in this exciting field over the next 5–10 years.

References

1. Knudtzon S. In vitro growth of granulocytic colonies from circulating cells in human cord blood. Blood 1974; 43:357–61.
2. Broxmeyer HE, Kurtzberg J, Gluckman E, et al. Umbilical cord blood hematopoietic stem and repopulating cells in human clinical transplantation. Blood Cells 1991; 17:313–29.
3. Gluckman E, Broxmeyer HA, Auerbach AD, et al. Hematopoietic reconstitution in a patient with Fanconi's anemia by means of umbilical-cord blood from an HLA-identical sibling. N Engl J Med 1989; 321:1174–8.
4. Lansdorp PM, Dragowska W, Mayani H. Ontogeny-related changes in proliferative potential of human hematopoietic cells. J Exp Med 1993; 178:787–91.
5. Vaziri H, Dragowska W, Allsopp RC, Thomas TE, Harley CB, Lansdorp PM. Evidence for a mitotic clock in human hematopoietic stem cells: loss of telomeric DNA with age. Proc Natl Acad Sci USA 1994; 91:9857–60.
6. Cairo MS, Wagner JE. Placental and/or umbilical cord blood: an alternative source of hematopoietic stem cells for transplantation. Blood 1997; 90:4665–78.
7. Wagner JE, Kernan NA, Steinbuch M, Broxmeyer HE, Gluckman E. Allogeneic sibling umbilical-cord-blood transplantation in children with malignant and non-malignant disease. Lancet 1995; 346:214–9.
8. Szabolcs P, Park KD, Reese M, Marti L, Broadwater G, Kurtzberg J. Coexistent naive phenotype and higher cycling rate of cord blood T cells as compared to adult peripheral blood. Exp Hematol 2003; 31:708–14.
9. Loetscher P, Uguccioni M, Bordoli L, et al. CCR5 is characteristic of Th1 lymphocytes. Nature 1998; 391:344–5.
10. Alfani E, Migliaccio AR, Sanchez M, Passarelli AM, Migliaccio G. Characterization of the T cell receptor repertoire of neonatal T cells by RT-PCR and single strand conformation polymorphism analysis. Bone Marrow Transplant 2000; 26:83–9.
11. Bone Marrow Donors Worldwide, Annual Report. 2006.
12. National Marrow Donor Program, Facts and Figures, 2007
13. Hurley CK, Setterholm M, Lau M, et al. Hematopoietic stem cell donor registry strategies for assigning search determinants and matching relationships. Bone Marrow Transplant 2004; 33:443–50.

14. Barker JN, Krepski TP, DeFor TE, Davies SM, Wagner JE, Weisdorf DJ. Searching for unrelated donor hematopoietic stem cells: availability and speed of umbilical cord blood versus bone marrow. Biol Blood Marrow Transplant 2002; 8:257–60.
15. Ballen KK, Hicks J, Dharan B, et al. Racial and ethnic composition of volunteer cord blood donors: comparison with volunteer unrelated marrow donors. Transfusion 2002; 42: 1279–84.
16. Ballen KK, Kurtzberg J, Lane TA, et al. Racial diversity with high nucleated cell counts and CD34 counts achieved in a national network of cord blood banks. Biol Blood Marrow Transplant 2004; 10:269–75.
17. Cairo MS, Wagner EL, Fraser J, et al. Characterization of banked umbilical cord blood hematopoietic progenitor cells and lymphocyte subsets and correlation with ethnicity, birth weight, sex, and type of delivery: a Cord Blood Transplantation (COBLT) Study report. Transfusion 2005; 45:856–66.
18. Ballen KK. New trends in umbilical cord blood transplantation. Blood 2005; 105:3786–92.
19. Ballen KK. Advances in Umbilical Cord Blood Transplantation. Curr Stem Cell Res Ther 2006; 1:317–24.
20. Locatelli F, Rocha V, Chastang C, et al. Factors associated with outcome after cord blood transplantation in children with acute leukemia. Eurocord-Cord Blood Transplant Group. Blood 1999; 93:3662–71.
21. Locatelli F, Rocha V, Reed W, et al. Related umbilical cord blood transplantation in patients with thalassemia and sickle cell disease. Blood 2003; 101:2137–43.
22. Rocha V, Wagner JE, Jr., Sobocinski KA, et al. Graft-versus-host disease in children who have received a cord-blood or bone marrow transplant from an HLA-identical sibling. Eurocord and International Bone Marrow Transplant Registry Working Committee on Alternative Donor and Stem Cell Sources. N Engl J Med 2000; 342:1846–54.
23. Kurtzberg J, Laughlin M, Graham ML, et al. Placental blood as a source of hematopoietic stem cells for transplantation into unrelated recipients. N Engl J Med 1996; 335:157–66.
24. Wagner JE, Barker JN, DeFor TE, et al. Transplantation of unrelated donor umbilical cord blood in 102 patients with malignant and nonmalignant diseases: influence of CD34 cell dose and HLA disparity on treatment-related mortality and survival. Blood 2002; 100:1611–8.
25. Staba SL, Escolar ML, Poe M, et al. Cord-blood transplants from unrelated donors in patients with Hurler's syndrome. N Engl J Med 2004; 350:1960–9.
26. Laughlin MJ, Barker J, Bambach B, et al. Hematopoietic engraftment and survival in adult recipients of umbilical-cord blood from unrelated donors. N Engl J Med 2001; 344:1815–22.
27. Long GD, Laughlin M, Madan B, et al. Unrelated umbilical cord blood transplantation in adult patients. Biol Blood Marrow Transplant 2003; 9:772–80.
28. Cornetta K, Laughlin M, Carter S, et al. Umbilical cord blood transplantation in adults: results of the prospective Cord Blood Transplantation (COBLT). Biol Blood Marrow Transplant 2005; 11:149–60.
29. Laughlin MJ, Eapen M, Rubinstein P, et al. Outcomes after transplantation of cord blood or bone marrow from unrelated donors in adults with leukemia. N Engl J Med 2004; 351: 2265–75.
30. Rocha V, Labopin M, Sanz G, et al. Transplants of umbilical-cord blood or bone marrow from unrelated donors in adults with acute leukemia. N Engl J Med 2004; 351:2276–85.
31. Takahashi S, Iseki T, Ooi J, et al. Single-institute comparative analysis of unrelated bone marrow transplantation and cord blood transplantation for adult patients with hematologic malignancies. Blood 2004; 104:3813–20.
32. Khouri IF, Saliba RM, Giralt SA, et al. Nonablative allogeneic hematopoietic transplantation as adoptive immunotherapy for indolent lymphoma: low incidence of toxicity, acute graft-versus-host disease, and treatment-related mortality. Blood 2001; 98:3595–9.
33. Daly A, McAfee S, Dey B, et al. Nonmyeloablative bone marrow transplantation: Infectious complications in 65 recipients of HLA-identical and mismatched transplants. Bio Blood Marrow Transplant 2003; 9:373–82.

34. Yuji K, Miyakoshi S, Kato D, et al. Reduced-intensity unrelated cord blood transplantation for patients with advanced lymphoma. Biol Blood Marrow Transplant 2005; 11: 314–18.
35. Miyakoshi S, Yuji K, Kami M, et al. Successful engraftment after reduced-intensity umbilical cord blood transplantation for adult patients with advanced hematological diseases. Clin Cancer Res 2004; 10:3586–92.
36. Narimatsu H, Kami M, Miyakoshi S, et al. Graft failure following reduced- intensity cord blood transplantation for adult patients. Br J Hematol 2005; 132:36–41.
37. Chao NJ, Koh LP, Long GD, et al. Adult recipients of umbilical cord blood transplants after nonmyeloablative preparative regimens. Biol Blood Marrow Transplant 2004; 10:569–75.
38. Weinreb S, Delgado JC, Clavijo OP, et al. Transplantation of unrelated cord blood cells. Bone Marrow Transplant 1998; 22:193–6.
39. Barker JN, Weisdorf DJ, DeFor TE, et al. Transplantation of 2 partially matached HLA-matched umbilical cord blood units to enhance engraftment in adults with hematologic malignancy. Blood 2005; 105:1343–7.
40. Mao P, Wang S, Zhu Z, et al. Umbilical cord blood transplant for adult patients with severe aplastic anemia using anti-lymphocyte globulin and cyclophosphamide as conditioning therapy. Bone Marrow Transplant 2004; 33:33–8.
41. Barker JN, Weisdorf DF, Defor TE, et al. Rapid and complete donor chimerism in adult recipients of unrelated donor umbilical cord blood transplantation after reduced-intensity conditioning. Blood 2003; 102:1915–19.
42. Brunstein C, Barker J, DeFor T, et al. Non-myeloablative (NMA) umbilical cord blood transplantation (UCBT): promising disease-free survival in 95 consecutive patients. Blood 2005; 106:166a.
43. Verneris, M.R., Brunstein, C., DeFor, T.E., et al. Risk of relapse (REL) after umbilical cord blood transplantation (UCBT) in patients with acute leukemia: marked reduction in recipients of two units. Blood 2005; 106:93a.
44. Majhail NS, Weisdorf DJ, Wagner JE, et al. Comparable results of umbilical cord blood and HLA-matched sibling donor hematopoietic stem cell transplantation after reduced-intensity preparative regimen for advanced Hodgkin lymphoma. Blood 2006; 107:3804–7.
45. Ballen KK, Spitzer TR, Yeap BY, et al: Double unrelated reduced intensity umbilical cord blood transplantation in adults. Biol Blood Marrow Transplant 2007; 13:82–9.
46. Haspel R, Ballen KK: Double Cord Blood Transplants: filling a Niche? Stem Cell Rev 2006; 2:81–6.
47. DeLima M, St. John LS, Wieder ED, et al. Double-chimerism after transplantation of two human leucocyte antigen mismatched, unrelated cord blood units. Br J Hematol 2002; 119:773–76.
48. Haspel RL, Kao GS, Yeap BY, et al: Pre-infusion variables predict the predominant cord blood unit in the setting of reduced intensity double cord blood transplant. Bone Marrow Transplant, 2008, in press.
49. Fernandez MN, Regidor C, Cabrera R, et al. Unrelated umbilical cord blood transplants in adults: early recovery of neutrophils by supportive co-transplantation of a low number of highly purified peripheral blood CD34+ cells from an HLA-haploidentical donor. Exp Hematol 2003; 31:535–44.
50. Kim DW, Chung YJ, Kim TG, Kim YL, Oh IH. Cotransplantation of third-party mesenchymal stromal cells can alleviate single-donor predominance and increase engraftment from double cord transplantation. Blood 2004; 103:1941–8.
51. Ramirez M, Regidor C, Marugan I, Garcia-Conde J, Bueren JA, Fernandez MN. Engraftment kinetics of human CD34+ cells from cord blood and mobilized peripheral blood co-transplanted into NOD/SCID mice. Bone Marrow Transplant 2005; 35:271–5.
52. Nash RA, Bowen D, McSweeney PA, et al. High-dose immunosuppressive therapy and autologous peripheral blood stem cell transplantation for severe multiple sclerosis. Blood 2003; 102:2364–72.

53. Burt RK, Traynor A, Oyama Y, Craig R. High-dose immune suppression and autologous hematopoietic stem cell transplantation in refractory Crohn's disease. Blood 2003; 101: 2064–6.
54. Goodwin HS, Bicknese AR, Chien SN, Bogucki BD, Quinn CO, Wall DA. Multilineage differentiation activity by cells isolated from umbilical cord blood: expression of bone, fat, and neural markers. Biol Blood Marrow Transplant 2001; 7:581–8.
55. Ma N, Stamm C, Kaminski A, et al. Human cord blood cells induce angiogenesis following myocardial infarction in NOD/scid-mice. Cardiovasc Res 2005; 66:45–54.
56. Vendrame M, Cassady J, Newcomb J, et al. Infusion of human umbilical cord blood cells in a rat model of stroke dose-dependently rescues behavioral deficits and reduces infarct volume. Stroke 2004; 35:2390–5.

Section III
Transfusion of Cord Blood

Chapter 10
Placental Umbilical Cord Whole Blood Transfusion: A True Blood Substitute to Combat Anemia in the Background of Chronic Disease – A Study Report (1999–2006)

Niranjan Bhattacharya

Introduction

All over the world, millions of people are saved every year as a result of blood transfusions. At the same time, many, particularly in the developing countries, still die because of inadequate supply of safe blood and blood products. A reliable supply of safe blood is essential to improve health standards at several levels, especially for women and children, and particularly in the poorer sections of society anywhere in the world. Half a million women still die of complications related to pregnancy and childbirth, and 99% of them are in the developing countries. Hemorrhage accounts for 25% of complications and is the most common cause of maternal death [1]. Malnutrition, thalassemia, and severe anemia are prevalent diseases in children, which require blood transfusion, apart from other complicated diseases. Over 80 million units of blood are collected every year, but the tragedy is that only 39% of this is collected in the developing world which comprises 82% of the global population.

Blood and blood derivatives are used not only as a treatment but also as a preventive measure. For instance, immunoglobulins are used to treat abnormal functions of the immune system, and Factor VIII is given routinely to hemophiliacs to enable them to live normal lives. Blood transfusion is routine in cases of surgery, trauma, gastrointestinal bleeding and, sometimes, in childbirth. Some genetic diseases like thalassemia and sickle cell disorder require regular blood transfusions.

The detection of human immunodeficiency viruses (HIV) in the 1980 s and Hepatitis B and C in the 1990 s highlighted the importance of safe blood to prevent transfusion-transmissible diseases (TTDs). Risks from transfusion of adult blood also include Parovirus 19, especially during pregnancy, hemolytic anemia and immunocompromised background, syphilis, kalaazar, malaria, etc. There are also problems associated with rare blood groups that are not screened normally but have

N. Bhattacharya (✉)
Advanced Medical Research Institute (AMRI) Hospitals, BP Poddar Hospital, Apollo Gleneagles Hospital, Vidyasagore Hospital, Calcutta, India

N. Bhattacharya, P. Stubblefield (eds.), *Frontiers of Cord Blood Science*,
DOI 10.1007/978-1-84800-167-1_10,

the potential to trigger hemolytic reactions. There could also be, although rarely, transfusion-induced lung, liver or kidney injuries. There are also problems associated with immunomodulation [2]. Lymphocytes can also be a source of infection even after leucodepletion [3].

Proper selection of donors still remains the most fundamental strategy towards minimizing the risk of TTDs. But, in some developing countries, it has been reported that 80% of blood supply comes from paid donors and replacement donors (family, friends or acquaintances), even though the percentage of population infected with communicable diseases is high. Moreover, an estimated 13 million units of blood worldwide are not tested against HIV or hepatitis viruses [4]. Since safe blood is required in adequate amounts to ensure that lives are saved, there is an ongoing search for a genuine blood substitute. Actually this search began over 70 years earlier after the publication of the report of Amberson et al. [5]. Since 1988–1989, after the first reports of the successful use of umbilical cord blood transplantation [6, 7], there has been growing interest in cord blood as an alternative source of hematopoietic stem cells (CD34) to treat cancer and certain genetic diseases, because they cause less graft-vs.-host reaction. Cord blood stem cells have a unique ability to regenerate blood production and the immune system, and have the potential to treat diseases. Cord blood banks claim that these stem cells are important in the treatment of certain cancers like Hodgkin's disease, non-Hodgkin's lymphoma, neuroblastoma, and refractory anemia; autoimmune diseases like multiple sclerosis, rheumatoid arthritis, and systemic lupus erythematosus; blood disorders like B thalassemia and sickle cell anemia; bone marrow failure syndromes like aplastic anemia, Kostmann syndrome and Fanconi's anemia; and inborn errors of metabolism like Hurler's syndrome, osteopetrosis, histiocytic disorders, Krabbe disease, etc. [8].

However, the same interest was not shown on the use of cord blood itself as a genuine and easily available alternative source of blood. Hematopoietic stem cells from cord blood are now harvested in many laboratories all over the world and stored in cord blood banks, but they constitute only 0.01% of the nucleated cells of the cord blood. The rest, that is 99.99% of blood, which is wasted, is rich in fetal hemoglobin, growth factors, and cytokine-filled plasma. Moreover, in the womb, the fetus benefits from the mother's in-built defenses against diseases, and the placental environment is basically infection-free in the case of a healthy newborn.

This chapter will first explain the benefits of cord blood as a true blood substitute, and then analyze the effects of its clinical use in a variety of diseases like thalassemia, leprosy, cancer, arthritis, etc., and discuss its potential for future use.

Other Blood Substitutes and Cord Blood

A continuous supply of donated blood is essential for the practice of modern medicine. In the absence of safe and adequate blood, blood substitutes are also becoming important sources of supply. These include RBC substitutes to provide the respiratory functions of hemoglobin, platelet substitutes, and coagulation factors. Hemoglobin has been extracted from human RBC, bovine RBC, and even from sea creatures like the sea worm (Arenicola marina) [9]. The most promising among the RBC substitutes is hemoglobin extracted from the lysis of the RBC from human and bovine sources, or a chemically modified hemoglobin, or a genetically modified hemoglobin molecule. These hemoglobin-based oxygen carriers have the intrinsic advantage of universal compatibility and storability at room temperature. However, they are expensive, and, therefore, prohibitive for the poor, particularly in the developing world. Moreover, specific problems arising from hypertensive impact, gastric irritability, and even sudden unexplained deaths have also been reported [10]. Other hemoglobin substitutes which are of less importance include perflurocarbons, i.e., fluorine substituted with linear or cyclic carbon atoms with high oxygen-carrying capacity, and liposome-encapsulated hemoglobin [11].

It is in this connection that the potential of transfusion of placental umbilical cord blood becomes important. It is a general norm among female animals to swallow the afterbirth; even herbivorous animals like cows follow this practice. They seem to have an intrinsic knowledge, which has not been given to human beings, except in some Chinese systems of traditional medicine, of the value of placenta, which nurtures the baby for so long in the womb. Actually, aseptically collected placental umbilical cord blood is a rich source of fetal hemoglobin. Fetal hemoglobin is a natural stress response to hemoglobin synthesis. Hypoimmune fetal cells, with their altered metabolic profile, are a gift of nature entrapped inside the placenta, from which it can easily be extracted and used to combat diseases ranging from simple anemia to complicated cases of thalassemia and aplastic anemia. It can be used as a genuine blood substitute not only in the under-resourced world but also in any emergency or in any country where there is need for blood.

There is an abundant source of blood. In India alone, 20 million placentas are produced every year in afterbirth, which could be a source of cord blood. This blood has some intrinsic advantages. Adult hemoglobin consists of 2 alpha and 2 beta polypeptide chains, each bound to a heme group, capable of binding with one molecule of O_2 (1 gm hemoglobin binds with 1.39 ml of oxygen). Therefore, 14% of adult hemoglobin can carry, on an average, 19.46 ml of oxygen. On the other hand, cord blood at term carries, on an average, 16.8 gm% hemoglobin, of which 20% belongs to the adult hemoglobin type (3.36 gm), and 80% belongs to the fetal hemoglobin type (13.44 gm) [12]. The concentration of fetal hemoglobin may increase further depending on fetal stress, maturity, and several other feto-maternal factors. Fetal hemoglobin has the potential to carry 50–60% more oxygen than adult hemoglobin [13], that is, 1 gm of fetal hemoglobin may carry up to 2.08 ml of oxygen. If one calculates the oxygen-carrying capacity of 100 ml of cord blood theoretically, taking into account the fact that it contains 80% fetal hemoglobin and 20% adult hemoglobin, it would be around 32.62 ml. This means that cord blood has 67.62% more oxygen-carrying capacity than adult blood, which has around 19.46 O_2/100 ml. There are several factors which modify the oxygen-binding affinity; for instance, (a) concentration of hydrogen ion, (b) carbon dioxide concentration in blood, (c) body temperature, and (d) 2-3 diphosphoglycerate concentration. The point that needs to be emphasized is that placental umbilical cord whole blood has the potential to carry more oxygen to tissues vol/vol because of its fetal hemoglobin component.

The blood volume of a fetus at term is 80–85 ml/kg [14]. The placental vessel at term contains approximately 150 ml of cord blood [15]. Cord blood contains three types of hemoglobin – HbF, HbA, and HbA2, of which HbF constitutes the major fraction [12]. HbA accounts for 15–40% and HbA2 is present only in trace amounts at birth [16]. HbF, which is a major component, has greater oxygen–binding affinity than HbA [17]. The oxygen tension at which cord blood hemoglobin is 50% saturated is 19–20 mm of Hg, that is, 6–8 mm Hg lower than that of normal adult blood. This shift to the left of the hemoglobin oxygen dissolution curve results from poor binding of 2-3 diphosphoglycerate by HbF [18, 19]. Fetal hemoglobin can carry more oxygen than the mother's blood, and also there is another potential advantage by which fetal hemoglobin (Bohr's effect) can carry more oxygen at low PCO_2 than at high PCO_2 [13]. Cord blood also has rich cytokine and growth factor filled plasma content, and this has a positive therapeutic implication for distressed or emaciated patients receiving placental umbilical cord whole blood transfusion.

As will be shown later in this chapter, transfusion of cord blood normally does not lead to any immunological or non-immunological reactions, which cannot be said of other blood substitutes. Immunological reactions are related to the stimulation of antibody production by foreign anti-allogens that are contained in the different components of blood, for instance, RBC, leucocytes, platelets, and plasma protein. Alloimmunization could also lead to immunological reactions in future through stimulation by a similar antigen. Commonly encountered immunological reactions are hemolytic reactions due to RBC incompatibility. Febrile or pulmonary reactions result from antigens of leucocytes and platelets. Allergic and anaphylactoid reactions are related to antibodies, and rarely graft-vs.-host reactions are encountered due to the engraftment of transfused lymphocytes in case of immunosuppression. Non-immunological reactions occur when the physical and chemical properties of blood/blood products are contaminated by bacteria or viruses, or because of the circulatory load. Cord blood, which is protected in the placenta, is relatively free from such contamination. The placenta is a unique and formidable biological barrier. There are many substances like P-glycoprotein, which form a functional barrier between maternal and fetal blood circulation in the placenta, thus protecting the fetus from exposure [20]. Even HIV cannot cross this barrier easily. However, at or near term, there is an increase in the feto-maternal bi-directional traffic as some cells may have access to the maternal circulation depending on the viral load pathogenicity, the maternal immune condition, and other hitherto identified or non-identified factors. One group of investigators has suggested that the trophoblastic barrier remains uninfected in full term placenta of HIV-seropositive mothers undergoing anti-retroviral treatment. They have opined that if there is any HIV transmission *in utero* at all, it occurs at the end of gestation through alternative routes, for instance, chorioamnionitis with leakage of the virus into the amniotic cavity or trophoblast damage [21]. The point, however, is that the blood of a healthy newborn is relatively safer than that of adult blood or other blood substitutes.

Pre-clinical and Clinical Studies on Cord Blood

Among the early pre-clinical studies, the path-breaking work of Søren Knudtzon, which showed that neonatal and cord blood contain a high number of granulocyte-macrophage progenitor cells, is worth mentioning. Human umbilical cord blood cells from 26 newborn infants and peripheral blood cells from 18 adults were cultured *in vitro*. An increased concentration of colony-forming cells was seen in the cord blood cultures [22]. Broxmeyer et al. demonstrated through murine experiments that blood from neonatal mice contained adequate progenitor cells for bone marrow reconstitution in irradiated mice [23]. Human cord blood was also shown to have sufficient progenitor cells to support durable engraftment [24]. What these experiments demonstrated were significant: for instance, (a) cultures of cord blood $CD34^+$ cells increase in cell number every 7–10 days several 100-fold greater than the increase in cultures of similar cells from adult bone marrow [25]; and (b) compared with bone marrow cells, $CD34^+/CD38^-$ cord blood cells proliferate more rapidly and generate larger number of progeny cells [26]. The greater proliferative capacity of cord blood has been explained in terms of the longer telomere length of cord blood cells [27]. The immunologic properties of cord blood differ from mature bone marrow or peripheral blood stem cells (PBSC). Later clinical trials showed that cord blood contains a high proportion of T cells expressing the $CD45RA^+/CD45RO^-$, $CD62L^+$ 'naive' phenotype [28]. Compared with adult T cells, the chemokine receptor CCR5, expressed by T helper 1 T cells, is less abundant [29]. Some studies show that cord blood cells produce increased amounts of the anti-inflammatory cytokine interleukin-10 (IL-10), which may lower the incidence of graft-vs.-host disease(GVHD) [30].

The first reported clinical experience was the use of an identical sibling's umbilical cord blood stem cells for hematopoietic reconstitution in a patient with Fanconi's anemia [6]. Subsequently, a lot of work has been done in this area [31], but it should be pointed out that these researches have used only the hematopoietic progenitor cells [colony-forming unit–granulocyte macrophages (CFU–GMs)] and not umbilical cord whole blood.

It should also be mentioned that Paxson CL Jr. suggested the feasibility of autologous fetal blood collection as early in 1979 [32]. None of the blood cultures exhibited the growth of bacterial pathogens. His data also demonstrated that fetal blood can safely be given to infants subjected to shock or iotragenic blood loss. Almost 65% of premature neonates with a birthweight of less than 1500 g receive at least one erythrocyte transfusion during their first week of life. A group of investigators claimed the use of this method of transfusion on a newborn infant in 2000 [33]. The preterm infant received two portions of autologous blood (on days 5 and 7), and no untoward effects were noted. Subsequently, the investigators concluded that the preparation of autologous RBCs from the cord blood of preterm infants is technically feasible. Later, Brune et al. noted that, in their work with 52 newborns, a comparison of cord blood and adult blood transfusion in neonates showed no difference in safety and efficacy between placental blood transfusion and allogeneic RBC transfusion [34]. In another report on neonatal surgery, Tagachi and his colleagues have reported that, although allogeneic blood transfusions have a risk of infection owing to unknown organisms, graft-vs.-host reaction, and immunosuppression, there is overall safety. Moreover, autologous cord blood transfusions have been reported to be effective in the treatment of anemia in premature infants. They have also examined the efficacy of autologous cord blood transfusion in neonatal surgical patients and concluded that it has the potential to become a useful alternative to homologous transfusion in newborns requiring surgery [35]. Hassal O et al. also reported on the use of allogeneic cord blood transfusion to combat severe anemia in the background of malaria in a sub-Saharan area of Africa, and noted that there was no transfusion-related complications in their series [36].

The importance of these findings lies in the fact they prove that the use of umbilical cord blood is safe and effective. In Calcutta, India, investigators have used umbilical cord whole blood (which also contains hematopoietic progenitor cells) not only as an emergency alternative to adult blood but also to combat anemia in malaria, leprosy, thalassemia, tuberculosis (TB), diabetes with early renal involvement, cancer, HIV, and arthritis. Not only there was no immunological or non-immunological reaction in any of the patients, there was a general betterment in their condition, which may be related to the growth factors, cytokine, and other components of umbilical cord whole blood [37]. The cord blood was transfused to patients with matching blood group of any age. These clinical studies were undertaken between 1 April 1999 and July 2005. The findings of these studies indicate that cord blood has an immunotherapeutic potential and positive prognostic implications, particularly in malignancy-induced immunosuppression, structural or functional, which is evidenced in the transient rise of CD34 in the peripheral blood of some patients.

Material and Methods

The material and methods used in all cases are similar, although there were variations on some of the tests done on patients prior to transfusion, depending on the kind of disease. The method of collecting cord blood was the same. Umbilical cord blood was collected from consenting mothers aseptically after lower uterine caesarian section (LUCS) under general or regional anesthesia. In case of gross prematurity or dysmaturity, or if the projected weight of the fetus was less than 2 kg, or if the mother suffered from any specific disease like hepatitis, HIV, etc., the cord blood collection was abandoned. Cord blood was collected only from informed, healthy mothers with their consent, after their healthy babies were born. The collection was started only after the baby was safely removed from the operation field, and the anesthetist verified that the physical condition of the mother was stable. The decision to proceed with umbilical cord collection was taken by the obstetrician only after that. The cord was immediately disinfected by spirit/Betadine solution at the site of the proposed puncture of the umbilical vein. A 16-g needle was attached to a standard pediatric collection bag, which contained 14 ml anti-coagulant citrate phosphate dextrose adenine solution, and this was used for the collection of cord blood. A second bag was used if the collection exceeded or neared 100 ml, and a second prick was made at a proximal region after using a clamp at the first prick site. Blood flowed by gravity, and generally within a minute 90% of the collection was ready. In most cases, blood flow ceased completely within 2 min due to clot formation. If there was any confusion regarding the condition of the baby, a decision was taken immediately to preserve the blood in consultation with the pediatrician for future use by the baby, or it was stamped "Unsafe for Transfusion". No risk was ever taken whatsoever vis-à-vis any future recipient of the blood.

When the collection was completed, the blood bag was closed, sealed, necessary identification markings were made, and then stored at 1–4°C. A sample from the collected blood was immediately tested for blood group (Rh and ABO), HIV (1 and 2), hepatitis B and C, VDRL, and malaria as per standard blood transfusion protocol [38]. Our study for osmotic fragility with .45% NaCl (N = 40) at 4°C, 35°C, and 40°C, with a time gap of 24 h, 48 h, 7 days, and 14 days, along with oxyhemoglobin (mmole/ml) and plasma hemoglobin (mg/ml) assessment in identical schedule, showed that the cord blood was reasonably stable at room temperature (Table 10.1). In case of any contamination or confusion, the culture was put aside for the identification of the pathogen, if any, through appropriate protocol, and the blood bag that matched the sample was marked unfit for transfusion.

The collection of cord blood varied from 50 ml to 146 ml; mean 86 ± 7.6 ml SD; median 80 ml; mean packed cell volume 48 ± 4.1 SD; mean hemoglobin concentration 16.2 ± 1.9 gm% SD. After the collection, the blood was immediately preserved in a refrigerator and transfused within 72 h of collection. Donation of cord

Table 10.1 Study results on the stability of cord blood at temperature and time

	Time			
Temperature	24 h	48 h	7 days	14 days
Mean fragility (% hemolysis in 0.45% NaCl) with standard deviation ($N = 50$)				
4°C	12.5 + 3.3	32.8 + 4.4	45.7 + 2.9	82.5 + 4.5
35°C	16.4 + 2.8	20.6 + 4.4	53.4 + 3.8	100
40°C	45.0 + 6.5	77.6 + 3.9	92.7 + 4.7	100
Mean oxyhemoglobin (mmole/ml) with standard deviation ($N = 74$)				
4°C	0.32 + .12	0.31 + .15	0.27 + .04	0.26 + .13
35°C	0.31 + .06	0.29 + .04	0.24 + .07	–
40°C	0.16 + .04	0.09 + .02	–	–
Mean plasma hemoglobin (mg/ml) with standard deviation ($N = 54$)				
4°C	6.07 + .83	6.35 + .76	7.04 + .88	9.69 + 1.8
35°C	4.49 + .55	7.65 + .87	10.0 + 2.4	–
40°C	10.2 + 1.7	13.4 + 2.4	–	–

blood to the recipients followed strict guidelines of the human ethical committee of the hospital, which is headed by an Emeritus Professor of Medicine.

As a rule, a volunteer who wishes to enroll to the cord blood transfusion program had to have a hemoglobin count below 8 gm%. Patients with cancer or some other critical illness were given priority. Before the transfusion of umbilical cord blood, a thorough clinical examination of the patient was done, including monitoring of the BP/pulse/respiration rate and other cardinal and presenting features. Prior to transfusion, little blood was drawn from the patient for blood grouping and tests including Tc, Dc, Hb, ESR, platelet count, Coombs test, C-reactive protein, sugar, urea, creatinine, and bilirubin. Other investigations were also carried out as per individual case requirement. For instance, Hb electrophoresis was done in the case of thalassemia, before as well as after transfusion, to determine the impact of transfusion. Little blood was re-drawn from each patient receiving cord blood transfusion after 24 h, 72 h, 7 days, 1 month, 2 months, and 3 months for similar testing. Subsequently, clinical follow-up continued at the OPD from time to time to study the effects of transfusion and to note adverse reactions, if any.

The actual transfusion procedure began after necessary cross-matching of the specimens and checking the identity of the patient. Cord blood was transfused through a blood transfusion set containing a filter (230 um). The patient was observed carefully for the initial 15 min or so in case there was any transfusion-related reaction. Thereafter, if no problem persisted, the transfusion rate was increased until completion.

Disease, Age, and Sex Distribution of Patients

Data regarding the first 413 units of cord blood aseptically collected from consenting mothers will be given here. Blood was transfused to 129 informed, consenting volunteers after the cases had been scrutinized and approved by the institution-based ethical committee. There were 54 male and 75 female patients in this group. The age of the patients ranged between 2 years and 86 years. Seventy-three patients were suffering from advanced cancer (56.58%), and 56 were suffering from other diseases (43.42%). Three pediatric patients were less than 10 years old, while one geriatric patient was over 80 years of age. Twenty-two patients (17.05%) were in the 60–80 years age bracket. However, the majority (50.38%) were in the 40–60-year age group. B+ was the most common blood group (31.78%), followed by O+ (28.68%) and A+ (24.03%), and finally, AB+ (13.95%). There was only one patient each in the O and B groups.

A patient with advanced cancer with hemoptysis received the highest number of units of cord blood. He received a total of 33 units, with 10 units being transfused at a time. A patient with aplastic anemia received 23 units (9 units of cord blood at a time); 16 units were given to a patient with transfusion-dependent thalassemic syndrome (8 units of cord blood at a time); and a patient with stage-IV cancer with metachronous metastasis received 15 units (7 units of cord blood at a time). Among the other recipients of cord blood transfusion, those who received more than

3 units at a time included one patient who received 10 units of cord blood, three who received 9 units each, two who received 8 units each, and 18 who received 7 units each. In addition, seven patients received 6 units each and another seven patients received 5 units each of umbilical cord whole blood transfusion. All patients presented with anemia (8 gm% or less of hemoglobin) and distress, be it in the background of ankylosing spondylitis, lupus erythematosus, rheumatoid arthritis, aplastic anemia, thalassemia major, bleeding per rectum, or hemoptysis due to malignancy. All cases responded clinically to cord blood transfusion. Not a single episode of immunological or non-immunological reaction was encountered.

Cord Blood in the Treatment of Anemia in the Background of Malaria

Malaria caused by infection with *Plasmodium falciparum* results in a million deaths each year [39], and anemia due to malaria is a major health problem in endemic areas, particularly among young children and pregnant women. *Plasmodium vivax* can also cause anemia and thrombocytopenia, although to a lesser extent. Anemia is the result of excess removal of non-parasitized erythrocytes, in addition to the immune destruction of parasitized red cells and an impaired compensation for this loss by bone marrow dysfunction. To combat anemia, concentrated fresh RBC transfusion or erythropoietin injection or blood substitutes (oxygen carriers like perfluro-carbon compounds, etc.) could be used, or the option of dietary supplementation of hematinics with other essential nutrient support needed for proper erythropiesis could be taken. The problem, however, is the availability of properly screened blood in the developing world, where malaria is largely prevalent. As has been mentioned earlier, about 13 million units of blood are not tested against HIV or hepatitis. Moreover, a large portion of the population in underdeveloped and developing countries cannot afford a proper diet, let alone erythropoietin therapy.

In one series of the present study, cord blood was given to 39 randomly selected patients with confirmed malaria and anemia between April 1999 and April 2005, following the voluntary patient consent protocol, after approval from the institutional ethical committee. The age of the patients varied from 8 to 72 years (mean 39.4 years). Twenty-four were males and 15 were females. In this series, 22 were infected with *P. falciparum* and 17 had *P. vivax* infection. A total of 94 units of cord blood (52–143 ml in volume; mean 81 $\pm$ 6.6 ml SD; median 82 ml; mean packed cell volume 48.9 $\pm$ 4.1 SD; mean hemoglobin concentration 16.4 $\pm$ 1.6 gm% SD) were transfused to these patients, with 2 units at a time to individual patients, with a maximum of 6 units to one patient. The amount of transfusion depended on the severity of anemia and the availability of compatible and screened cord blood.

The pathophysiology [40], iron metabolism [41, 42], and erythropoietin production [43] are different in the case of anemia in chronic disease. Hepcidin, an

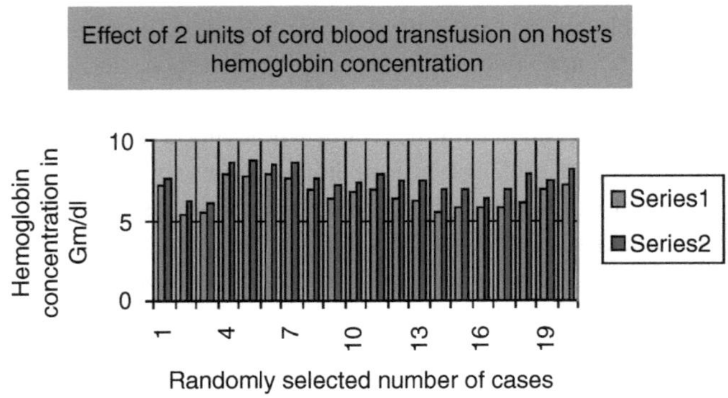

Fig. 10.1 Graphical impact of 2 units of cord blood transfusion on the host after 72 h. Series 1 shows the pre-transfusion hemoglobin in gm/dl; series 2 shows the post-transfusion hemoglobin in gm/dl (after 72 h). Source: Malar J. 2006; 5: 20. Published online 2006 March 23. doi: 10.1186/1475-2875-5-20. Copyright © 2006 Bhattacharya; licensee BioMed Central Ltd.

iron-regulated acute-phase protein that is composed of 25 amino acids, has helped to shed light on the relationship of the immune response to iron homeostasis and anemia of chronic disease [41, 42].

The pre-transfusion hemoglobin in malaria patients in this study varied from 5.4 to 7.9 gm/dl for those with *P. falciparum* infection, and from 6.3 to 7.8 gm/dl in those with *P. vivax.* The rise in hemoglobin, as estimated after 72 h of transfusion of 2 units of cord blood, was from 0.5 to 1.6 gm/dl (Fig. 10.1). What is noteworthy was that there was a slow but sustained rise in hemoglobin on the seventh day after transfusion (Series 3). A univariate analysis using Fisher's exact test was performed on the results of Series 2 (rise of hemoglobin after 7 days from pre-transfusion value). The difference between Series 2 and Series 3 values and their comparison

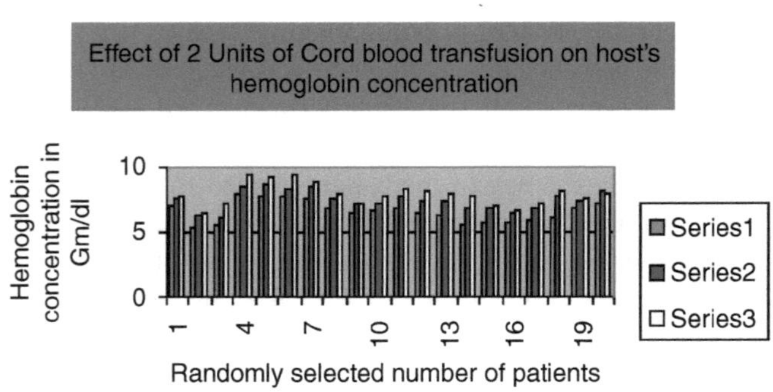

Fig. 10.2 Graphical impact of 2 units of cord blood transfusion on the host after 72 h and 7 days. Series 1 shows the pre-transfusion hemoglobin in gm/dl; series 2 shows the post-transfusion hemoglobin in gm/dl after 72 h; series 3 shows the post-transfusion hemoglobin in gm/dl after 7 days. Source: Malar J. 2006; 5: 20. Published online 2006 March 23. doi: 10.1186/1475-2875-5-20. Copyright © 2006 Bhattacharya; licensee BioMed Central Ltd.

with the pre-transfusion values appeared to be significant ($P < 0.003$). The observed effect could be due to the bone marrow stimulating impact of the different cytokine systems in placental blood (Fig. 10.2). As mentioned, no unfavorable immunological or non-immunological reaction or adverse metabolic impact on the recipient was encountered in the follow-up. There was no detected rise in serum creatinine (Fig. 10.3), urea (Fig. 10.4), glucose (Fig. 10.5), or bilirubin (Fig. 10.6) levels from the pre-transfusion levels. There was also an improvement in appetite and a sense of well-being in all the recipients of cord blood, which could be due to the high oxygen affinity and growth factor components of umbilical cord whole blood.

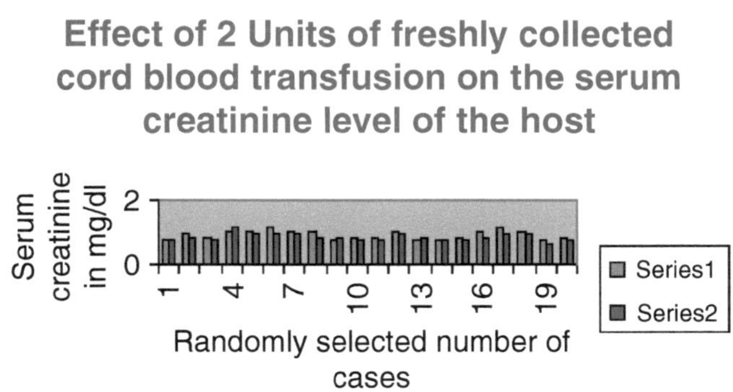

Fig. 10.3 Graphical impact of 2 units of cord blood transfusion on the host's creatinine level as seen after 72 h. Series 1 shows the pre-transfusion creatinine in mg/dl; series 2 shows the post-transfusion creatinine in mg/dl after 72 h. Source: Malar J. 2006; 5: 20. Published online 2006 March 23. doi: 10.1186/1475-2875-5-20. Copyright © 2006 Bhattacharya; licensee BioMed Central Ltd.

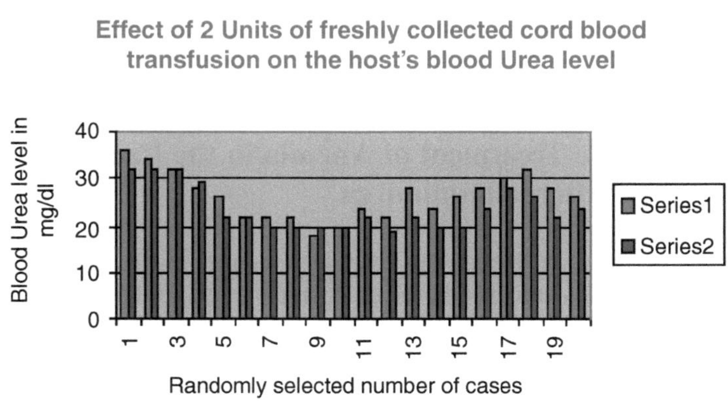

Fig. 10.4 Graphical impact of 2 units of cord blood transfusion on the host's urea level as seen after 72 h. Series 1 shows the pre-transfusion urea level in mg/dl; series 2 shows the post-transfusion urea level in mg/dl after 72 h. Source: Malar J. 2006; 5: 20. Published online 2006 March 23. doi: 10.1186/1475-2875-5-20. Copyright © 2006 Bhattacharya; licensee BioMed Central Ltd.

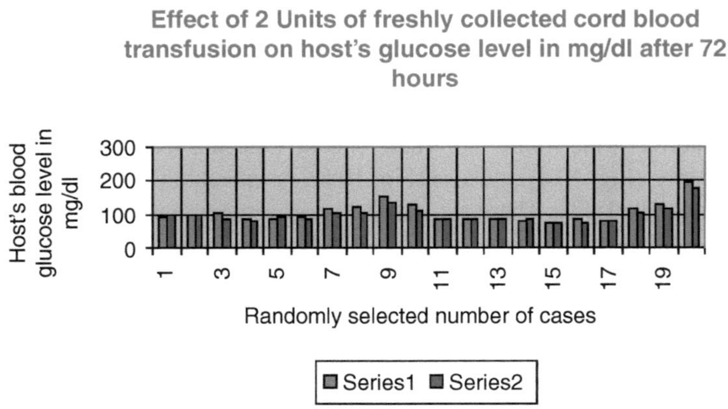

Fig. 10.5 Graphical impact of 2 units of cord blood transfusion on the host's glucose level as seen after 72 h. Series 1 shows the pre-transfusion glucose in mg/dl; series 2 shows the post-transfusion glucose in mg/dl (after 72 h). Source: Malar J. 2006; 5: 20. Published online 2006 March 23. doi: 10.1186/1475-2875-5-20. Copyright © 2006 Bhattacharya; licensee BioMed Central Ltd.

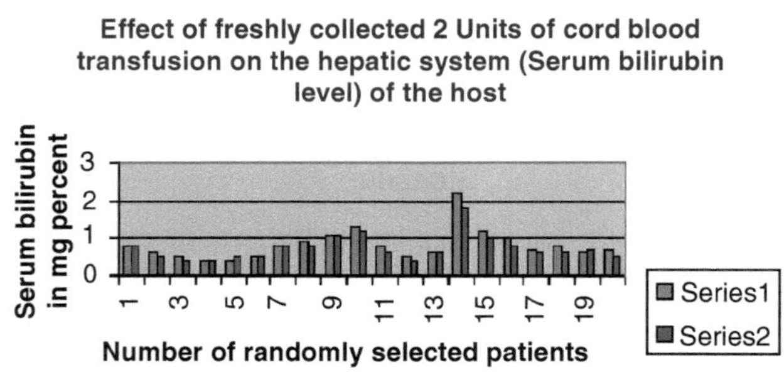

Fig. 10.6 Graphical impact of 2 units of cord blood transfusion on the host's bilirubin level as seen after 72 h. Source: Malar J. 2006; 5: 20. Published online 2006 March 23. doi: 10.1186/1475-2875-5-20. Copyright © 2006 Bhattacharya; licensee BioMed Central Ltd.

Cord Blood in the Treatment of Anemia in the Background of Diabetes and Microalbuminurea

As mentioned earlier, cord blood was given in a number of diseases with anemia as a common feature. Anemia is a familiar accompaniment of diabetes, particularly in patients with albuminurea or reduced renal function. The estimated prevalence of anemia depends on an essentially arbitrary criterion to define the presence or absence of anemia. Anemia in chronic diseases like diabetes is mostly immune-driven, where cytokines and cells of the reticuloendothelial system participate in altering iron homeostasis. Adequate proliferation of erythroid progenitor cells is also prevented along with dysregulation of erythropoietin (Epo) production and sensitivity, and there is an additional problem of altered life span of red cells [44].

Many factors have been suggested for the onset of anemia in a chronic metabolic disease like diabetes. A lower Hb count is associated with a more rapid decline in the glomerular filtration rate (GFR) [45]. It has been noted that early treatment of anemia in renal failure slows the rate of decline in renal function [46]. One of the most potent causes of suboptimal response to Epo is chronic and overt inflammation, associated with an increased production of cytokines, such as tumor necrosis factor-α (TNF-α), IL-1, or interferon-γ (INF-γ) [47], which might suppress erythrocyte stem cell proliferation [48]. Anemia also has a negative impact on patient survival, and is considered to be an important cardiovascular risk factor associated with renal disease. It appears more likely that proteinuria is a marker of tubulointerstitial injury in diabetes [49], perhaps more so than in non-diabetic conditions associated with proteinuria, which is considered to be primarily glomerular in origin. It has been suggested that the widespread use of ACE inhibitors may contribute to anemia in patients with diabetes [50]. The excretion of growth factors in urine has been implicated in the pathogenesis of tubulointerstitial disease that characterizes proteinuric renal disease. In some cases of uncontrolled diabetes, there is an unexplained anemia which, apart from blunted response to erythropoietin as a result of interstitial damage, could also be due to low serum level, abnormal glycosilation of the cytokine system, dysautonomia, or presence of infection or some other cause [50, 51, 52, 53, 54, 55, 56, 57, 58, 59, 60, 61]. Bleeding episodes, vitamin deficiencies (of cobalamin and folic acid, for instance), hypersplenism, helminthiasis, and malnutrition may all contribute to the anemic process as well. Independent predictors of anemia in diabetes are transferring saturation, glomerular filtration rate, sex, albumin excretion rate, glycosilation status, etc. [62].

Understanding the pathogenesis of anemia associated with diabetes and nephropathy may, therefore, lead to opportunities for developing interventions to optimize outcomes in these patients.

In this study, too, there were 49 informed, consenting patients (22 male and 27 female, aged 48–74 years, mean 59.6 years) randomized into two groups. Group A was the control group ($N = 15$: male = 8, female = 7), and Group B was the study group ($N = 24$: male = 14, female = 10). Group A patients were treated as per the standard regime of act rapid insulin, ace-inhibitor, combating dyslipidaemia, hyperuricemia, and transfusion of 2–4 units of fresh adult RBC. Group B patients were treated with an identical regime with one exception: freshly collected cord blood was transfused instead of adult blood, depending on the availability after cross-matching and fulfiling other essential criteria.

The pre-transfusion Hb of the patients varied from 5.2 to 7.8 gm/dl. They had Type-2 diabetes (fasting sugar 200 mg or more) with features of microalbuminurea (albumin secretion 30–299 mg/g creatinine). These patients were clinically examined, and standard indices like creatinine, albumin, fasting blood glucose, fasting lipid profile, HbA_{1c}, C-reactive protein, and ferritin levels were recorded. Urinary creatinine, urea, albumin, and protein obtained from a 24-h collection were also tested and recorded. Medical records of these patients showed no evidence of advanced diabetic nephropathy (creatinine clearance $\geq 30\,mg/kg/1.7\,m^2$).

For transfusion to Group B, 78 units of human placental umbilical cord blood were collected from consenting mothers after LUCS under general or regional anesthesia. The collected blood varied from 56 to 138 ml; in this series, mean 82 ± 5.6 ml SD; median 84 ml; mean packed cell volume 49.7 ± 4.2 SD; mean hemoglobin concentration 16.6 ± 1.5 gm% SD. Cord blood was transfused at the earliest (within 72 h at the latest) to the study group patients, following the standard WHO adult blood transfusion protocol. In all cases, there was strict adherence to the institutional committee guidelines and the patient consent protocol.

The data showed an increase from 1.5 to 1.8 gm/dl in the Hb count of Group A patients after transfusion of 2 units of cord blood and estimation of hemoglobin after 72 h of transfusion. In Group B patients, the increase in Hb after 72 h following the transfusion of 2 units of cord blood was between .5 and 1.6 gm/dl. Like in the case of malaria patients, there was a subjective improvement in appetite and a feeling of well-being among the patients who received cord blood transfusion.

Microalbuminurea was assessed in both groups after 1 month of treatment with transfusion and other identical support. In Group A, the mean value of albumin excretion in 24 h urine was 152 ± 18 mg SD of albumin per gram of creatinine (pre-transfusion mean value was 189 ± 16 mg). In Group B, it was 103 ± 16 mg SD per gram of creatinine (pre-transfusion mean value was 193 ± 21 mg). A univariate analysis using Fisher's exact test was performed for the results of Groups A and B, and the difference in the microalbuminurea values between the two groups ($P < 0.003$) appeared statistically significant.

The exact etiopathogenesis behind the improvement of the microalbuminurea in Group B patients is not clear, apart from the fact that freshly collected cord blood is rich in cytokine and many growth factors, whose individual impact is currently under study. Fetal hemoglobin-rich cord blood with its altered viscosity may have a positive impact on renal circulation. As mentioned earlier, this blood also has a high WBC and platelet content, is hypoantigenic in nature, and has altered metabolic profile. It may also have the potential to play a role in immune response modification in chronic anemia due to its rich cytokine and growth factor content. The impact of these cytokines and growth factors on the recipients' bone marrow and kidney may possibly antagonize chronic and inflammatory anemia and erythropoietin deficiency, or receptor sensitivity caused by tubulointerstitial injuries in diabetic patients. In this context, it should be remembered that proteinurea is not only a major correlate of declining renal function, but may also directly lead to disease progression by contributing to tubulointerstitial injury through the release of inflammatory and vasoactive substances into the interstitium [63]. The enhanced ultrafiltration of growth factors that occurs in proteinuric states has also been implicated as pathogenetically linked to the development of tubulointerstitial disease [64, 65]. The improvement of microalbuminurea in Group B patients may be the result of the positive effect of pregnancy-specific growth factors and cytokines on the renal derangement caused by diabetes. It appears that freshly collected cord whole blood transfusion is not only a transfusion of fetal hemoglobin-rich, high oxygen-affinity blood, but also an infusion of serum that is rich in pregnancy-specific growth factors and cytokines. In diabetic patients with anemia, its promise could be immense, not only in cash-strapped under-resourced countries but also in developed countries where patients may benefit from the extra potentials of cord blood.

Cord Blood in the Treatment of Anemia in the Background of Tuberculosis and Emaciation

In TB, too, umbilical cord whole blood has a similar potential to act as an immunoadjuvant therapy. TB is a major health hazard world wide, with the WHO reporting that one person gets infected every second, and that currently about one-third of the world population is infected. In a report of 1996, WHO estimated that, in the following decade, 300 million more people will be infected, 90 million will develop the disease, and 30 million will die from it [66]. Among those aged over 5 years, TB kills more people than AIDS, malaria, diarrhea, leprosy, and all other tropical diseases combined. An estimate of the WHO puts death due to TB at 3–4 million (around 2004) [67]. In India, about 500,000 people die of TB each year, and it has far more cases than any other country, amounting to two million new cases per annum [68].

The prevalence of TB infection and clinical diseases varies widely in different age groups. It is higher among children in household contact with adult patients, and the risk is higher for those in contact with sputum-positive patients [69]. The nutritional history of TB patients generally reveals that they have a higher level of anorexia, vomiting, nausea, and diarrhea, and consequently they suffer from a considerable degree of malnourishment. Directly Observed Treatment–Short Course (DOTS) has been a successful strategy in the global control of TB in adults. However, there are uncertainties of TB in extremes of ages, i.e., in the pediatric and geriatric age groups as well as in adults who receive steroids and other immunosuppressives, or in case of uncontrolled diabetes, or in nutritionally deprived patients in under-resourced regions. In such cases, patients can present to the physician with vague symptoms, unreliable tuberculin tests or TB score charts, non-specific hematological, biochemical or radiological evidences, difficulty in sputum expectoration, and non-availability or ill-affordability of specialized tests [70].

Anemia in TB is a serious co-morbidity, which is caused by various factors like hemoptysis in the case of pulmonary Kochs in an advanced stage, or lack of proper nutrition and micronutrients in the diet, or co-existent helminthiasis, or other co-existent diseases like HIV, and/or other pre-existing or compounding problems like gastrointestinal troubles, which can alter the available iron store or reserve or cause bone marrow dysfunction. Anemia in TB is anemia of chronic disease. There are disturbances of iron homeostasis, with increased uptake and retention of iron within the cells of the reticuloendothelial system, which subsequently limits the availability of iron for erythroid progenitor cells, and cause iron-restricted erythropoiesis. A report has shown that mice that are injected with pro-inflammatory cytokines IL-1 and TNF-α develop both hypoferremia and anemia [71]. In chronic inflammation, the acquisition of iron by macrophages takes place most prominently through erythrophagocytosis [72] and the transmembrane import of ferrous iron by the protein divant metal transporter 1 (DMT 1) [73]. INF-γ, lipopolysaccharide, and

TNF-α up-regulate the expression of DMT 1 with an increase of iron into activated macrophages [74]. The identification of hepcidin, as noted earlier, has helped in the recognition of the relationship of the immune response to iron homeostasis and anemia of chronic disease. Hepcidin expression is induced by lipopolysaccharide and IL-6 and inhibited TNF-α.

Anemia of chronic diseases like TB is the result of acute or chronic immune activation due to inflammation. This anemia is the second most prevalent anemia after anemia caused by iron deficiency [75]. In South Asia, malnutrition and anemia are a typical presentation of persons with TB, particularly in rural and semi-urban areas.

The rationale for the treatment of anemia in TB is, firstly, anemia can be generally deleterious by itself and may require a compensatory increase in cardiac output to maintain systemic oxygen delivery, and secondly, anemia is associated with poorer prognosis in a variety of conditions, including TB. In any case, when the hemoglobin count is less than 8 gm per deciliter or less, the decision to give packed-cell transfusion slowly is often taken. In anemia in the background of TB, too, cord blood has been proven to be not only effective, but an interesting phenomenon has been observed.

One hundred six units of cord blood were collected from consenting mothers after LUCS under general or local anesthesia. In this series, the volume varied from 48 to 148 ml $\pm$ 6.6 ml SD; median 82 ml; mean packed cell volume 49.4 $\pm$ 3.1 SD; mean hemoglobin concentration 16.3 gm% SD. Blood was transfused within 72 h of collection after due consent and following the ethical procedures of the institutional ethical committee.

In this series, 21 TB patients with anemia (8 gm or less per deciliter) were included. Sixteen cases were suffering from pulmonary Kochs', of whom four presented with cavitation. The other five had extra-pulmonary Kochs' involvement, i.e., intestinal Kochs' involvement was detected in four cases and skin involvement in one case. The criteria for clinical diagnosis of TB were typical clinical features like loss of weight, evening rise of temperature, weakness, and other constitutional symptoms depending on the primary involvement of the organ. For assessment of the Kochs' status, primary or reactivation, and to determine the background, X-rays were taken, and usual tests like Mantoux test, hemoglobin, total count of WBC, differential count of WBC, and erythrocyte sedimentation rate were done. However, in extra-pulmonary silent presentation of suspected Kochs' infection, Elisa TB IgA, IgM, IgG, and screening for HIV 1 and 2 were done routinely in patients of young age group. In case of clinical confusion, adenine deaminase, INF-γ, fine-needle aspiration cytology, and biopsy were used as supportive investigation. In two cases, we had to take the support of DNA (PCR) from ascitic fluid and also from serum for confirmation. In the pulmonary presentation group, in addition to Kochs' reactivation, two cases had HIV in the background and four cases had cancer. Cord blood was transfused to these patients to combat anemia due to hemoptysis-induced blood loss.

The study group included 13 female and 8 male patients aged between 18 and 74 years. The patients received 2–21 units of blood with 8 units in a row being transfused to one patient. All patients who received cord blood demonstrated positive clinical responses like less weakness, a sense of well-being, and weight gain, which was more obvious in patients who received more than 3 units of cord blood (16 cases).

Apart from general clinical improvement, a unique and interesting phenomenon was observed. There was a rise in the peripheral blood CD34 level in assessments done by flow analysis cytometry 72 h after transfusion. A search of published medical literature has not revealed any similar phenomenon reported elsewhere. This test was repeated after 3 months in consenting volunteers. The normal CD34 level in peripheral blood is 0.09%. In the present study, among those TB patients with an anemic background who received cord blood transfusion, the level of CD34 varied from 2.99 to 33%. This returned to individual base levels in 66.66% of the cases, at the 3-month CD34 level re-estimation.

The point at issue was why did this rise in the CD34 level occur in the first place, and why did it vary from individual to individual without provoking any graft-vs.-host reaction. No patient in this series (HLA and sex randomized) received any specific immunosuppressive drug therapy apart from the anti-tubercular drug. One possible explanation could be the interaction of (?) the hypoantigenic cord blood and the (?) immune mosaic condition in TB; another reason could be that freshly collected cord blood contains growth-stimulating cytokine, and this may have an impact on the hosts' bone marrow or some other specific system.

Another probable explanation can also be ventured. The placenta has a unique microenvironment and its sensitization impact on cord blood cells may play a role in a transient transplantation impact on the host system. One very important factor, apart from intrinsic differences, is the fact that hematopoietic stem cell (HSC) in umbilical cord blood cell (UCBC) have had a different set of microenvironmental exposures as compared to those of adult marrow or peripheral blood stem cell (PBSC). Examples of differences between sources include some of the observed changes in HSC cell cycle status, gene expression, and the adhesive and invasive properties induced by mobilization procedures used to generate PBSC, e.g., granulocyte colony-stimulation factor (G-CSF). The placenta is a complex organ that regulates maternal–fetal interactions. Many cytokines that can influence lymphohematopoietic development, e.g., G-CSF, c-kit ligand [stem cell factor (SCF)], granulocyte macrophage colony stimulated factor (GM-CSF), IL-15, and others, are produced by the placenta. The production of G-CSF by the placenta may be especially relevant to UCBT. G-CSF is produced both by the maternal decidua and by the fetal chorionic villi and enters the fetal circulation by a process that does not require a functional G-CSF receptor. G-CSF from the mother probably does not enter the fetal circulation, as administration of recombinant human G-CSF (rhG-CSF) to pregnant macaques did not result in detectable rhG-CSF in the fetuses [76]. The function of placental G-CSF production is unknown; however, it may serve as an immunoregulator that protects the mother and fetus from each other's allogeneic immune systems. G-CSF inhibits the ability of placental mononuclear cells to mediate cytotoxicity against allogeneic targets including choriocarcinoma cells.

Although precisely not clear yet, the rise of peripheral blood CD34 after cord blood transfusion to TB patients with anaemia may be due to functional hypoantigenecity of the freshly collected and immediately transfused cord blood antigen with its complex cytokine interaction. Freshly collected cord blood and its cytokines may have a role in immune-selective masking, i.e., immune mosaicism, in anemic patients with TB. Some degree of structural or functional immunosuppression may exist in TB due to drugs, chronic nature of the disease, or malnutrition with helminthiasis. The impact of growth factors or selective cytokine impact of the cord blood on the bone marrow of the recipient may alter the situation. Cord blood may have the potential to convert TH2 responses to TH1 responses due to its rich cytokines, which may have a role in immune response modification.

The detrimental effects of nutritional deficiencies on TB could result from alterations in the T lymphocytes and macrophages' functional regulation, which are the major cell types mediating anti-mycobacterial immunity. Cytokines play a central role in mediating anti-mycobacterial immunity. IL-2 is required to initiate and amplify immune responses. IFN-γ and TNF-α are important macrophage-activating cytokines and crucial in the immune response to TB. Other advances in our understanding of the pathophysiology of anemia of chronic diseases like TB, as mentioned earlier, suggest that disturbances of iron homeostasis, impaired proliferation of erythroid progenitor cells, and blunted erythropoietin response to anemia have made possible the emergence of new therapeutic strategies. There is no other published work on the use of umbilical cord whole blood in the treatment of anemia in the background of TB. The clinical improvement as a result of cord blood transfusion and the transient rise in the peripheral blood CD34 level stimulates us to think of the probable adjuvant immunopotentiating role or immunotherapeutic impact on the hosts' suppressed immune system, which were caused by malnutrition, chronic disease, or even drug impact. Hepatotoxicity occurs with isoniazid, rifampicin, pyrazinamide, and ethionamide. Risk factors include old age, malnutrition, and high alcohol consumption. If cord blood has an adjuvant immunotherapeutic impact, it may play a positive role in negating immunosuppression in TB patients.

Cord Blood in the Treatment of Anemia in the Background of Advanced Rheumatoid Arthritis

A similar effect was seen when cord blood was transfused to patients with anemia in the background of rheumatoid arthritis (RA). RA is the commonest form of arthritis and affects 1–3% of the population in the western hemisphere. The clinical presentation is heterogeneous with a wide variation of age at the onset, degree of joint involvement, and severity. Apart from causing disability in patients with severe disease or extra-articular symptoms, mortality is equal to that of patients with triple coronary artery disease or stage-IV Hodgkin's lymphoma [77]. There are recent therapeutic advances in the treatment of RA, but they are costly. In countries with inadequate resources, the problem is compounded by economic constraints, malnutrition, and a limited number of specialists [78].

Anemia is a common comorbidity in individuals with RA. In fact, anemia of the type characterized by low serum iron concentration in conjunction with adequate iron stores is frequently associated with RA and has served as a model for anemia of chronic disease. Investigators have suggested that RA patients who have anemia are more likely to have very severe joint disease. However, if anemia is treated successfully, the joint disease is likely to respond as well [79]. Antigen-activated CD4+ T cells stimulate monocytes, macrophages, and synovial fibroblasts to produce the cytokines IL-1, IL-6, and TNF-α, and to secrete matrix metalloproteinases through cell-surface signaling by means of CD69 and CD118 as well as through the release of soluble mediators, such as INF-γ and IL-17. IL-1, IL-6, and TNF-α are the key cytokines that drive inflammation in RA. Activated CD4+ T cells also stimulate B cells through cell-surface contact and through the binding of $\alpha_L\beta_2$ integrin, CD154 (CD40 ligand), and CD28 to produce immunoglobulins, including rheumatoid factor.

Patients with RA are also considered to be at nutritional risk. One cause of poor nutritional status in this patient population is thought to be the result of weight loss and cachexia linked to cytokine production [80]. In patients experiencing chronic inflammation, the production of cytokines, such as IL-1 and tumor necrosis factor, increases the resting metabolic rate and protein breakdown. The patient is then faced with the challenge of increasing both calorie and protein intake to meet the nutritional requirements of increased metabolic rate. This is frequently difficult partly because of the pain and swelling associated with RA, which make food preparation and purchasing difficult for those who live alone or have limited resources. In the Indian subcontinent, malnutrition and anemia, weakness, and emaciated look are a quite typical presentation in case of persons with arthritis reporting to state government hospitals for free treatment in the rural and semi-urban areas.

Diet may play a role in the management of RA, particularly in alleviating the symptoms of the disease, combating the side effects of therapy, and reducing the risk of complications. Proper antioxidant nutrients (vitamin A, vitamin C, and selenium) may provide an important defence against increased oxidant stress, and a supplementation of folate and vitamin B12 in patients treated with methotrexate (MTX) can reduce the incidence of side effects and offset the elevation in plasma homocysteine, which is frequent in these patients. Calcium and vitamin D, in patients treated with corticosteroids, can reduce bone loss, while a simple supplementation with iron may not always prevent anemia. But such a balanced diet containing all the micronutrients and protein is not affordable to under-resourced and marginalized people who report to government hospitals for free treatment. The cause behind anemia in arthritis is also not so simple that a properly balanced diet can fully alleviate the problem. Neither iron or folic acid nor B12 supplement can effectively reverse the condition of anemia in arthritis.

One Western study had suggested that the incidence of anemia was high: 49%, 46%, and 35% in RA, systemic lupus erythematosus (SLE), and psoriatic arthropathy (PsA), respectively. Low levels of serum B12 were also frequent (24%), with almost similar occurrence in the three disease groups [81]. During the active phase of the disease, elevated plasma concentrations of inflammatory cytokines, such as IL-6, IL-1β,

TNF-α, and acute-phase proteins, not only cause anemia but also lead to a reduction of fat free body mass (FFM) with a mean loss of 15% of cell body mass (CM) and a consequent reduction of muscle strength [82]. The common anemic form in arthritis is mainly normochromic, hypochromic, or normocytic; it can be even microcytic where iron deficiency is common. There is also associated thrombocytosis, raised ferritin, low serum iron, and iron-binding capacity [83]. The effect of erythropoietin on such anemia is controversial, and evidence exists that cytokines may affect hemopoiesis, possibly by affecting sensitivity to erythro-poietin [84].

In developing countries, the problem of treatment of RA is complicated because of the poor socioeconomic condition and educational background of a large majority of patients, who start non-compliance with prescribed drugs as soon as there is some relief. In the present series, the patients who were enrolled for cord blood transfusion were unable to afford erythropoietin injections or fresh packed cells. They included marginalized homeless persons, alcoholics, drug abusers, landless laborers, and others who came from the poverty background.

The patients were enrolled with their consent, and the institutional ethical committee approved each case. The American College of Rheumatology's (ACR) revised criteria for inclusion of arthritis patients were followed. However, although helpful, the ACR criteria are not optimal in distinguishing between early RA and undifferentiated polyarthritis and SLE. Yet, as per the ACR suggestions, 1–3 years of the disease process was considered early disease.

In this study, 78 units of human umbilical cord whole blood were collected from consenting mothers after LUCS (42–136 ml; mean 80.6 ± 3.6 ml SD in the present series; median 82.4 ml; mean packed cell volume 48.2 ± 2.1 SD; mean hemoglobin concentration 16.4 ± 1.5 gm% SD). This was transfused to 28 RA patients with anemia (plasma hemoglobin 8 gm or less per deciliter). Pre-transfusion and three days after the transfusion, blood was drawn from the patients for peripheral blood hematopoietic stem cell (CD34) estimation at Ranbaxy Laboratory.

The age of patients varied from 4 to 62 years. Eighteen were female and 10 were male. O (Rh+) was the commonest blood group (11 cases), followed by A (Rh+) in seven patients and B (Rh+) in six cases. Four patients had AB (Rh+) blood group. The background pre-transfusion hemoglobin varied from 5.6 to 7.9 gm per deciliter. Each patient received 2–6 units of blood within a span of 15 days, depending on availability and need. Blood was transfused immediately after collection after grouping and cross-matching. The study, which began in April 1999, was followed up to April 2005. Not a single post-transfusion patient suffered from any immediate or late complication of blood transfusion, i.e., immunological or non-immunological reaction. There was an increase of body weight of 3–5 lb in 75% of patients. A sense of well-being, both subjective and objective, as noted when cord whole blood was transfused to patients suffering from anemia in the background of other diseases like malaria or diabetes, was also noted in these cases. There was also an improvement in appetite in all the patients.

Peripheral blood CD34 study was done by flow analysis cytometry, pre-transfusion, 72 h post-transfusion, and after 3 months. The pre-transfusion peripheral blood hematopoietic stem cell (CD34) level was 0.09%. This showed an increase of

5.3–21% in the 72-h post-transfusion report. This returned to the base level in most cases in the 3-month estimation, without provoking any graft-vs.-host reaction in any of the patients.

The basic reason for non-rejection of the conceptus is the fact that pregnancy and neoplasm are two outstanding examples of natural tolerance to homograft. In order to avoid maternal HLA systems' recognition, there is non-cytopathic antibody inside the placenta apart from the hypoantigenic fetal cells. At or near term, however, a slow bi-directional traffic of cells at the fetal–maternal interface slowly develops. Moreover, fetal progenitor cells have been found to persist in maternal peripheral blood for decades after childbirth. Progenitor cells can differentiate into mature immune-competent cells. Chimerism is used to indicate a body that contains cell populations derived from different individuals; microchimerism indicates low levels of chimerism. Male DNA, of presumed fetal origin, can be detected in maternal circulation decades after delivery, and is referred to as fetal microchimerism (FM) [85]. Lymphohemopoietic cytokines are now recognized to be central participants in the cellular communication events underlying the complex and dynamic remodeling processes required to accommodate the semi-allogeneic conceptus during mammalian reproduction. Cytokines are identified to be of particular importance in mediating communications between the conceptus and the maternal cells, particularly the uterine epithelium and infiltrating leukocytes, both prior to implantation and as the placenta develops.

However, the issue of the rise of CD34 in peripheral blood remains intriguing. Here, too, one can venture the argument that the placenta has a unique microenvironment and its sensitization impact on cord blood cells may play a role in transient impact on the host system. One very important factor is that hematopoietic stem cells in UCBC have a different set of microenvironmental exposures as compared to that of adult bone marrow or PBSC. Examples of differences between sources include some of the observed changes in HSC cell cycle status, gene expression, and the adhesive and invasive properties induced by mobilization procedures used to generate PBSC, e.g., G-CSF. The placenta is a complex organ that regulates maternal–fetal interactions [86]. This placental environmental exposure of cord blood cells along with immune suppression(?)/immune mosaic in the host, either due to drugs, the chronic nature of the disease, malnutrition with helminthiasis, or other associated factors like the impact of growth factors or selective cytokine impact of the cord blood on the bone marrow of the recipient, may help in the transient rise in CD34 in the host. Preliminary bone marrow studies also suggested a positive impact on the host bone marrow cellularity in these patients.

Cord Blood in the Treatment of Anemia in the Background of Leprosy

Leprosy is a chronic infectious disease caused by acid-fast mycrobacterium known as *Mycrobacterium leprae*. It affects the skin, the peripheral nerves, the eyes, the upper respiratory tract, etc. Leprosy is still a major problem in most developing countries, with India and Brazil topping the list with a prevalence rate of 4.3–4.5 per 10,000 persons. India alone accounted for 78% of the 690,830 newly detected cases in 2001 [87, 88, 89]. There are several effective chemotherapeutic agents against *M. leprae*, of which Dapsone (diaphenylsulfone, DDS), rifampicin, clofazimine, ofloxacin, and minocycline constitute the backbone of the multidrug therapy as recommended by the WHO. Gastrointestinal toxicity and skin discoloration are the major side effects in long-term treatment with clofazimine, and rifampicin is known for its hepatotoxicity. However, the most important side effect, which is prominent, is the hematological problems with Dapsone [90]. The common hematological side effects with Dapsone therapy are hemolytic anemia, methamoglobinaemia, reticulocytosis, and reduction of cell resistance as seen in osmotic fragility studies. These effects are much more pronounced in Lepromatous leprosy patients with blunted erythropoietin response, low serum iron, and mildly raised serum ferritin concentration. The problem of Dapsone therapy is complicated further in endemic areas where, because of low nutrition, malaria, and intestinal parasitism, the hemoglobin concentration is already compromised.

Varying degrees of anemia, in any case, are prevalent in leprosy patients, which could be due to background malnutrition; coexistent diseases like helminthiasis; or drug impact on the immune system (including the bone marrow); poor red cell survival; and sometimes, though rare, glucose-6-phophate deficiency (Dapsone therapy).

In order to combat anemia in leprosy patients, with varying degrees of refractoriness due to the drug on the disease or the host reaction [91, 92, 93, 94, 95, 96] Dharmendra [97], a noted leprosy specialist from India, many years back, suggested blood transfusion from other consenting leprosy patients. However, in the current study, umbilical cord whole blood was transfused to consenting leprosy patients to combat anemia.

In the present series, 16 cases were enrolled (15 male + 1 female; age 12–72 years, mean 48.4 years). Five cases were of the pausibacillary type (PB), and 11 cases had the multibacillary type (MB) of leprosy. The clinical spectrum varied widely from the tuberculoid to the Lepromatous type, and one patient presented with gangrene of the leg preceding auto-amputation and was infested with maggots. MB patients received rifampicin 600 mg once monthly and clofazimin 200 mg initially, followed by 50 mg daily along with Dapsone 100 mg daily for 12 months uninterrupted. PB patients received 600 mg rifampicin once monthly along with Dapsone 100 mg daily for 6 months.

In the present series, 74 units of placental umbilical cord whole blood (52–142 ml, mean 83 ml, and 14 ml SD) were collected after LUCS from consenting mothers, which were transfused to leprosy patients with anemia within 3 days of collection (the blood being kept in a refrigerator earlier). In that, 2–8 units of placental blood was transfused to each patient without encountering any immunological to non-immunological reactions so far. Immediate reactions due to transfusion, viz., fever, chill and rigor, flank pain, back pain, blood in urine, fainting, and dizziness, were not seen in any of the cases. Even late reactions like mild or progressive renal complications were not encountered. Feto-maternal cell traffic has been implicated for the cause of scleroderma in mothers in case of male babies. In the present series, no such rare and unusual complication due to neonatal blood transfusion in the adult system was observed, excepting one unusual reaction, which was seen in post-transfusion cases relating to the other diseases discussed earlier.

In some leprosy patients, 7 days after the completion of cord blood transfusion, the flow analysis cytometry study showed a rise (pre-cord blood transfusion peripheral blood CD34 normal range is up to 0.09%) of peripheral blood CD34 level, from the pre-transfusion level, varying from 3.6 to 16.2% in 75% of cases. This effect became normal after 3 months. There was no clinical sign of graft-vs.-host reaction in any of the patients. There was no growth factor- or bone marrow-stimulating or -suppressing drug utilized during the transfusion protocol for cord blood.

The functional hypoantigenecity of the cord blood antigen with its complex cytokine interaction may have a role in immune-selective masking in leprosy, i.e., immune mosaicism, in anemic patients with leprosy either due to drugs like Dapsone, disease, nutrition or helminthiasis, or other associated factors like the impact of growth factors or selective cytokine impact of the cord blood on the bone marrow of the recipient. All the patients, irrespective of their background, tolerated the procedure well, and there was a sense of well-being in most of the cases.

Cord Blood in the Treatment of Anemia in the Background of HIV

Anemia is a frequent complication of HIV infection. Anemia that does not resolve is associated with the progression of the disease and a shorter survival rate for HIV patients. Recovery from anemia has been linked to improvement in survival outcomes. In general, as the disease progresses, the severity of anemia increases. Recently, the use of highly active anti-retroviral therapy has been associated with a significant increase in hemoglobin concentrations and a decrease in the prevalence of anemia.

However, some investigators have also claimed an acceleration of disease progression and mortality in patients with HIV infection after blood transfusions, and a review of related literature suggests that the mechanism for negative transfusion-associated outcomes may be transfusion-related immunomodulation.

Apart from the problem of immunosuppression, blood transfusion in severe anemia may trigger cardiac overload and failure unless adequate care and precautions are taken. The other alternative could be once-weekly epoetin alpha along with anti-retroviral therapy. However, this is expensive, and patients in under-resourced countries cannot afford erythropoietin. Transfusion of cord blood, however, proved to be safe, and there was general improvement with no signs of immunosuppression.

In the present series, 16 cases with severe anemia (hemoglobin less than 8 gm/dl) in the background of HIV were admitted for cord blood transfusion after getting necessary donor and recipient consent and approval of the institutional ethical committee. Seventy-five percent of the cases had full blown AIDS. None of them were intravenous drug users. All the patients had heterosexual transmission, and there was no case of homosexual mode of transmission.

Six patients had had B+ blood group, five were O+, three were A+, and two patients were AB+. The age group varied from 20 to 40 years. Eight were males and eight were females. One hundred twenty-three units of freshly collected umbilical cord whole blood were transfused to the 16 patients. One patient received 22 units, with 5 units at a time in a row. Among the others, one received 17 units, another 16 units, and a third 10 units. Two patients received 9 units each. The rest received lesser amounts. Blood was transfused within 72 h of collection on the basis of clinical priority, availability, cross-matching, and after proper screening as per the standard WHO blood transfusion protocol. Between the first and last blood transfusions, there was a gap of 4–10 months, and periodic clinical investigations were carried out. Patients who received more than 3 units of cord blood showed subjective and objective improvement in the form of less weakness, improved appetite, and a sense of well-being. A gain of 3–5 lb was also perceived in these patients during clinical observation. It should be noted that, here too, there was no immunological or non-immunological reaction observed in any of the HIV patients who received cord blood transfusion, thus again proving the safety of umbilical cord whole blood.

In some patients, too (randomly selected), pre-transfusion and 72-h post-transfusion CD34 studies from peripheral blood were undertaken, and again, a substantial rise, i.e., 3.6–23% (pre-transfusion value 0.09%) was noted in the post-transfusion reports, which subsequently returned to normal after 3 months of cessation of the last transfusion of cord blood.

Cord Blood in the Treatment of Anemia in the Background of Cancer

Anemia is the commonest abnormality seen in patients with cancer. Certain types of chemotherapy trigger anemia through bone marrow suppression. Radiation and rapid tumor progression can also trigger anemia through marrow suppression and/or infiltration or refraction. If existing anemia is not corrected before radiation, subsequent tumor cell hypoxia in conjunction with anemia can reduce the tumorocidal effect of radiation [98]. Anemia increases with the progression of the disease, and correction of anemia often improves the quality of life of cancer patients [99]. In any case, physiological adjustment to chronic and acute anemia has a limit, particularly in elderly patients with myocardial vascular disease. Treatment options include administration of different hematopoietic growth factors, red cell transfusion, various erythropoietin preparations, and dietary enrichment and regulations. A report published from USA, which noted that chemotherapy increases anemia, with 37% of the study group who were anemic (hemoglobin less than 12 gm%) increasing to 41% post-chemotherapy, suggested that these patients should be treated with RBC transfusions or erythropoietin. However, as has been noted, there are problems of cost, inconvenience of frequent injections, limitation of efficacy, bone marrow refraction, and other indication restrictions involved in erythropoietin therapy [100]. It also has the potential to trigger thromboembolic manifestations [101].

Due to the disease or the treatment, cancer patients often become immunocompromised, and thus become predisposed to a variety of bacterial, viral and fungal infections, and allied cellular-mediated immune response [102]. Advanced cancer patients, by virtue of their frequent exposure to transfusion, develop HLA alloantibodies, which can have an adverse effect on therapy, e.g., refractoriness of platelet transfusion. Ideally, therefore, cancer patients should receive specially processed blood products, such as leucoreduced, irradiated cytomegalovirus seronegative blood products. Leucoreduction can prevent febrile non-hematological reactions, including HLA alloimmunization, antibody platelet reaction and subsequent refractoriness of platelet transfusion, prevention of cytomegalovirus transfusion, etc. Blood components are irradiated to reduce transfusion-related graft-vs.-host reaction, which can be potentially lethal, by interfering with the ability of lymphocytes to proliferate. The standard guideline for good practice is the implementation of the recommendation to use RBCs, platelets, and granulocytes with a minimum dosage of 2500 cGi radiation [103].

Cord blood not only serves as a safe alternative to adult blood for transfusion in cancer patients, but it also has multifaceted advantages. Two hundred and thirteen units of cord blood were transfused to 72 consenting volunteers with anemia (hemoglobin less than 8 gm/dl) in the background of cancer, after following the same protocol used in the transfusion of cord blood in all the other diseases mentioned previously, and with the consent of the institutional ethical committee. Of the 72 volunteers who opted for cord blood transfusion, 30 patients were males and 42 were females. The age of the patients ranged from 14 to 86 years (1.38% belonged to the age group of 21–30 years and another 1.38% belonged to the age group of >80 years). The majority, however, belonged to the age group of 41–50 years, i.e., 41.66%, followed by 25% belonging to the 51–60-year age bracket. Of the total, 9.72% suffered from stage I cancer and 19.44% had stage 2 cancer. The rest, i.e., 70.84%, were in an advanced stage of the disease. In this study, 69 patients were suffering from carcinoma and three patients were suffering from sarcoma. Breast cancer was the most common (28 cases), followed by head and neck cancer (11 cases), gastrointestinal cancer (10 cases), gynecological cancer (8 cases), lung cancer (5 cases), urological cancer (4 cases), and blood cancer (3 cases).

In the present series, the collection of blood varied from 54 to 128 ml (Fig. 10.1); mean 82 ± 7.6 ml SD; mean packed cell volume 48 ± 4.1 SD; and mean hemoglobin concentration 16.4 ± 1.6 gm% SD. In one instance, 1–33 units (2706 ml on the basis of mean volume calculation of 82 ml per unit) of cord blood were transfused very slowly to the same patient, with 10 units (mean 82 × 10 = 820 ml) at a time in a row. There was no single episode of nausea, vomiting or any other specific gastrointestinal problem or hypertensive response during transfusion of umbilical cord whole blood. Once again, no instance of immunological or non-immunological reaction was observed.

On the other hand, the rise of hemoglobin within 72 h of the transfusion of 2 units of freshly collected cord blood was 0.5–1.7 gm/dl. Also, the extra oxygen and the rich cytokine- and growth factor-filled plasma in the cord blood may have a positive effect on cancer patients, since in this study all the patients who received cord blood transfusion demonstrated subjective and objective improvement.

Spontaneous Transient Rise of CD34 Cells in Peripheral Blood after 72 h in Patients Suffering from Advanced Malignancy with Anemia: Effect and Prognostic Implications of Treatment with Placental Umbilical Cord Whole Blood Transfusion

In diseases like HIV, a transient rise in CD34 cells was noticed 72 h after transfusion of umbilical cord whole blood in patients with anemia. Anemic patients in the advanced stage of malignancy were also given the same treatment, and here, too, the same phenomenon was observed. But, the prognostic implications of cord blood transfusion in some types of advanced malignancy may be even more positive.

Six cases of stage IV malignancy were enrolled in the protocol for the study of hematopoietic stem cells (CD34) after cord blood transfusion (as assessed from peripheral blood CD34 levels, 72 h after transfusion). All cases of transfusion-related CD34 of the peripheral blood were analyzed between 16 August 1999 and 16 May 2001.

The study group included three male and three female patients suffering from clinical stage IV malignancy. The hemoglobin count of each of the patients was <8 gm per deciliter. Apart from standard malignancy-related treatment like surgery, radiation, and chemotherapy (as per stage and grade of illness), they also received cord blood for the treatment of anemia.

Case 4 was suffering from sarcoma breast. She received 6 units of cord blood, which was the lowest amount transfused in this group. Case 6, suffering from cancer breast received the largest amount, i.e., 32 units. The youngest patient (case 1) was a 16-year-old boy suffering from non-Hodgkin's lymphoma, and he received 8 units of cord blood. Case 5 (metachronous metastasis lymph node neck) received 15 units; case2 (cancer breast) received 14 units; and case 3 (cancer lung) received 7 units. As noticed in other diseases, there were no transfusion-related clinical, immunological, or non-immunological reactions.

Periodic assessment of the CD34 levels from the peripheral blood revealed the trends as shown below:

Case 1: In case of non-Hodgkin's lymphoma, the peripheral blood CD34 level showed an apparent rising trend up to 24%. The patient died within 3 months after the last transfusion, due to bronchopneumonia.

Case 2: In case of the patient with cancer breast, the peripheral blood CD34 level showed a declining trend from an initial rise after the first transfusion of cord blood. The patient died within 2 months after the last transfusion.

Case 3: In case of the patient with cancer lung, the peripheral blood CD34 level never crossed the base line. The patient died within 15 days after the last transfusion.

Case 4: In case of the patient with sarcoma breast, after an initial hike, the CD34 level came down to the base level with slight marginal variation. The patient died within 7 months after the last transfusion.

Case 5: In case of the patient with metachronous metastatic bilateral neck nodes, there was marginal variation from the base line. The patient died within 21 days after the last transfusion of cord blood.

Case 6: In case of the patient with cancer breast, there was a substantial rise after practically every unit of transfusion, reaching up to 99% of the peripheral blood CD34 level (the normal level of peripheral blood CD34 is less than 0.09%). This patient is surviving today without any clinical disease.

The comparison and follow-up at the OPD till date show that the only patient who is surviving today without clinical disease is UB (case 6). She received the highest number of cord blood transfusions, and it was in her that we noted a steep rise in the CD34 level after transfusion. In four other cases, there was very little variation or a downward trend in the CD34 level after an initial rise. In case 1 (non-Hodgkin's lymphoma), there was a slow increase, but the level never crossed 24%. On the other hand, in case 6, it actually reached up to 99%.

There are many important factors that decide the fate of malignancy and the host, i.e., stage and grade of the disease, type of malignancy and organ involved, age, background nutrition, modalities of treatment offered, and finally, the immune status of the host.

New approaches include immunotherapeutic strategies, but the type and extent of spontaneous immune responses against tumor antigens remains unclear. A dominance of TH2 cytokines in the patients' sera, reported previously, suggests systemic tumor-induced immunosuppression, which potentially inhibits the induction of tumor-reactive T cells [104]. Whether the effect on bone marrow of the freshly collected cord blood growth factor cytokine systems, or bone marrow rejuvenation by the CD34 rich cord blood transfusion, causes a transplantation effect due to background immune suppression in advanced disease, is a matter under present study and follow-up.

The persistence of donor leukocytes in the transfusion recipient is termed microchimerism. It is likely that microchimerism reflects the engraftment of the recipient with donor hematopoietic stem cells. This is very uncommon in transfusion for elective surgery, sickle cell anemia, thalassemia, and HIV[105]. Long-term white blood cell (WBC) microchimerism of at least 2 years has been reported in trauma patients receiving fresh non-leukoreduced (non-LR) blood [106]. A better understanding of factors determining clearance vs. chimerism of transfused leukocytes is critical to the prevention of alloimmunization and transfusion-induced GVHD and, potentially, to the induction of tolerance for transplantation [107].

As mentioned earlier, pregnancy and neoplasm represent the most interesting examples of immune accommodation seen in mammalian biology. Cytokines of maternal origin act on placental development. At the same time, antigen expression on the placenta determines maternal cytokine patterns [108]. In case of tumors, the expression of HLA-G protein on the surface of primitive melanoma and metastatic cells confers protection from natural killer (NK) cells and cytopathic T lymphocyte (CTL) lytic activity [109, 110].

It has been mentioned further that the placenta is a complex organ that regulates maternal–fetal interactions [76]. It has a unique microenvironment, and its sensitization impact on cord blood cells may play a role in transient transplantation impact on the host system. Trophoblast cells of the placenta invade deep into the maternal uterine tissue to establish a life-giving connection with the maternal blood supply [111, 112].

This exposure of the hypoantigenic cord blood cells in the placental environment (or this exposure to the hypoantigenic cord blood cells nurtured in the placental environment) along with the immune suppression(?)/immune mosaic state existing in the host system, either due to drugs, chronic nature of the disease in advanced cancer, malnutrition with helminthiasis, reactivation of bacterial, viral or fungal diseases, or other associated causes like the impact of growth factors or selective cytokine impact of the cord blood on the bone marrow of the recipient, may help in the transient rise in CD34 in the host. There was no clinical GVHD in any of the cases. The preliminary bone marrow study also suggested a positive impact on the host bone marrow with improved cellularity in those patients.

For continuation of the tolerance state, a certain degree of chimerism (coexistence of cells of genetically different individuals) is needed. This is best achieved if the inoculation contains cells capable of self-renewal, i.e., stem cells [113]. In the present report, the results of freshly collected umbilical cord blood transfusion have been noted, and it has been recognized that there is a transient rise of peripheral blood CD34 level (much higher than its normal level, i.e., up to 0.09%). The positive prognostic significance of this hitherto unreported unique phenomenon may be due to (a) non-specific killing of the cancer cells by the CD34 cells of the donated cord blood, or (b) through induction of the dendritic cells (DC) of the cord blood, which are important accessory cells capable of initiating an immune response. The generation of functional DC from mononuclear cells isolated from human umbilical cord blood cells has already been reported. It has been shown that the cord blood-derived antigen-specific CTL can cause killing of human leukemic cells (K562) and breast cancer cells (MDA-231) [114]. The other possibility (c) is the impact of the growth factor content or other specific cytokine components of freshly collected and transfused cord blood on the hosts' bone marrow or immune system.

Whatever the trigger be, there was a transient rise of CD34 cells in the peripheral blood up to 99% in one case in the bone marrow without provoking clinical GVHD. This phenomenon has visible prognostic connotations as can be seen particularly from case 6 who is surviving today (September 2007). On the other hand, it was noted that, in cases where there was no significant fluctuation in the CD34 level after cord blood transfusion, early death occurred (cases 3 and 5). The pathophysiology and clinical significance of this phenomenon are being currently scientifically scrutinized.

Cord Blood in the Treatment of Anemia in the Background of Thalassemia

Thalassemia, also known as Cooleys' anemia, is an autosomal recessive genetic disorder affecting the hematopoietic system. It is characterized by anemia and compromised hemoglobin transport throughout the body. It has various clinical ramifications depending on the stage and grade of the disease. For the most part, the disease is due to decreased production of the beta component of hemoglobin, which is the primary carrier of O_2 in the blood. This disorder affects people of the Mediterranean, the Middle East, and South Asia in a large measure. Beta thalassemia can be of three different types. Type A is mainly asymptomatic (trait) and is also known as thalassemia minor, which can present with mild anemia. Type B presents with hepatosplenomegaly and anemia along with growth failure features. Type C is the major variety of beta thalassemia, which presents with severe anemia and complications of excessive iron load in the body, generally within 1 year of birth. In a general estimation, about 300,000 victims of thalassemia major can be detected globally. Treatment of beta thalassemia is essentially symptomatic with RBC transfusion to maintain a sufficient level of hemoglobin along with the treatment of side effects of iron load by iron chelation therapy to remove excess iron. Life-long transfusion dependence can create many problems for the unfortunate thalassemic patient, although there are global attempts for making blood transfusions safer with stricter vigilance. There are also protocols for inactivation of microbes in platelet units, use of plasma with reduced viral activity, and liberalization of the use of red cell substitutes [102]. However, the risks associated with the transfusion of adult blood or blood substitutes have been detailed earlier. Therefore, cord blood transfusion was also attempted in the case of thalassemic patients.

In the present series, 92 units of human umbilical cord blood were collected following the same protocol as in the treatment of anemia in the other diseases noted earlier. The collection varied from 57 to 136 ml; mean 84 $\pm$ 7.2 ml SD; median 87 ml; mean packed cell volume 45 $\pm$ 3.1 SD; mean hemoglobin concentration 16.4 $\pm$ 1.6 gm% SD. Donation of cord blood followed the guidelines of the human ethical committee of the hospital. The hemoglobin count of the recipient had to be below 6 gm% for enrollment to the cord blood transfusion program for thalassemia patients. Apart from usual investigations as per case-related requirements, Hb electrophoresis was done before and after the transfusion to examine the impact of transfusion.

Fourteen patients were enrolled for cord blood transfusion after due informed consent and authorization of the ethical committee. The age of the patients ranged from 6 months to 38 years with a sex ratio of 1:1. One patient received 23 units of cord blood transfusion (receiving 6 units at a time) because she started to have sudden menarche. Another patient received 16 units of cord blood (receiving 8 units at a time) due to bleeding P/R (hemorrhoid that was treated with ligation and interruption). All other patients received 2–8 units of cord blood, receiving at least 2 units at a time. They had universal complications of malnutrition along with growth retardation in four cases, impaired liver function in four cases, and hypofunction of the marrow in three cases. Osteodystrophy, Elisa Tb positivity for IgA and IgM (two cases), mitral stenosis and incompetence, irregularity of periods, and hypothyroid were some of the other complications. The hemoglobin concentration of patients in the present series varied from 3.5 to 5.9 gm%; mean 4.36 gm%. All the patients tolerated the procedure, and not a single episode of immunological or non-immunological reaction was encountered. Yet another interesting finding was that there was a definite subjective sense of well-being in the recipients, much more than the previous episodes of transfusion with concentrated RBC from adult sources.

Apart from not encountering any immunological or non-immunological complication in the aftermath of cord blood transfusion, and the general improvement in the subjective condition of the 14 patients, the hemoglobin electrophoresis study of one of the patients, a two-year-old boy with thalassemia major and impaired liver function, revealed an increase in fetal hemoglobin from 10.4 to 22.4% after the transfusion of a single unit of cord blood. It has been pointed out earlier that 14 gm% of adult hemoglobin can carry 19.46 ml of oxygen on an average, while cord blood at term generally carries on an average 16.8 gm% of hemoglobin, of which 20% belongs to the adult hemoglobin type (3.36 gm) and 80% belongs to the fetal hemoglobin type (13.44 gm). Fetal hemoglobin has the potential to carry 50% more hemoglobin than adult hemoglobin. Moreover, it has been said that, of the three types of hemoglobin contained in cord blood (HbF, HbA, and HbA2), HbF constitutes the major part (50–85%) and has greater oxygen affinity than HbA. The oxygen tension at which the hemoglobin of cord blood is 50% saturated is 19–20 mm of Hg, which is 6–8 mm Hg lower than that of normal adult blood. This shift to the left of the hemoglobin oxygen dissolution curve results from poor binding of the 2-3 diphosphoglycerate by HbF [18, 19]. An increase in fetal hemoglobin can have positive potentials for thalassemic patients.

Follow-up Study

The patients in the cord blood study were advised to report for follow up every third month to the OPD for clinical follow-up in the first year, followed by six monthly reviews to report on any untoward clinical reaction, i.e., late reactions like progressive detection of renal problems or delayed anemia. They were also cautioned to report immediately in case of any rare or unknown complications like the triggering of an autoimmune disease or unexpected problems resulting from the clinical impact of microchimerism like scleroderma or similar unknown skin or intestinal disorders. However, not a single patient who reported for the follow-up complained of any immunological or non-immunological reaction.

Future Implications of the Work

The findings of the present study on the use of cord blood (1999–2005) has shown that freshly collected cord blood after adequate screening can act as a true adult blood substitute. Moreover, placental umbilical cord whole blood can play a role in neurology, cardiology, nephrology, and other branches of medicine as a concentrated source of fetal hemoglobin-rich RBC, which has the potential to improve oxygen perfusion involving the ischemic cells of the recipient's system. It may also play a part in the subsequent repair of the system due to the interaction with a host of primitive cells found in cord blood, which have a regenerative capability. These cells are the hematopoietic stem cells, endothelial progenitors and angiogenesis-stimulating cells, mesenchymal stem cells, unrestricted somatic stem cells with activities resembling embryonic stem cells, and other cells. It should be underscored that ABO-matched cord blood transfusion may have a transplant impact, as noted earlier in various cases where there was a rise in CD34 in the peripheral blood.

Cord blood is currently under intense experimental investigation in pre-clinical models of pathophysiologies that range from myocardial ischemia, to stroke, to muscle regeneration. Cord blood mesenchymal stem cells appear to be capable of expansion to approximately 20 times, whereas adipose-derived cells expand on average eight times and bone marrow-derived cells expand five times [115].

Cord blood has some immunological properties involving both stem cell and non-stem cell fractions. The possibility of utilizing allogeneic cells for regenerative applications without fully compromising the recipient's immune system should not be dismissed. There are interesting similarities between cord blood transplantation and fetal–maternal cell trafficking during normal pregnancy.

Lymphocytes from cord blood, in contrast to adult blood, are generally immature. Numerous trials have been conducted administering doses of up to 2×10^9 paternal lymphocytes into pregnant mothers who have had recurrent miscarriages [116]. These doses are higher than the $1.5–3 \times 10^7$ nucleated cells per kilogram administered during a cord blood transplant [117]. Interestingly, no GVHD has ever been observed in pregnant women who were administered these high doses of completely allogeneic cells, although Th2 immune deviation has been reported by some groups [118].

The pertinent question here is: why is there a reduced incidence of GVH disease in case of cord blood transplantation than in adult blood? One reason may be that cytokine cascade is claimed to be responsible for GVHD. An interesting study by I.M.H. Chalmers et al. showed that cord blood lymphocytes (CBL) actually produce less IL-2, IL-4, IFN-γ, and TNF-α than adult peripheral blood lymphocytes (ABL). A further subset study by the same group hinted that the majority of cytokine-producing cells were CD4 + CD45RA+, whereas in adult blood, the cytokine-producing cells were both CD4 + CD45RO+ and CD8 + CD45RO+ [119].

In the present study on the use of cord blood transfusion in different diseases, ABO-matched HLA-randomized cord blood was administered to the extent of as many as 32 units to an individual, without encountering any clinical features of GVHD. The basic fact appears to be that the homeostatic proliferation in lymphopenic environment actually causes GVHD following ablation of host T cells. This creation of an "empty compartment" allows for homeostatic expansion of the newly introduced T cells, which primes them for aggressive immune reactions and alleviates their requirement for costimulation [120]. A group of contemporary researchers has even proposed that GVHD is not an intrinsic property of the allogeneic cells introduced into the host, but a result of lymphoablation induced in the recipient prior to cellular administration [121].

References

1. World Health Organization. International Federation of Red Cross and Red Crescent Societies, *Safe Blood Starts with Me*. Geneva; World Health Organization. 2000:12.
2. Goodnough LT, et al. Blood transfusion. *N Engl J Med.* 1999;340(6):438–7.

3. Mortimer PP. Editorial making blood safer. *BMJ*. 2002;325:400–401.
4. Sloand EM, Pitt E, Klein G. Safety of blood supply. *JAMA*. 1995;274:1368–73.
5. Amberson WR, Mulder AG, Steggerda FR, et al. Mammalian life without blood corpuscles. *Science*. 1993;78:106–7.
6. Gluckman E, Broxmeyer HA, Auerbach AD, et al. Hematopoietic reconstitution in a patient with Fanconi's anemia by means of umbilical-cord blood from an HLA-identical sibling. *N Engl J Med*. 1989;321:1174–8.
8. See for instance, the website of Healthcord Cryogenics Corporation, Canada. http://www.healthcord.com accessed on 2 September 2006.
9. Hannah Hoag. Blood Substitute from Worm Show Promise – Hemoglobin from Sea Creature could Replace Red Cells. http://www.nature.com/nsu/030602/030602-7 html, 4 June 2003.
10. Sloan EP, Koenigsburg M, Gens D, et al. Diasprin cross linked hemoglobin (DCLHb) in the treatment of severe hemoohagic shock: a randomized controlled efficacy trial. *JAMA*. 1999;282:1857–64.
11. Klein HG. The prospect of red blood substitute. *N Eng J Med*. 2000;342(22):1666–8.
12. Oski A, Naiman JL. *Hematologic Problems in the Newborn*. 3rd Ed. Philadelphia; WB Saunders. 1992.
13. Guyton AC, Hall JE. *Textbook of Medical Physiology*. Bangalore; WB Saunders. 1996:1036.
14. Usher R, Shephard M, Lind J. The blood volume of the newborn infants and the placental transfer. *Acta Pediatr.* 1963;52:497.
15. Haselhorst G, Allmeling A. Die gewichtszunahme von neugeborenen infolge postnataler transfusion. *Z Geburtshilfe Perinatol.* 1930;98:103.
16. Karaklis A, Fessas P. The normal minor components of fetal hemoglobin. *Acta Haematol.* (Basel). 1963;29:267.
17. Davis JA, Dobbing J. *Scientific Foundation of Pediatrics*. Int. Ed. London; William Heineman Medical Books. 1996:514.
18. Killmartin JV. Interaction of hemoglobin with protein, CO and 2-3 diphosphoglycerate. *Br Med Bull*. 1976;32:209.
19. Delivoria Padopoulos M, Roncevic NP, Oski FA. Post-natal changes in the oxygen transfer of term, premature and sick infants: the role of 2-3 diphosphoglycerate and the adult hemoglobin. *Pediatr Res*. 1971;5:235.
20. Molsa M, Heikkinen T, Hakala K, Wallerman O, Wadelius M, Wadelius C, Laine K. Functional role of P-glycoprotein in the human blood-placental barrier. *Clin Pharmacol Ther.* 2005;78(2):118–22.
21. Tscherning-Casper C, Papadogiannakis N, Anvert M, Stolpe L, Lindgern S, Bohlin AB, Albert J, Fenyo EM. Trophoblastic epithelial barrier is not infected in full term placentae of human immunodeficiency virus-seropositive mothers undergoing antiretroviral therapy. *J Virol*. 1999;73(11):9673–8.
22. Knudtzon S. In vitro growth of granulocytic colonies from circulating cells in human cord blood. *Blood*. 1974;43:357–61.
23. Broxmeyer HE, Kurtzberg J, Gluckman E, et al. Umbilical cord blood hematopoietic stem and repopulating cells in human clinical transplantation. *Blood Cells*. 1991;17:313–29.
24. Broxmeyer HE, Douglas GW, Hangoc G, et al. Human umbilical cord blood as a potential source of transplantable hematopoietic stem/progenitor cells. *Proc Natl Acad Sci U S A*. 1989;86:3828–32.
25. Lansdorp PM, Dragowska W, Mayani H. Ontogeny-related changes in proliferative potential of human hematopoietic cells. *J Exp Med*. 1993;178:787–91.
26. Hao QL, Shah AJ, Thiemann FT, Smogorzewska EM, Crooks GM. A functional comparison of CD34 + CD38– cells in cord blood and bone marrow. *Blood*. 1995;86:3745–53.
27. Vaziri H, Dragowska W, Allsopp RC, Thomas TE, Harley CB, Lansdorp PM. Evidence for a mitotic clock in human hematopoietic stem cells: loss of telomeric DNA with age. *Proc Natl Acad Sci U S A*. 1994;91:9857–60.

28. Szabolcs P, Park KD, Reese M, Marti L, Broad-water G, Kurtzberg J. Coexistent naive phenotype and higher cycling rate of cord blood T cells as compared to adult peripheral blood. *Exp Hematol.* 2003;31:708–14.
29. Loetscher P, Uguccioni M, Bordoli L, et al. CCR5 is characteristic of Th1 lymphocytes. *Nature.* 1998;391:344–5.
30. Bacchetta R, Bigler M, Touraine JL, et al. High levels of interleukin 10 production in vivo are associated with tolerance in SCID patients transplanted with HLA mismatched hematopoietic stem cells. *J Exp Med.* 1994;179:493–502.
31. Ballen KK. New trends in umbilical cord blood transplantation. *Blood.* 2005;105(10): 3786–92.
32. Paxson CL Jr. Collection and use of autologous fetal blood. *Am J Obstet Gynecol.* 1979;134(6):708–10.
33. Eichler H, Schaible T, Richter E, Zieger W, Voller K, Leveringhaus A, Goldmann SF. Cord blood as a source of RBCs for transfusion to preterm infants. *Transfusion.* 2000;40(9): 1111–7.
34. Brune T, Garritsen H, Hentschel R, Louwen F, Harms E, Jorch G. Efficacy, recovery and safety of RBCs from autologous placental blood: clinical experience in 52 newborns. *Transfusion.* 2003;43(9):1210–6.
35. Taguchi T, Suita S, Nakamura M, Yamanouchi T, Ogita K, Taguchi S, Uesugi T, Nakano H, Inaba S. The efficacy of cord blood transfusions in neonatal surgical patients. *J Pediatr Surg.* 2003;38(4):604–7.
36. Hassal O, Bedu-Addo G, Danso K, Bates I. Umbilical-cord blood for transfusion in children with severe anaemia in under-resourced countries. *Lancet.* 2003;361(9358):678–9.
37. Bhattacharya N, Mukherjee KL, Chettri MK, et al. A study report of 174 units of placental umbilical cord whole blood transfusion in 62 patients as a rich source of fetal hemoglobin supply in different indications of blood transfusion. *Clin Exp Obstet Gynecol.* 2001;28: 47–52.
38. Bhattacharya N. Placental umbilical cord whole blood transfusion. [Letter]. *J Am Coll Surg.* 2004;1992:347–8.
39. World Health Organization. Severe falciparum malaria. *Trans R Soc Trop Med Hyg.* 2000;94(Suppl 1):Sl–90.
40. Weiss G. pathogenesis and treatment of anaemia of chronic disease. *Blood Rev.* 2002;16: 87–96.
41. Nemeth E, Rivera S, Gabayan V, Keller C, Taudorf S, Pedersen BK, Ganz T. IL-6 mediates hypoferremia of inflammation by inducing the synthesis of the iron regulatory hormone hepcidin. *J Clin Invest.* 2004;113:1271–6.
42. Nicolas G, Bennoun M, Porteu A, Mativet S, Beaumont C, Grandchamp B, Sirito M, Sawadogo M, Kahn A, Vaulont S. Severe iron deficiency anaemia in transgenic mice expressing liver hepcidin. *Proc Natl Acad Sci U S A.* 2002;99:4596–601.
43. Jelkmann W. Preinflammatory cytokines lowering erythropoietin production. *J Interferon Cytokine Res.* 1998;18:555–9.
44. Weiss G, Goodnough LT. Anemia of chronic disease. *N Engl J Med.* 2005;352:1011–23.
45. Rossing K, Christensen PK, Hovind P, Tarnow L, Rossing P, Parving HH. Progression of nephropathy in type 2 diabetic patients. *Kidney Int.* 2004;66:1596–605.
46. Gouva C, Nikolopoulos P, Ioannidis JP, Siamopoulos KC. Treating anemia early in renal failure patients slows the decline of renal function: a randomized controlled trial. *Kidney Int.* 2004;66:753–60.
47. Goicoechea M, Martin J, de Sequera P, Quiroga JA, Ortiz A, Carreno V, Caramelo C. Role of cytokines in the response to erythropoietin in hemodialysis patients. *Kidney Int.* 1998;54:1337–43.
48. Zanjani ED, McGlave PB, Davies SF, Banisadre M, Kaplan ME, Sarosi GA. In vitro suppression of erythropoiesis by bone marrow adherent cells from some patients with fungal infection. *Br J Haematol.* 1982;50:479–90.

49. Katz A, Caramori ML, Sisson-Ross S, Groppoli T, Basgen JM, Mauer M. An increase in the cell component of the cortical interstitium antedates interstitial fibrosis in type 1 diabetic patients. *Kidney Int*. 2002;61:2058–66.
50. Dikow R, Schwenger V, Schömig M, Ritz E. How should we manage anaemia in patients with diabetes? *Nephrol Dial Transplant*. 2001;17:67–72.
51. Symeonidis A, Kouraklis-Symeonidis A, Psiroyiannis A, Leotsinidis M, Kyriazopoulou V, Vassilakos P, Vagenakis A, Zoumbos N. Inappropriately low erythropoietin response for the degree of anemia in patients with noninsulin-dependent diabetes mellitus. *Ann Hematol.* 2006;85(2):79–85. Epub 2005 Aug 31.
52. Biesenbach G, Schmekal B, Eichbauer-Sturm G, Janko O. Erythropoietin requirement in patients with type 2 diabetes mellitus on maintenance hemodialysis therapy. *Wien Klin Wochenschr*. 2004;116(24):844–8.
53. Craig KJ, Williams JD, Riley SG, Smith H, Owens DR, Worthing D, Cavill I, Phillips AO. Anemia and diabetes in the absence of nephropathy. *Diabetes Care*. 2005;28(5):1118–23.
54. Bosman DR, Winkler AS, Marsden JT, Macdougall IC, Watkins PJ. Anemia with erythropoietin deficiency occurs early in diabetic nephropathy. *Diabetes Care*. 2001;24(3): 495–9.
55. Kuriyama S, Tomonari H, Yoshida H, Hashimoto T, Kawaguchi Y, Sakai O. Reversal of anemia by erythropoietin therapy retards the progression of chronic renal failure, especially in nondiabetic patients. *Nephron*. 1997; 77(2):176–85.
56. Cotroneo P, Maria Ricerca B, Todaro L, Pitocco D, Manto A, Ruotolo V, Storti S, Damiani P, Caputo S, Ghirlanda G. Blunted erythropoietin response to anemia in patients with Type 1 diabetes. *Diabetes Metab Res Rev*. 2000;16(3):172–6.
57. Yun YS, Lee HC, Yoo NC, Song YD, Lim SK, Kim KR, Hahn JS, Huh KB. Reduced erythropoietin responsiveness to anemia in diabetic patients before advanced diabetic nephropathy. *Diabetes Res Clin Pract*. 1999;46(3):223–9.
58. Kario K, Matsuo T, Kodama K, Nakao K, Asada R. Reduced erythropoietin secretion in senile anemia. *Am J Hematol*. 1992;41(4):252–7.
59. Vogeser M, Schiel X. Serum erythropoietin concentrations in patients with anemia – preliminary hemoglobin-related reference ranges. *Clin Lab*. 2002;48(11–12):595–8.
60. Thomas MC, Cooper ME, Tsalamandris C, MacIsaac R, Jerums G. Anemia with impaired erythropoietin response in diabetic patients. *Arch Intern Med*. 2005;165(4):466–9.
61. Thomas MC, Tsalamandris C, MacIsaac R, Medley T, Kingwell B, Cooper ME, Jerums G. Low-molecular-weight AGEs are associated with GFR and anemia in patients with type 2 diabetes. *Kidney Int*. 2004;66(3):1167–72.
62. Thomas MC, MacIsaac RJ, Tsalamandris C, Power D, Jerums G. Unrecognized anemia in patients with diabetes: a cross-sectional survey. *Diabetes Care*. 2003;26(4):1164–9.
63. Remuzzi G, Bertani T. Patho-physiology of progressive nephropathies. *N Engl J Med.* 1998;339:1448–56.
64. Wang SN, Hirschberg R. Growth factor ultrafiltration in experimental diabetic nephropathy contributes to interstitial fibrosis. *Am J Physiol Renal Physiol.* 2000;278:F554–60.
65. Gilbert RE, Akdeniz A, Weitz S, Usinger WR, Molineaux C, Jones SE, Langham RG, Jerums G. Urinary connective tissue growth factor excretion in patients with type 1 diabetes and nephropathy. *Diabetes Care*. 2003;26(9):2632–6.
66. World Health Organization. Tuberculosis. Fact sheet No. 104 (revised). Available at: http://www.who.ch/. Accessed March 1996.
67. World Health Organisation. *TB – A Global Emergency. WHO report on the TB epidemic*. Geneva; WHO. 1994.
68. Tuberculosis control — India. New Delhi, India: Directorate General of Health Services, 2002. (Accessed October 7, 2002, at http://www.tbcindia.org).
69. Singh M, Mynak ML, Kumar L, Mathew JL, Jindal SK. Prevalence and risk factors for transmission of infection among children in household contact with adults having pulmonary tuberculosis. *Arch Dis Child*. 2005;90(6):624–8.

70. Arora VK, Gupta R. Directly observed treatment for tuberculosis. *Indian J Pediatr.* 2003;70(11):885–9.
71. Alvarez-Hernandez X, Liceaga J, McKay IC, Brock JH. Induction of hypoferremia and modulation of macrophage iron metabolism by tumor necrosis factor. *Lab Invest.* 1989;61:319–22.
72. Moura E, Noordermeer MA, Verhoeven N, Verheul AF, Marx JJ. Iron release from human monocytes after erythrophagocytosis in vitro: an investigation in normal subjects and hereditary hemochromatosis patients. *Blood.* 1998;92:2511–9.
73. Andrews NC. The iron transporter DMT1. *Int J Biochem Cell Biol.* 1999;31:991–4.
74. Ludwiczek S, Aigner E, Theurl I, Weiss G. Cytokine-mediated regulation of iron transport in human monocytic cells. *Blood.* 2003;101:4148–54.
75. Hopewell PC. Impact of human immunodeficiency virus infection on the epidemiology, clinical features, management, and control of tuberculosis. *Clin Infect Dis.* 1992;15:540–47.
76. McCracken S, Layton JE, Shorter SC, Starkey PM, Barlow DH, Mardon HJ. Expression of granulocyte-colony stimulating factor and its receptor is regulated during the development of the human placenta. *J Endocrinol.* 1996;149:249–58.
77. Buckley CD. Science, medicine, and the future: treatment of rheumatoid arthritis. *BMJ.* 1997;315:236–8.
78. Bhattacharya N, Chhetri MK, Mukherjee KL, et al. Human fetal adrenal transplant: a possible role in relieving intractable pain in advanced rheumatoid arthritis. *Clin Exp Obstet Gynecol.* 2002;29:197–206.
79. Wilson A, Yu HT, Goodnough LT, Nissenson AR. Prevalence and outcomes of anemia in rheumatoid arthritis: a systematic review of the literature. *Am J Med.* 2004;116 Suppl 7A:50S–57S.
80. Roubenoff R, Freeman LM, Smith DE, Abad LW, Dinarello CA, Kehayias JJ. Adjuvant arthritis as a model of inflammatory cachexia. *Arthritis Rheum* 1997;40(3):534–9.
81. Segal R, Baumoehl Y, Elkayam O, Levartovsky D, Litinsky I, Paran D, Wigler I, Habot B, Leibovitz A, Sela BA, Caspi D. Anemia, serum vitamin B12, and folic acid in patients with rheumatoid arthritis, psoriatic arthritis, and systemic lupus erythematosus. *Rheumatol Int.* 2004;24(1):14–9. Epub 2003 April 29.
82. Miggiano GA, Gagliardi L. Diet, nutrition and rheumatoid arthritis. *Clin Ter.* 2005;156(3): 115–23
83. Akil M, Amos RS. ABC of rheumatology: rheumatoid arthritis – I: clinical features and diagnosis. *BMJ.* 1995;310:587–90.
84. Smith MA, Knight SM, Maddison PJ, Smith JG. Anaemia of chronic disease in rheumatoid arthritis: effect of blunted response to erythropoietin and of interleukin-1 production by marrow macrophages. *Ann Rheum Dis.* 1992;51:753–7.
85. Lambert NC, Lo YM, Erickson TD, Tylee TS, Guthrie KA, Furst DE, Nelson JL. Male microchimerism in healthy women and women with scleroderma: cells or circulating DNA? A quantitative answer. *Blood.* 2002;100(8):2845–51.
86. Chao NJ, Emerson SG, Weinberg KI. Stem cell transplantation (cord blood transplants). *Hematology Am Soc Hematol Educ Program.* 2004:354–71 Review.
87. World Health Organization. *World Health Assembly – Resolution WHA44.9.* Geneva; WHO. 1991.
88. Sasaki S, Takeshita F, Okuda K, Ishii N. *Mycobacterium leprae* and leprosy: a compendium. *Microbiol Immunol.* 2001;45:729–36.
89. Ishii N, Onoda M, Sugita Y, Tomoda M, Ozaki M. Survey of newly diagnosed leprosy patients in native and foreign residents of Japan. *Int. J. Lepr.* 2000; 68:172–6.
90. Ishii N. Recent advances in the treatment of leprosy. *Dermatol Online J.* 2003;9(2):5.
91. Halim NK, Ogbeide E. Haematological alterations in leprosy patients treated with dapsone. *East Afr Med J.* 2002;79(2):100–2.

92. Queiroz RH, Melchior Junior E, de Souza AM, Gouveia E, Barbosa JC, de Carvalho D. Haematological and biochemical alterations in leprosy patients already treated with dapsone and MDT. *Pharm Acta Helv.* 1997;72(4):209–13.
93. Jollow DJ, Bradshaw T, McMillan DC. Dapsone-induced hemolytic anemia. *Drug Metab Rev.* 1995;27(1–2):107–24. Review.
94. Byrd SR, Gelber RH, Byrd SR, Gelber RH. Effect of dapsone on haemoglobin concentration in patients with leprosy. *Lepr Rev.* 1991;62(2):171–8.
95. Puavilai S, Chutha S, Polnikorn N, Timpatanapong P, Tasanapradit P, Charuwichitratana S, Boonthanom A, Wongwaisayawan H. Incidence of anemia in leprosy patients treated with dapsone. *J Med Assoc Thai.* 1984;67(7):404–7.
96. Khaire DS, Magar NG. Haemolytic effects of DDS in leprosy patients. *Indian J Med Res.* 1972;60(10):1510–9.
97. Dharmendra, Dharmendra. Transfusion of blood from leprosy patients. *Lepr India.* 1979; 51(2):176–81.
98. Steensma DP. Management of anemia in patients with cancer. *Curr Oncol Rep.* 2004; 6(4):297–304.
99. Smith RE Jr, Tchekmedyian S. Practitioners'practical model for managing cancer related anemia. *Oncology (Huntingt).* 2002;16(9 Suppl 10):55–63.
100. Pirker R, Wiesenberger K, Pohl G, Minar W. Anemia in lung cancer: clinical impact and management. *Clin Lung Cancer.* 2003;5(2):90–7.
101. Tchekmedyian NS. Anemia in cancer patients: significance, epidemiology, and current therapy. *Oncology (Huntingt).* 2002;16(9 Suppl 10):17–24.
102. Goodnough LT. Transfusion medicine –blood conservation –second of two parts. *N Engl J Med.* 1999;340(7):525–33.
103. Guideline for the gamma irradiation of the blood components for the prevention of the transfusion associated graft vs host disease. BCSH blood transfusion task force. *Transfus Med.* 1996;6(3):261–71. No abstract available PMID: 8885157 [PulMed-indexed for MEDLINE].
104. Schmitz-Winnenthal FH, Volk C, Z'graggen K, Galindo L, Nummer D, Ziouta Y, Bucur M, Weitz J, Schirrmacher V, Buchler MW, Beckhove P. High frequencies of functional tumor-reactive T cells in bone marrow and blood of pancreatic cancer patients. *Cancer Res.* 2005;65(21):10079–87.
105. Lee TH, Paglieroni T, Ohto H, Holland PV, Busch MP. Survival of donor leukocyte subpopulations in immunocompetent transfusion recipients: frequent long-term microchimerism in severe trauma patients. *Blood.* 1999;93(9): 3127–39.
106. Lee TH, Paglieroni T, Utter GH, Chafets D, Gosselin RC, Reed W, Owings JT, Holland PV, Busch MP. High-level long-term white blood cell microchimerism after transfusion of leukoreduced blood components to patients resuscitated after severe traumatic injury. *Transfusion.* 2005;45(8):1280–90.
107. Lee TH, Paglieroni T, Ohto H, Holland PV, Busch MP. Survival of donor leukocyte subpopulations in immunocompetent transfusion recipients: frequent long-term microchimerism in severe trauma patients. *Blood.* 1999;93(9):3127–39.
108. Szekeres-Bartho J. Immunological relationship between the mother and the fetus. *Int Rev Immunol.* 2002;21(6):471–95.
109. Carosella ED. HLA-G: fetomaternal tolerance. *C R Acad Sci III.* 2000;323(8):675–80.
110. Ishitani A, Sageshima N, Lee N, Dorofeeva N, Hatake K, Marquardt H. Geraghty DE. Protein expression and peptide binding suggest unique and interacting functional roles for HLA-E, F, and G in maternal-placental immune recognition. *J Immunol.* 2003;171:1376–84.
111. Sargent IL. Maternal and fetal immune responses during pregnancy. *Exp Clin Immunogenet.* 1993;10:85.
112. Le Bouteiller P, Rodriguez AM, Mallet V, Girr M, Guillaudeux T, Lenfant F. Placental expression of HLA class I genes. *Am J Reprod Immunol.* 1996;35:216.
113. Roitt I, Brostoff J, Male D. *Immunology*, 6th Edition, Chapter 12. Mosby Publisher. 2001:205–6.

114. Joshi SS, Vu UE, Lovgren TR, Lorkovic M, Patel W, Todd GL, Kuszynski C, Joshi BJ, Dave HP. Comparison of phenotypic and functional dendritic cells derived from human umbilical cord blood and peripheral blood mononuclear cells. *J Hematother Stem Cell Res.* 2002;11(2):337–47.
115. Kern S, Eichler H, Stoeve J, Kluter H, Bieback K. Comparative analysis of mesenchymal stem cells from bone marrow, umbilical cord blood or adipose tissue. *Stem Cells.* 2006; 24(5):1294–301. Epub 2006 Jan 12. PMID: 16410387 [PulMed-indexed for MEDLINE].
116. Ito K, Tanaka T, Tsutsumi N, Obata F, Kashiwagi N. Possible mechanisms of immunotherapy for maintaining pregnancy in recurrent spontaneous aborters: analysis of anti-idiotypic antibodies directed against autologous T-cell receptors. *Hum Reprod.* 1999;14:650–55. doi: 10.1093/humrep/14.3.650.).
117. Porter D, Levine JE. Graft-versus-host disease and graft-versus-leukemia after donor leukocyte infusion. *Semin Hematol.* 2006;43:53–61. doi: 10.1053/j.seminhematol.2005.09.005.
118. Szpakowski A, Malinowski A, Glowacka E, Wilczynski JR, Kolasa D, Dynski M, Tchorzewski H, Zeman K, Szpakowski M. The influence of paternal lymphocyte immunization on the balance of Th1/Th2 type reactivity in women with unexplained recurrent spontaneous abortion. *Ginekol Pol.* 2000;71:586–92.
119. Chalmers IMH, Janossy G, Contreras M, Navarrete C. Intracellular cytokine profile of cord and adult blood lymphocytes. *Blood.* 1998;92(1):11–8.
120. Marleau AM, Sarvetnick N. T cell homeostasis in tolerance and immunity. *J Leukoc Biol.* 2005;78:575–84. doi: 10.1189/jlb.0105050.
121. Riordan NH, Chan K, Marleau AM, Ichim TE. Cord blood in regenerative medicine: do we need immune suppression? *J Transl Med.* 2007;5:8.

Chapter 11
Umbilical Cord Blood Therapy in Neurology

Abhijit Chaudhuri and Niranjan Bhattacharya

Introduction

Neurological diseases are responsible for significant disability all over the world. Based on the epidemiological data presented in the Global Burden of Disease 2000 study by the World Health Organization [1], it was calculated that in Europe, brain diseases account for a third of all disabilities [2]. The cost of brain disease in Europe is €386 billion, or €829 per European resident at present [3]. With an aging global population, the socio-economic cost of chronic disability from brain diseases is likely to increase in the coming years especially in the absence of any effective and established therapy for neuronal regeneration and repair. It is therefore imperative that potential strategies to minimize the burden of brain disease are rapidly developed and tested by ethical research and clinical trials.

Stem cell therapy has become a major focus of research for neuronal repair because of the ability of these cells for self-renewal and potential to differentiate into specialist cell types in the central nervous system. Transplantation of stem cells or mobilization of endogenous stem cells within the adult brain has been proposed as future therapies for neurodegenerative disorders [4]. There is some evidence from clinical trials, particularly in patients with Parkinson's disease [5, 6], that cell replacement therapy (CRT) leads to symptomatic improvement. However, there are ongoing ethical debates regarding the source of stem cells, which may be used in human research and possible therapy.

Challenges Involving Stem Cell Replacement Therapy

Even if stem cell research develops the technology to generate large number of functional neuronal cell lines, the delivery of effective CRT in neurodegenerative disorders will have to overcome three other major obstacles. First, the precise

A. Chaudhuri (✉)
Consultant Neurologist, Essex Centre for Neurological Sciences, Queen's Hospital, Romford, England
e-mail: abhijitchaudhuri@btinternet.com

N. Bhattacharya, P. Stubblefield (eds.), *Frontiers of Cord Blood Science*,
DOI 10.1007/978-1-84800-167-1_11,

pathogenesis of human neurodegenerative diseases is not clearly known at present. For example, the concept of idiopathic Parkinson's disease as a selective degeneration of dopaminergic striatonigral neurons is really an oversimplification. The disease pathology is much wider and consequently, transplanting dopaminergic cell lines in the substantia nigra would not be a cure. Although human trials with intrastriatal transplantation of fetal striatal tissue support the concept of CRT in Huntington's disease, the clinical benefit of treatment was unclear [7]. The issue becomes more complex with other neurodegenerative disorders as there are no specific targets for CRT in patients with multiple sclerosis, fronto-temporal dementia, Alzheimer's disease or multiple system atrophy. The characterization and therapeutic replacement of appropriate neuronal cell lines in these disorders will remain a formidable challenge.

Second, selection of patients for therapy is not likely to be straightforward. While Parkinson's disease and Huntington's disease may be relatively easily and specifically diagnosed, conditions like fronto-temporal dementia and multiple system atrophy select heterogeneous population and have no diagnostic biomarker. In patients with Parkinson's disease and dementia, the disease pathology extends well beyond striatum and these cases would not benefit from striatal CRT.

Third, technology for survival and functionality of transplanted cells requires significant improvement before CRT can be advocated for large clinical trials. Treatment protocol for neuronal CRT requires better standardization. As an example, it is not clear if immunosuppressive treatment should be routinely recommended after human stem cell grafts. Failure of differentiation of the transplanted cells and of the resident precursor cells at the site of injury in the human brain and spinal cord is probably also contributed by unfavorable microenvironment at the site of injury. Attempts to block these inhibitory local factors with monoclonal antibodies (such as anti-Nogo antibody) in order to promote local repair mechanism have shown early promise in the experimental models. Treatment will also be required for suppression of unwanted neural differentiation and function after CRT. The ideal strategy for minimizing risk of teratoma from embryonic stem cell grafts and graft-induced dyskinesias in striatal transplants is still being developed.

Of all these, probably, the most important question regarding disease-specific CRT is whether the present explanation of neurodegenerative diseases offers a true representation of the underlying pathogenic processes.

Neurodegenerative Disorder as a Possible Systemic Disease

The established view is that in each of the conditions like Parkinson's disease, Huntington's disease or motor neuron disease (amyotrophic lateral sclerosis), the spectrum of cell types involved is highly specific, and consequently, different types of neuronal cell lines would be necessary for successful stem cell therapy, which would be specific for individual diseases. This may be true, but there is a second, more unifying concept of neurodegeneration. The common pathway underlying disorders as diverse as Alzheimer's disease, Parkinson's disease and Cruetzfeldt-Jakob disease is the aggregation and deposition of misfolded proteins, leading to progressive central nervous system amyloidosis [8]. Deposits of insoluble amyloid fibrils lead to fibrous aggregates in the form of extracellular amyloid plaques, neurofibrillary tangles and/or intracytoplasmic or intranuclear inclusions. Many of the amyloidogenic proteins associated with neurodegenerative disease are expressed systemically. What protects the nervous system during the period of asymptomatic, preclinical phase and the rest of the systems during the symptomatic neurological disease is unknown, but may reflect unique vulnerability of specific neuroanatomical systems to protein misfolding in a time-dependent fashion are due to aging-related changes and metabolic influences. An emerging and key research area in neurodegenerative diseases is the kinetics of protein misfolding and fibrillization and how this process is linked to aging-related metabolic impairments affecting the nervous system [9].

Common examples of brain diseases where systemic factors can significantly influence neurodegeneration are stroke and multiple sclerosis. In stroke, the clinical event itself is precipitated by focal ischemia due to reduced regional brain blood flow, which is directly related to the nature of vascular pathology at the given time point. However, neuronal injury in stroke is also influenced by oxygenation, temperature, blood glucose and the severity of inflammatory response. Patients with multiple sclerosis experience relapsing symptoms due to the regional breakdown of the blood-brain-barrier in parallel with neurodegeneration. The rate of relapse and neurodegeneration in multiple sclerosis is influenced by infection, local inflammatory response, and neuronal metabolic rate. The pathological hallmark of the disease is multi-focal demyelination around veins due to a local breakdown of the blood-brain-barrier. The mechanism of neurodegeneration in multiple sclerosis is not known but is believed to be primarily neuronal, axonal or both [10]. There is an emerging view that infection and systemic inflammatory response accelerate cognitive decline in patients with Alzheimer's disease and other neurodegenerative diseases [11, 12]. Influence of age, infection or inflammation on brain metabolism may target vulnerable neuronal pools in genetically predisposed individuals, and accelerated protein misfolding and apoptosis at these sites could lead to the clinical manifestations of system-specific neurodegenerative diseases. Prion diseases provide an excellent proof of this concept, which is also supported by the experimental murine model [13].

Scope of Umbilical Cord Blood Therapy in Neurology

Since the first successful umbilical cord transplant in a patient with Fanconi's anemia in 1989, nearly 5,000 cord blood transplants have been performed worldwide to date, with particular success in areas like thalassemia, sickle cell disease, falciparum malaria, and acute leukemia. Cord blood cells have been recently used, with success, to treat Hurler's syndrome, a metabolic disorder caused by reduced activity of lysosomal enzyme α-L iduronidase [14]. Seventeen of the 20 treated children improved their neurocognitive performance after treatment with umbilical cord blood cells, with median follow-up of 905 days [14].

The biology of umbilical cord blood has been reviewed in detail elsewhere in this monograph and would not be discussed here. However, there are three main properties of umbilical cord blood, which are of potential value. First, umbilical cord blood has a high concentration of fetal hemoglobin (Hb F), which has greater oxygen binding capacity than normal adult hemoglobin. This has been shown to be of considerable therapeutic importance in sickle cell disease and hemoglobinopathy, and holds promise for improving oxygenation in ischemic tissue. Provided there is partial blood flow either from subtotal vaso-occlusion or collateral circulation to the area of injury, Hb F can deliver better oxygenation to the surviving neurons in the ischemic penumbra.

Second, umbilical cord blood has more undifferentiated stem cell population compared to adult hematopoietic tissue in the bone marrow. These primitive stem cells in the umbilical cord are multi-potent and have the ability to transdifferentiate into multiple lineage, including neural tissue. The cell population expresses adhesion molecules CD 13+, CD 29+, and CD 44+ [15]. Exposure of cord blood cells to basic fibroblast growth factor and human epidermal growth factor in culture was found to induce expression of neural and glial markers [16]. Glial fibrillary acidic protein and neuron-specific neural protein were expressed by cord blood cells 10 days after culture with brain-derived neurotrophic factor [17]. In addition, mesenchymal stem cells in human umbilical cord blood may be cultured to transdifferentiate into neural cell lines rapidly [18]. Umbilical cord blood therefore offers a potential source of stem cells for CRT comparable to embryonic and fetal tissue-based cell therapy.

Third, both T- and B-lymphocyte populations in the umbilical cord blood are immature. Most T cells in the umbilical cord blood express CD45 RA+/CD45 RO−/CD62 L+ and the suppressor and cytotoxic T-cell subsets are virtually absent [19]. Consequently, HLA-matching requirements for umbilical cord blood are less restrictive and as compared to bone marrow grafts, the risk of graft versus host disease is substantially less after cord transplantations [20]. Umbilical cord transplants, therefore, has therapeutic advantage over adult bone marrow-derived hematopoietic tissue in the treatment of select neurological diseases (neuronal storage disorders and multiple sclerosis).

Experiments of Umbilical Cord Blood in Brain Diseases

Experiments on umbilical cord blood cell therapy for brain diseases have been limited. The approach so far has been to either to use umbilical cord blood (which contains stem cells) or umbilical cord stem cells.

Stroke: Intravenous infusion of human umbilical cord blood in rats with middle cerebral artery occlusion significantly improved functional recovery after 24 hours [21]. Analysis of the ischemic tissue showed significant migration of cord cells to the ischemic injury area as compared to normal brain tissue. Intravenous delivery of a purified fraction of CD 34+ human umbilical cord blood cells 48 hours after ischemic injury to immunocompromised mice was found to induce neovascularization and endogenous neurogenesis in the ischemic zone [22]. In a comparative study of intravenous versus intrastriatal administration of umbilical cord stem cell therapy in a rodent model of stroke, behavioral recovery was found to be similar with both methods, but greater functional recovery was associated with the intravenous route [23].

Traumatic brain injury: Twenty-four hours after traumatic brain injury, umbilical cord blood was administered intravenously in the rats. Treated animals showed significant improvement in the neurological deficit compared with the control animals by the 4th week [24]. Histological study showed that the infused cells had preferentially entered brain, migrated to the injured area and expressed neuronal markers. In addition, some cord blood cells were also found to be integrated within the vascular walls of the injured area. Improvement in neurological outcome with a reduction in the volume of injured tissue was also reported in experimental studies of spinal cord injury [25].

Neurodegenerative diseases: In an experimental mouse model (G 93A) of motor neuron disease (amyotrophic lateral sclerosis), intravenous administration of umbilical cord blood in pre-symptomatic animals resulted in a delay of the disease progression by 2–3 weeks and increased life span in the diseased mice [26]. The transplanted cells survived for 10–12 weeks after administration and enter into the areas of motor neuron degeneration in the brain and spinal cord, where they were found to express neural markers. In addition, the transplanted cells were widely distributed in the peripheral circulation and in the spleen [26]. High volumes of human umbilical cord blood mononuclear cell infusion in a mice model of Huntington's disease (B6CBA-TgN 62 Gpb mice) reduced the rate of weight loss, which appears before the onset of chorea, and total duration of survival [27]. These workers also found improved survival of mice overexpressing amyloid precursor protein (a model of Alzheimer's disease) with high-dose cell therapy [28].

Future of Umbilical Cord Blood in Brain Diseases

Clearly, there are several possible therapeutic indications where clinical trials of umbilical cord blood therapy require consideration (Table 11.1). The limited evidence so far supports the view that cord blood transplantation is effective after intravenous administration, and selective cell infusions from pooled blood may not have any significant additional benefit. There may be an advantage to use whole blood containing red cells for transplants in acute ischemic stroke for better carriage of oxygen in poorly perfused brain areas because of high-affinity binding of oxygen with Hb F. In theory, progenitor stem cells from the transplanted umbilical cord blood can enter the central nervous system relatively easily in diseases where blood-brain-barrier breaks down, and stroke, traumatic brain injury and multiple sclerosis appear to be appropriate indications to test the hypothesis. The ease of peripheral administration gives umbilical cord blood (or cells) a logistic advantage over

Table 11.1 Therapeutic areas of umbilical cord blood therapy

Very likely to benefit
Acute ischemic stroke (combined with anti-platelet therapy)
Likely to benefit
Traumatic brain injury
Multiple sclerosis
Neuronal storage disorders
Cruetzfeldt-Jakob disease
Possible benefit
Motor neuron disease
Huntington's disease
Alzheimer's disease
Parkinson's disease

site-specific CRT with embryonic or fetal tissue transplants in neurodegenerative disorders. However, umbilical cord cells have been found to migrate to non-brain sites, and the peripheral effects of transplants may be important in modifying systemic influence on neurodegenerative diseases about which our current knowledge is admittedly limited.

Umbilical cord transplants may also be useful for neuronal storage disorders. Although rare, most neuronal storage disorders are untreatable. Even in selected forms of lysosomal storage diseases where effective enzyme replacement therapy has become available in the recent years, neuronal function is not influenced by treatment because of the inability of the recombinant enzymes to cross the blood-brain-barrier. Umbilical cord transplant offers a possible alternative in the neuronal form of Gaucher's disease or exceptional cases of multiple sclerosis where bone marrow transplantation has been advocated previously.

Potential Risks of Therapy with Umbilical Cord Blood

Infection and in case of whole blood therapy, transfusion reaction from ABO blood group incompatibility are likely to be the most common risks of using umbilical cord blood, which are probably similar to the risks associated with blood products in current practice. One complication of the umbilical cord transplantation in unrelated adult donors appears to be early infection because of the delay in the immune reconstitution (compared to bone marrow transplantation) after therapy [29].

The cost of umbilical cord blood collection, storage and purification is high. At present, the trend is to store cord blood at commercial centers, with the intention of providing the individual their own umbilical cord blood cells for future use in the event of traumatic injury or age-related neurodegenerative disease. Autologous umbilical cord transplant is not a cost-effective option and it does not provide a practical solution in the foreseeable future for patients who currently have or are at a risk of brain disease. Consequently, voluntary donation of umbilical cord blood is essential for this kind of research to progress and benefit mankind.

Conclusion

Umbilical cord blood therapy in brain diseases may have the potential to reduce the burden of disability. To be sure, there are many unanswered questions regarding its therapeutic value and the practicality of its use in neurological patients. However, only research and controlled clinical trials, rather than skepticism [30], can answer these questions. Umbilical cord blood can be obtained in large quantities at birth, can be used without risking the ethical objections of embryonic and fetal stem cell therapy, and because the collection of cord blood will parallel population increase, populous countries would be able to use their own resources effectively to treat brain diseases at a lower cost. There is no other therapy that can bring the beginning and the end of life together into the same circle: "FROM JOY ALL BEINGS HAVE COME, BY JOY THEY ALL LIVE AND UNTO JOY THEY ALL RETURN" – Taittriya Upanishad, 3.1–6 (500 B.C.)

References

1. Mathers CD, Stein C, Fat DM, et al. Global Burden of Disease 2000: Version 2, Methods and Results. Global Programme on Evidence for Health Policy Discussion Paper No. 50: World Health Organisation 2002, Geneva, 2002.
2. Olesen J, Leonardi M. The burden of brain diseases in Europe. Eur J Neurol 2003; 10: 471–7.
3. Andlin-Sobocki P, Jansson B, Whittchen HU, et al. Cost of disorders of the brain in Europe. Eur J Neurol 2005; 12 (Suppl. 1): 1–27.
4. Lindvall O, Kokaia Z, Martinez-Serrano A. Stem cell therapy for human neurodegenerative disorders-how to make it work. Nat Med 2004; 10: S42–S50.
5. Freed CR, et al. Transplantation of embryonic dopamine neurons for severe Parkinson's disease. N Engl J Med 2001; 344: 710–9.
6. Olanow CW, et al. A double-blind controlled trial of bilateral fetal nigral transplantation in Parkinson's disease. Ann Neurol 2003; 54: 403–14.
7. Hauser RA, et al. Bilateral human fetal striatal transplantation in Hungtington's disease. Neurology 2002; 58: 687–95.
8. Forman MS, Trojanowski JQ, Lee VM. Neurodegenerative diseases: a decade of discoveries paves the way for therapeutic breakthrough. Nat Med 2004; 10: 1055–63.
9. Chaudhuri A, Shahni U, Gibbs J. From bovine spongiform encephalopathy and Creutzfeldt-Jakob disease to prions and normal brain protein homeostasis. In: Olesen J, Baker MG, Freund T, et al. Consensus Document on European Brain Research. J Neurol Neurosurg Psychiatr 2006; 7: i28–9.
10. Chaudhuri A. Neurodegeneration and neuroprotection in multiple sclerosis. Int J Neuroprot Neuroregener 2006; 2: 86–9.
11. Cunningham C, Wilcockson DC, Campion S, Lunnon K, Perry VH. Central and systemic endotoxin challenges exacerbate the local inflammatory response and increase neuronal death during chronic neurodegeneration. J Neurosci 2005; 25: 9275–84.
12. Perry VH, Anthony DC, Bolto SJ, Brown HC. The blood-brain barrier and the inflammatory response. Mol Med Today 1997; 3: 335–41.
13. Combrink MI, Perry VH, Cunningham C. Peripheral infection evokes exaggerated sickness behaviour in preclinical murine prion disease. Neuroscience 2002; 112: 7–11.
14. Staba SI, Escolar ML, Poe M, et al. Cord blood transplants from unrelated donors in patients with Hurler's syndrome. N Engl J Med 2004; 350: 1960–9.

15. Goodwin HS, Bichnese AR, Chien SN, Bogucki BD, Quinn Co, Wall DA. Multilineage differentiation activity by cells isolated from umbilical cord blood: expression of bone, fat and neural markers. Biol Blood Marrow Transplant 2001; 7: 581–8.
16. Bicknese AR, Goodwin HS, Quinn CO, et al. Human umbilical cord blood cells can be induced to express markers for neurons and glia. Cell Transplant 2002; 11: 261–4.
17. Zhao ZM, Lu SH, Zhang QJ, et al. The preliminary study on in vitro differentiation of human umbilical cord blood cells into neural cells. Zhonghua Xue Ye Xue Za Zhi 2003; 24: 484–7.
18. Fu YS, Shih YT, Cheng YC, Min MY. Transformation of human umbilical mesenchymal cells into neurons in vitro. J Biomed Sci 2004; 11: 652–60.
19. Szabolcs P, Park KD, Reese M, et al. Coexistent naïve phenotype and higher cycling rate of cord blood T cells as compared to adult peripheral blood. Exp Hematol 2003; 31: 708–14.
20. Fasouliotis SJ, Schenker JG. Human umbilical cord blood banking and transplantation: a state of the art. Eur J Obstet Gynecol Reprod Biol 2000; 90: 13–25.
21. Li Y, Wang L, Lu M, et al. Intravenous administration of umbilical cord blood reduces behavioural deficits after stroke in rats. Stroke 2001; 32: 2682–8.
22. Taguchi A, Soma T, Tanaka H, et al. Administration of CD 34+ cells after stroke enhances neurogenesis via angiogenesis in a mouse model. J Clin Invest 2004; 114: 330–8.
23. Willing AE, Lixian J, Milliken M, et al. Intravenous versus intrastriatal cord blood administration in a rodent model of stroke. J Neurosci Res 2003; 73: 296–307.
24. Lu D, Sanberg PR, Mahmood A, et al. Intravenous administration of human umbilical cord blood reduces neurological deficit in the rat after traumatic brain injury. Cell Transplant 2002; 11: 275–81.
25. Saporta S, Kim JJ, Willing AE, et al. Human umbilical cord blood stem cells infusionin spinal cord injury: engraftment and beneficial influence on behaviour. J Hematother Stem Cell Res 2003; 12: 271–78.
26. Garbuzova-Davis S Willing AE, Zigova T, et al. Intravenous administration of human umbilical cord blood cells in a mouse model of amyotrophic lateral sclerosis: distribution, migration and differentiation. J Hematother Stem Cell Res 2003; 12: 255–70.
27. Ende N, Chen R. Human umbilical cord blood cells ameliorate Huntington's disease in transgenic mice. J Med 2001; 32: 231–40.
28. Ende N, Chen R, Ende-Harris D. Human umbilical cord blood cells ameliorate Alzheimer's disease in transgenic mice. J Med 2001; 32: 241–7.
29. Saavedra S, Sanz GI, Jarque I, et al. Early infections in adult patients undergoing unrelated donor cord blood transplantation. Bone Marrow Transplant 2002; 30: 937–43.
30. Schwartz R. The politics and promise of stem cell research. N Engl J Med 2006; 355: 1189–91.

Chapter 12
Cord Blood: Opportunities and Challenges for the Reconstructive Surgeon

Andrew Burd, T. Ayyappan, and Lin Huang

A significant proportion of the activities of a plastic and reconstructive surgeon is directed toward the healing of wounds and the reconstruction of defects in the skin and soft tissue. In this chapter, we look at some of the opportunities and challenges presented by the stem cells and, in particular, those derived from cord blood in the fields of chronic wound healing, and skin repair and regeneration. It should be stated at the outset that our perspectives on new waves of biological evolution are influenced by experience, disappointments and frustrations: a fundamental problem being a consistent underestimation of the biological complexity of the human body not only just in terms of the genetic source and cellular structure but also in terms of the extracellular matrix and composition of organs and tissues. When Rheinwald and Green described the serial cultivation of strains of human epidermal keratinocytes with the formation of keratinizing colonies from single cells over 30 years ago, naive claims were made by the laboratory scientists that the burns care of the future would be a simple matter of quick and easy cover after the excision of burn wounds. Unfortunately, this is far from reality [1]. The next decade brought the concept of tissue engineering.

When the term "tissue engineering" was officially coined at a National Science Foundation Workshop in the United States in 1988, it was understood to mean "the application of principles and methods of engineering and life sciences toward fundamental understanding of structure–function relationships in normal and pathological mammalian tissues and the development of biological substitutes to restore, maintain, or improve tissue function." This *concept* has unfortunately led to some serious *misconceptions* that have resulted in the early promise of skin tissue engineering being slow to be realized in clinical practice. The misconception was that skin was a tissue, like cartilage, and would be relatively simple to address as a tissue engineering challenge. Skin however is *not* a tissue but an extremely complex organ that brings into conjunction cells from three different embryological

A. Burd (✉)
Chief of Plastic & Reconstructive Surgery, Department of Surgery, Prince of Wales Hospital, Shatin, Hong Kong
e-mail: andrewburd@surgery.cuhk.edu.hk

N. Bhattacharya, P. Stubblefield (eds.), *Frontiers of Cord Blood Science*,
DOI 10.1007/978-1-84800-167-1_12,

origins: ectoderm, mesoderm, and neural crest. It subserves multiple functions. The original futuristic claims of producing "off-the shelf" skin replacements have become far more restrained in their expectation and now tissue engineering skin products are being described as skin substitutes to aid healing and repair, temporary skin replacements, and occasionally aids to regeneration.

Structure and Function of Skin

Skin is the largest immunologically competent organ in the body [2, 3]. It extends to over 1.6 m^2 in the adult and weighs approximately 3000 gm. The skin has two layers: epidermis and dermis (Fig. 12.1). The epidermis is rich in cells and is of ectodermal origin. The cells are specialized in the formation of keratin and are called keratinocytes. The basal keratinocytes adhere to the basement membrane, which forms part of the zone between epidermis and dermis: the dermo-epidermal junction (DEJ). Basal keratinocytes are unique, in that they are capable of proliferating to form either new basal cells or terminally differentiating keratinocytes. The terminally differentiating keratinocyte moves up through several layers and undergoes certain changes: the cytoplasm becomes increasingly packed with keratin and the nucleus shrinks. The outermost layer – the stratum corneum – contains dead keratinocytes packed with keratin, forming a barrier between the living tissues and the external environment.

The area of the basement membrane far exceeds that of the surface of the stratum corneum, because multiple dermal papillae project from the surface of the dermis

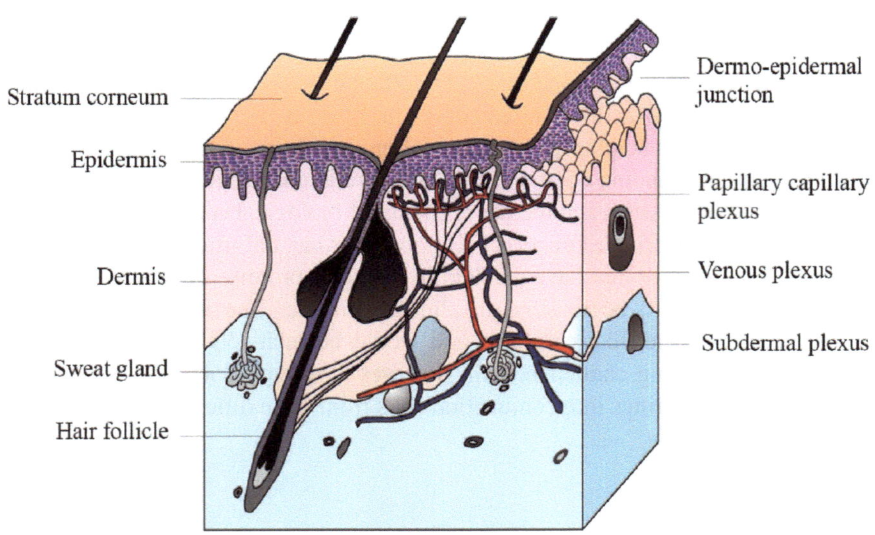

Fig. 12.1 A diagrammatic section of skin

and only about 12% of the basal cells are proliferating at any one time. These papillae are formed by loose approximations of collagen bundles referred to as the papillary dermis, which lies on the relatively much thicker reticular dermis. Collagen bundles in the reticular dermis are thicker and more condensed.

Between the organized structure of elastin and collagen fibers is a thick, viscous fluid made up of glycosaminoglycans and hyaluronan. This arrangement of the dermis gives the skin its major biomechanical properties, allowing stretching and recoil and deformation without destruction.

The dermis contains a complex vascular arrangement of capillary and venous plexuses. Within the dermis are adnexeal structures of ectodermal origin-hair follicles, sweat glands, and sebaceous glands – which are lined with keratinocytes. This arrangement becomes particularly important when considering the mechanisms of wound healing.

Multifunctional Langerhan's cells found in the epidermis have an important role as antigen-presenting cells in cutaneous immune reactions. Skin color is determined principally by the pigment melanin, produced by melanocytes. These cells package the melanin into melanosomes, which are then transferred to keratinocytes.

The skin is richly endowed with sensory nerve endings that enable the skin to play its vital role as a tactile interface between the body and the environment. Other sensory functions provide important stimuli for behavioral modification, e.g., the withdrawal reflex associated with pain or excessive temperature.

Healing: Regeneration and Repair

Healing in the skin takes place by two principle processes: regeneration and repair (Fig. 12.2). Regeneration is the capacity of a tissue to renew itself so that the end result is indistinguishable from the pre-injured tissue. Regeneration is a feature seen in superficial partial-thickness burns, in which the injury involves the loss of epidermis and basement membrane and the papillary dermis. There may be a highly exudative and painful wound.

The exudative phase persists for several days, and as it decreases the nature of the exudate changes. The viscosity and relative protein content increase, and eventually a fibrin layer seals the wound. In the meantime, the basal keratinocytes at the margin of the wound begin to undergo mitosis. In the normal resting state, only approximately 12% of basal keratinocytes are proliferating at any one time, giving the skin a tremendous reserve capacity. Re-epithelialization begins not only just at the wound margin, but also from the appendageal structures. The rate of keratinocyte proliferation and migration is extremely high, and when the exposed dermis is completely covered with a new keratinocyte layer, contact inhibition stops migration and redirects the cells to stratification. A superficial partial-thickness burn or abrasion will heal with a stratified squamous epithelium in a matter of days. Disturbance in normal pigment expression can occur, even with no scarring.

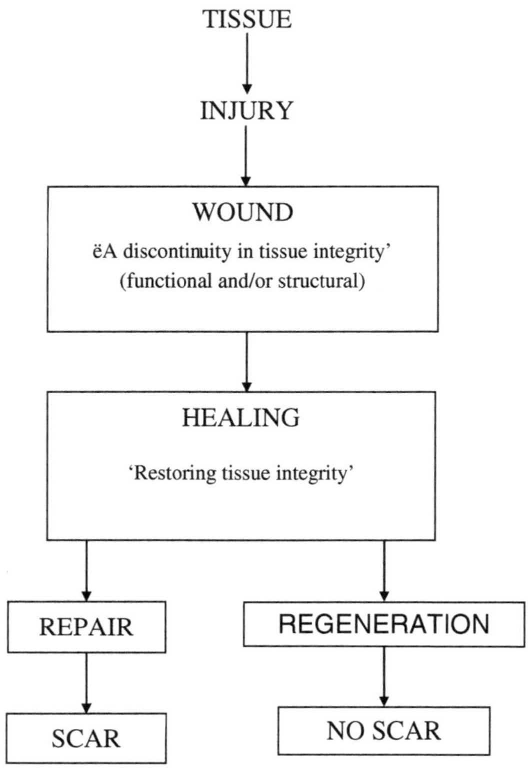

Fig. 12.2 Wound healing – the pathways

In people with darker pigmentation, areas of absent pigment can have major social and psychological sequelae.

As the wound becomes deeper, the nature of the healing changes. In a burn, damage to the dermis involves irreversible denaturation of the collagen. The inert collagen has to be removed for re-epithelialization to take place. Removal involves an autolytic process with enzymatic degradation and phagocytosis, augmented by an inflammatory response (Fig. 12.3). Healing takes longer. As the depth of injury increases through the thickness of the dermis, the phenomenon of inflammation plays an even more important role in the healing process. Typically, inflammation initiates a cascade of events, with polymorphonuclear leucocytes being attracted to the wound site. Their principal role is proteolysis and phagocytosis of debris. The leucocytes release cytokines which cause macrophage activation. The activated macrophages enter the wound site to undertake a more detailed assessment of the damage and through further cytokine signaling, they recruit fibroblasts to begin the process of replacing the damaged collagen. Fibroblasts involved in wound healing have the capacity to produce abundant amounts of collagen, but they have lost the capacity to place and organize it in a highly structured way. The end result of dermal repair is the deposition of disorganized collagen, which is physically

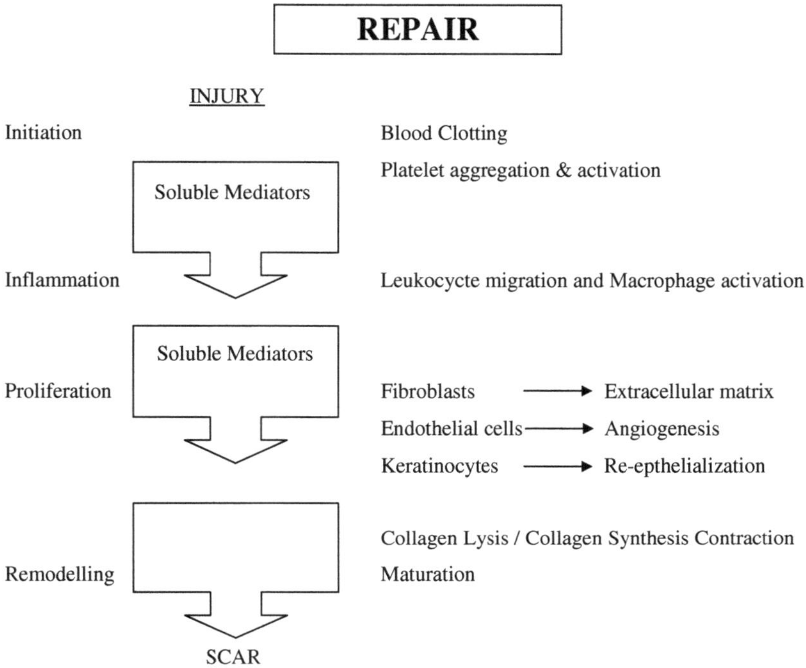

Fig. 12.3 Wound healing – repair

apparent as scar tissue. Scarring represents a very complex biological phenomenon. Hypertrophic and keloid scars represent clinical descriptions of a heterogeneous group of disorders with various etiologies and pathological mechanisms that result in the production of a disorganized connective tissue [4]. The duration of the phase of wound closure (i.e., re-epithelialization) and the incidence of adverse scarring increase as the depth of injury increases.

Fetal Wound Healing

Early in gestation, fetal wounds are capable of healing without scarring. That is to say that there is regeneration of tissue. The nature and mechanism of this scarless repair has been intensively investigated as the achievement of regeneration in the post-natal wound would have overwhelming benefits for mankind. The cellular mediators of fetal skin repair have been studied including platelets, inflammatory mediators, and fibroblasts. The extracellular matrix has also been extensively studied as well as the effects and influence of cytokines such as TGF-β, PDGF, fibroblast growth factors, and vascular endothelial growth factor. Despite intensive research, it appears that the ability to heal scarlessly is intrinsic to fetal skin [5]. Nevertheless, this is another area where the potential control and interaction of stem cells is and will be the focus of considerable research.

The Need for Skin Substitutes

Skin substitutes are needed to augment the healing process of chronic wounds such as diabetic and vascular ulcers [6]. The abnormalities associated with these ulcers include systemic factors (advanced age, malnutrition, diabetes, and renal disease), local factors (prolonged infection, ischemia), and decreased synthesis of collagen, increased levels of proteinases and defective macrophage function [7].

Skin substitutes are also needed for wounds that arise from extensive tissue loss or damage. These may result from trauma, in particular burns, and in pathological conditions such as epidermolysis bullosa and acute exfoliative skin conditions. Such wounds may need either temporary or permanent closure with substitutes.

The ideal skin substitute should be as following [8, 9, 10]:

(1) Protect the wound, and maintain a moist healing environment and control protein and electrolyte loss.
(2) Prevent local infection and provide an environment for accelerated wound healing.
(3) Reduce pain and allow early mobilization.
(4) Be easy to handle and cost-effective.
(5) Must be safe in terms of virus transmission and not provoke a strong immunological reaction.
(6) Should be readily available.

Strategy of Skin Tissue Engineering

Strategies used to construct skin substitutes in tissue engineering are generally considered to be either ex vivo tissue manufacturing with guided generation or in vivo regeneration [11]. These are shown in Table 12.1. The strategy of ex vivo tissue manufacturing is the technique initially most commonly associated with tissue engineering. In this approach, fibroblasts and/or keratinocyte are seeded into dermal matrix or scaffold and co-cultured in a bioreactor or specialized culture system with some growth factors. The matrix provides a scaffold combining with the bioreactor providing cellular nutrients, allowing the cells to proliferate and differentiate in the ex vivo environment. When the procedure is completed, the skin substitute is implanted into the wound and further matures and integrates into the recipient

Table 12.1 Comparison of ex vivo and in vivo strategies

Ex vivo	In vivo
Laboratory based tissue manufacturing	Guided generation or regeneration of tissue
Complex and tissue consuming technical processes	Need for significant understanding of biological processes and gene control
No intrinsic blood supply	Develops blood supply in situ
One stage procedure but usually temporary	Multiple stage procedure but can be permanent

tissues. Such available products include: Epicel^{TM}-cultured epidermal sheet [12], Dermagraft® [13], Apligraf® [14], and cultured skin substitute [15].

The other strategy is to guide the "bioengineering" of skin in situ. Such a strategy needs an understanding of the cellular and molecular interactions in tissue healing and development. Examples are Alloderm® and Integra®, which can act as "dermal generation templates" in vivo to direct the formation of a new autocollagenous "dermal" matrix [16, 17, 18].

The Keratinocyte Layer

A major problem with the keratinocyte layer is its extreme antigenicity, mediated principally through Langerhans cells. This has presented a major obstacle in the restoration of epidermal cover by tissue engineering. The major contributions have been to develop materials to carry cells, cultured in the laboratory, onto the wound.

In 1975, when Rheinwald and Green first described the technique of producing keratinocyte cultures in vitro, it appeared that a new era of wounds management was about to commence [19]. Indeed it has, but the expectation of rapid wound closure with laboratory-produced cultured epithelial cell autografts (CEAs) has not been fulfilled in clinical practice. The process of preparation is expensive. Although it takes only a few weeks to create enough CEAs from a few square centimeters of original biopsy to cover the entire body, the actual take and survival of the CEAs on the body has been a disappointment. Keratinocyte delivery vehicles have been developed to facilitate the process and improve the rate of successful engraftment, but this has further increased the costs of this strategy while not significantly increasing the success [20].

There has been a tremendous amount of research and development in keratinocyte preparation and application, and there has been a parallel development in the area of dermal replacement and/or regeneration. One major problem that has faced workers in this field is how to combine the two layers of the skin. The DEJ is extremely complex. It is a combined unit with structural components produced by both keratinocytes and by dermal fibroblasts. In nature, a new DEJ is formed when proliferating keratinocytes migrate across the dermal collagen. This occurs in all superficial wounds and in healing donor sites. There is no problem in the function of a DEJ in these situations, and this focused attention on the role of the undifferentiated, proliferating keratinocyte cell suspensions in burn wound coverage. Fiona Wood, a pioneer in this field, has used cell suspensions of keratinocytes to treat burns in an increasing number of clinical applications, including dermal collagen remodeling, pigment expression, and keratin expression [21]. Thus, the interaction between the products of the keratinocytes and the dermal fibroblasts becomes as important as the speedy regeneration of the lost epidermis.

The Challenge

The 21st century tissue engineer faces the challenges of both possibility and practicality. Complex and costly products will not find commercial applications. In the meantime, the biological complexity of the skin has been appreciated and it is no

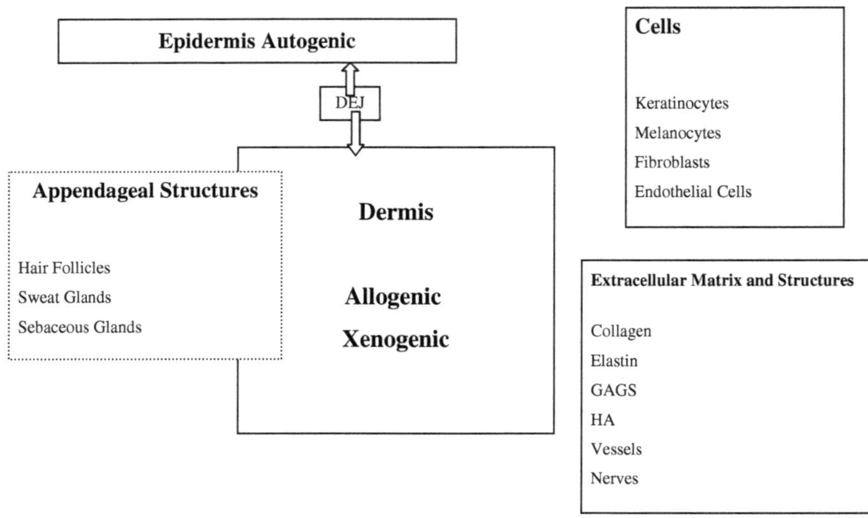

Fig. 12.4 Biological concepts of skin tissue engineering

longer viewed as a bilaminar tissue but a multidimensional organ. The tissue engineer must ask how much of this complex biological tissue is going to be constructed. (Fig. 12.4) shows the "biological" as opposed to the "engineering" concepts of the skin structure. The skin began in the embryonic stage as a conjunction of cells which integrated their specialized functions. The key cell of the epidermis is the keratinocyte which produces keratin. It is the outer layer of keratin-filled dead cells, the stratum corneum that is responsible for the principle protective functions of the skin. The mesodermal fibroblasts are principally involved in the formation and maintenance of the dermis. The problem for the tissue engineer is that the time scale for cellular matrix production is too slow in clinical application. A preformed matrix is required either as a permanent or temporary scaffold. The problem with the permanent scaffold is *biocompatibility* and the problem with the temporary scaffold is *stability*.

For the permanent replacement of lost skin, it will be necessary to use a dermal analogue which is slowly replaced by an autologous dermis. Such a product might be formed by an immune-modulated allogeneic or xenogenic dermis modified with mesenchymal stem cells, either of marrow or adipocyte origin. This layer would need to be seeded with a stem cell-enriched keratinocyte formulation possibly including melanocytes. The attachment is critical and will require a medium such as hyaluronic acid which can support the cells whilst promoting proliferation and attachment. These ex vivo-derived components would be combined for in vivo culture. Such a process can be simply conveyed diagrammatically (Fig. 12.5), but the practicality of such a construct presents considerable challenges. The history of the evolution of skin tissue engineering does suggest, however, that for permanent skin replacement the body's own "tissue engineering" capacity must be harnessed using stem cell technology with or without synthesized matrix support. For tissue

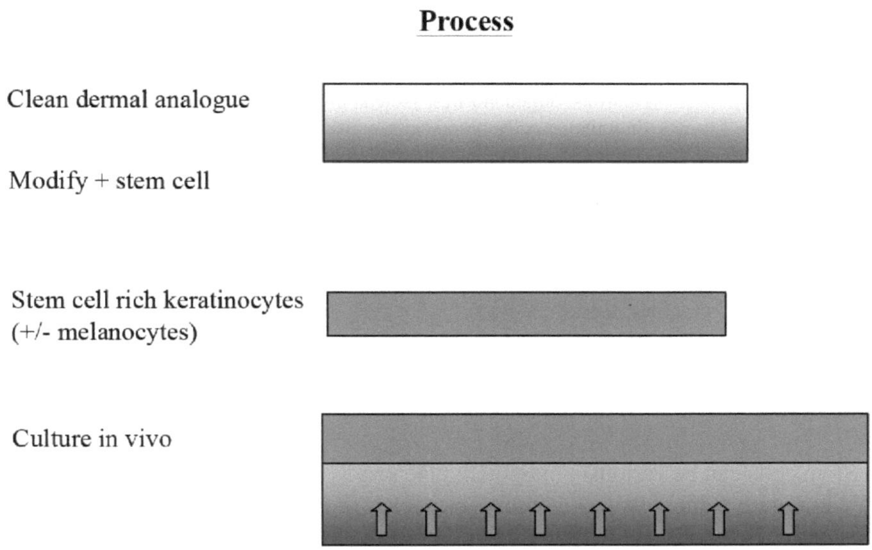

Fig. 12.5 The conceptual process of construction

engineered skin substitutes to provide temporary wound cover materials science and technology already shows promise but the challenge is to reduce costs. Again for products which are aimed at modulating wound healing, living cells can be genetically engineered to restore molecular balance to chronic wounds. Again knowledge and technology are available but the challenge is to develop products that are safe, effective, easy to use, and also affordable.

Stem Cells

From the foregoing it is apparent that the skin is indeed a complex structure incorporating a fusion of multiple cell types, integrated within a three-dimensional matrix containing both fibrillar and non-fibrillar elements. To synthesize such a complex structure by identifying the component parts and to put them together is neither practical nor realistic. It must be observed, however, that this integrative strategy has been the major one used in skin tissue engineering during its less productive phase [22]. The great attraction of stem cells in the construction of a complex tissue or organ is that the component parts can be simplified at the initial stage and a significantly greater proportion of the neogenerative process can be driven by the intrinsic bioengineering capacity of the cells and tissues. It is important to realize that cells by themselves cannot generate organs and the matrix provides a critical element in defining appropriate differentiation and three-dimensional organization. Stem cells are going to play an increasingly important role in tissue engineering and they will be derived from a range of sources.

Table 12.2 Potential plasticity of adult stem cells [adapted from Rosenthal N [24]]

Location of stem cell	Type of cells generated
Brain	Neurons, oligodendrites, skeletal muscle, blood cells
Bone marrow	Endothelial cells, blood cells, cartilage, bone, adipocytes, cardiac muscle, skeletal muscle, neuronal cells, dermal fibroblasts, oval cells, gastro-intestinal tract cells, thymus, pulmonary epithelial cells
Skeletal muscle	Skeletal muscle, bone, cartilage, fat, smooth muscle
Myocardium	Myocytes, endothelial cells
Skin	Keratinocytes
Liver	Liver cells
Tests and ovaries	Gonads
Pancreatic ducts	Islet cells
Adipose tissue	Fat, muscle, cartilage, bone

Stem cells can be variously classified. One way is to identify the source and thus we can regard stem cells to be embryonic, fetal, or adult in nature. An alternative perspective is to look at the future, the potential and to describe stem cells as being totipotent, pluripotent, and multipotent.

The totipotent cells contain all the complete genetic information needed to manufacture all the cells of the body as well as the placenta. These cells are present immediately after fertilization of the egg and for three to four divisions thereafter. As the cells become more specialized, they are described as pluripotent. The cells are extremely adaptable and can develop into any cell type with the exception of the placenta. Further division of the pluripotent cells will give rise to multipotent cells. These are far more specialized and can only generate a limited number of cell types [23].

The true stem cell must satisfy certain criteria: it must be clonogenic, i.e., capable of unlimited self-renewal by symmetric division; it must also be able to divide asymmetrically, with one daughter cell resembling the mother (to perpetuate the clone) but the other capable of giving rise to multiple types of differentiated cells which indeed represent derivatives of all three primitive embryonic-germ layers.

It is the concept of "plasticity" that makes the stem cell so attractive to the tissue engineer and so one critical aspect of stem cells will be the variable expression of plasticity related to source. In Table 12.2, the potential plasticity of some adult stem cells is detailed which does indicate the wide range of cells that have thus far been generated from bone marrow cells [24 It is evident, however, that this plasticity is limited in adult stem cells certainly as compared to stem cells derived from the inner cell mass of the early embryonic blastocyst (ES) cells, which can both proliferate indefinitely and also give rise to virtually any type of cell [25].

Adult Stem Cells

Adult stem cells have been incorporated into tissue engineered constructs used by reconstructive surgeons. A recent review has focused on the four components in developing tissue substitutes: gene therapy, growth factors and pharmalogical preparations, scaffolds, and cells. It is this last component, the cells, where increasing attention is focusing on stem cells particularly in true tissue as opposed to organ engineering. Bone, cartilage, tendon, and muscle have all been developed to some degree of success from adult stem cells. The preferred source of adult stem cells, however, remains uncertain and the functional plasticity of adult stem cells exists more as of scientific experimentation than clinical application [26, 27].

Cord Blood

In view of the many ethical and biological issues involved, it will be many years before embryonic stem cells reach the clinic. Research in this field has not been helped by the highly publicized claims of scientific fraud by some high-profile researchers [28]. Nevertheless, the attraction of supplies of pluripotent stem cells remains as a prized resource by scientist and clinicians. The annual global 100 million human birth rate underlines the possibility that umbilical cord blood (UCB) represents the world's largest untouched stem cell resource. The particular advantages of stem cells from this source include ethical acceptability, a naive-immune status, and relatively unshortened telomere length. Claims are already being made that stem cells with embryonic characteristics can be produced from human UCB [29]. Cord blood is being used for an increasing number of clinical and experimental applications that have highlighted the reduced incidence of graft-versus-host reaction when the hemopoietic fraction is used as an allogenic transplant [30].

As more uses are found for UCB, considerable attention has been addressed to expand the number of stem cells at differing stages of maturity. Expansion factor of 10 to more than 1000 have been claimed and one aspect of considerable significance is that undifferentiated stem cells can be expanded. Cell process engineering for expansion does rely in three-dimensional matrices in bioreactors [31].

Plasticity of Cord Blood

Cord blood and cells derived from the umbilical cord have been used in a variety of tissue engineering projects. Living patches of tissue fabricated from synthetic polymers (PGA/P4HB) seeded with fibroblasts harvested from umbilical cord tissue and endothelial progenitor cells have been cultured in a perfusion bioreactor and have the potential of being used in congenital cardiac conditions [32]. Attempts to engineer microvessels using similar endothelial progenitor cells and polyglycolic acid-poly-L-lactic acid (PGA-PLLA) scaffolds demonstrated a lack of vessel formation. However, when the same cells were co-cultured with human smooth muscle cells, microvessel formation was observed on the porous (PGA-PLLA) scaffolds [33]. Skeletal myogenic differentiation has been observed in mesenchymal cells isolated from UCB [34].

The response and interaction of stem cells and target cell differentiation is a focus of particular interest to the plastic surgeon. The review by Heng et al. discusses strategies for directing keratinocyte stem cell lineage in vitro using selective purification and proliferation [35]. A three-step process is described with the first step being to induce commitment of the (non-epidermal) stem cell into keratinocyte progenitors. These progenitors have to then be selected and purified and finally this purified population of committed keratinocyte progenitors has to be expanded by proliferation and allowed to differentiate.

Various strategies are discussed for committing stem cells to the keratinocyte lineage including induction with exogenous cytokines, growth factors, chemicals, and extracellular matrix. It is becoming obvious that stem cell biology is potentially very complex if such strategies are to be adopted to direct stem cell differentiation and maintain it.

It is evident, however, that there are going to be considerable challenges in the development of reliable protocols that can confidently preclude risks of teratoma formation and other, as yet unforeseen complications. This will certainly have an impact on the introduction of widespread clinical applications of mesenchymal stem cells in tissue engineering.

Wound Healing Modulation

One area of reconstructive practice that may be of more immediate clinical application is the use of stem cells to promote and modulate the healing of wounds. In this situation, the cells will be placed into a pathological environment, for example, a chronic non-healing wound. They will undertake an assessment of the physiological deficiencies in terms of matrix composition and cytokine milieu and correct these by producing the appropriate wound healing modulators. In a sense, this means that the cells are acting as a intelligent, interperative biofeedback control mechanisms that can autoregulate biological systems. Bone marrow, peripheral blood, and UCB have all been used in chronic wounds to modulate the healing response. Whilst the early experience is limited, the prospects are promising and some of the concerns about incorporating stem cell-derived tissue, into the body are unwarranted [36].

Of particular interest is the effect of topical applications of bone marrow-derived cells on chronic wounds. Although the reports are few, the consistent theme is that a chronic wound changes its nature to become an acute wound that heals or becomes healthy and can be closed with a skin graft [37, 38, 39]. Laboratory studies looking at cutaneous healing in a chimeric mouse model indicate that when marrow is transplanted it can contribute to the reconstitution of the dermal fibroblast population in the wound although local cutaneous cells reconstitute the epidermis [40]. An in vitro study indicated that collagen synthesis and levels of basic fibroblast growth factor (bFGF) and vascular endothelial growth factor (VEGF) were much higher in bone marrow stromal cells than those in dermal fibroblasts. This suggests the potential of topically applied bone marrow cells to accelerate wound healing [41]. A further study has looked at the effects of a bone marrow-impregnated collagen matrix and found a significantly increased angiogenic effect in an experimental mouse model.

This same group applied an autogenous bone marrow-impregnated collagen matrix to a patient with a chronic leg ulcer and observed a dramatic healing response [42].

In our own clinical experience, we have applied autologous bone marrow to a chronic unhealed burn wound, a donor site that had repeatedly failed to heal and a chronic wound at the extremity of latissimus dorsi-free muscle flap where the graft was being traumatized by footwear. The burn wound changed from being chronic and non-healing to re-epithelializing and was closed with a graft. The donor site that had failed to heal and also had repeatedly failed to take a graft, healed with no grafting necessary. The chronic heal wound became more vascular and was definitively closed with a skin graft. Another recent report describes the use of allogenic bone marrow mesenchymal stem cells for the treatment of a patient with deep skin burns [43].

It is in these cases that we see the great potential for topical application of cord blood as a biological wound healing modulator. It is of interest to note that amniotic membranes have been used in the past as biological dressings for wounds but concerns about risks of disease transmission have severely limited this practice in many parts of the world. Similarly, the question of potential risk of disease transmission when using cord blood may also be raised. However, there are already well-defined screening processes to reduce and/or eliminate such risks as applied in routine blood banking. Another consideration is that this use of cord blood is temporary and the relative lack of immunogenicity will limit adverse effects.

As the understanding of the range and nature of the stem cell composition in cord blood becomes more clear, it may be possible to apply more selective fractions onto wounds both chronic and acute to modulate the biological healing mechanisms. It would be a mistake to underestimate the complexity of stem cell biology and the clinical applications. Nevertheless, there is a hope that the resource provided by UCB will make a major contribution in the provision of cost-effective care of both acute and chronic wounds throughout the world.

References

1. Burd A. New skin. Transplantation 2000;70:1551–1552.
2. McGrath JA, Eady RAJ, Pope FM. Anatomy and Organization of Human Skin. In: Rook's Textbook of Dermatology. Eds: Burns T, Breathnach S, Cox N, Griffiths C. Vol 1, 7th Ed. UK: Blackwell Publishing. pp. 3.1–3.84.
3. Archer CB. Functions of the Skin. In: Rook's Textbook of Dermatology. Eds: Burns T, Breathnach S, Cox N, Griffiths C. Vol 1, 7th Ed. UK: Blackwell Publishing. pp. 4.1–4.12.
4. Burd A, Huang L. Hypertrophic response and keloid diathesis: two very different forms of scar. Plast Reconstr Surg 2005;116:150e–157e.
5. Dang C, Ting K, Soo C, Longaker MT, Lorenz HP. Fetal wound healing – Current perspectives. Clin Plastic Surg 2003;30:13–23.
6. Loots MA. Differences in cellular infiltrate and extracellular matrix of chronic diabetic and venous ulcers versus acute wounds. J Invest Dermatol 1998;111:850–857.
7. Fahey TJ III, Sadaty A, Jones WG. Diabetic impairs the late inflammatory response to wound healing. J Surg Res 1991;50:308–313.
8. Berthod F, Damour O. In vitro reconstructed skin models for wound coverage in deep burns. Br J Dermatol 1997;136:809–816.

9. Cooper ML, Spielvogel RL. Artificial skin for wound healing. Clin Dermatol 1994;12: 183–191.
10. Hansbrough JF, Cooper ML. Methods of skin coverage: achieving temporary and permanent coverage. Crit Care Rep 1990;2:50–62.
11. Sefton MV, Woodhouse KA. Tissue engineering. J Cutan Med Surg 1998;3 Suppl 1:18–23.
12. Carsin H, Ainaud P, Le Bever H, Rives J, Lakhel A. Cultured epithelial autografts in extensive burn coverage of severely traumatized patients: a five year single-center experience with 30 patients. Burns 2000;26:379–387.
13. Cooper ML, Hansbrough JF, Spielvogel RL, Cohen R. In vivo optimization of a living dermal substitute employing cultured human fibroblasts on a biodegradable polyglycolic acid or polyglactin mesh. Biomaterials 1991;12:243–248.
14. Falanga V, Margolis D, Alvarez O, Auletta M. Rapid healing of venous ulcers and lack of clinical rejection with an allogeneic cultured human skin equivalent. Arch Dermatol 1998;134:293–300.
15. Boyce ST. Skin substitutes from cultured cells and collagen-GAG polymers. Med Biol Eng Comput 1998;36:791–800.
16. Kearney JN. Clinical evaluation of skin substitutes. Burns 2001;27:545–551.
17. Burke JF. Observations on the development and clinical use of artificial skin – an attempt to employ regeneration rather than scar formation in wound healing. Jpn J Surg 1987;17: 431–438.
18. Wainwright D, Madden M, Luterman A. Clinical evaluation of an acellular allograft dermal matrix in full-thickness burns. J Burn Care Rehabil 1996;17:124–136.
19. Rheinwald JG, Green H. Serial cultivation of strains of human epidermal keratinocytes: the formation of keratinizing colonies from single cells. Cell 1975;6:331.
20. Boyce ST. Design principles for composition and performance of cultured skin substitutes. Burns 2001;27:523–533.
21. Navarro FA, Stoner ML, Lee HB, Park CS, Wood FM, Orgill DP. Melanocyte repopulation in full-thickness wounds using a cell spray apparatus. J Burn Care Rehabil 2001;22:41–46.
22. Metcalfe AD, Ferguson MWJ. Harnessing wound healing and regeneration for tissue engineering. Biochem Soc Trans 2005;33:413–417.
23. http://serendip.brynmawr.edu/bb/neuro/neuro04/web2/abruce.html (accessed 29/12/2005).
24. Rosenthal N. Prometheus's vulture and the stem-cell promise. N Engl J Med 2003;349:267–274.
25. Fodor WL. Tissue engineering and cell based therapies, from the bench to the clinic: the potential to replace, repair and regenerate. Reprod Biol Endocrinol 2003;1:1–6.
26. Hedrick MH, Daniels EJ. The use of adult stem cells in regenerative medicine. Clin Plastic Surg 2003;30:499–505.
27. Quesenberry PJ, Dooner G, Colvin G, Abedi M. Stem cell biology and the plasticity polemic. Exp Hematol 2005;33:389–394.
28. Jones N, Cyranoski D. Investigation says Hwang lied. News (doi:10.1038/news051219-17)
29. McGuckin CP, Forraz N, Baradez MO, Navran S, Zhao J, Urban R, Tilton R, Denner L. Production of stem cells with embryonic characteristics from human umbilical cord blood. Cell Prolif 2005;38:245–255.
30. Lewis ID. Clinical and experimental uses of umbilical cord blood. Intern Med J 2002;32: 601–609.
31. Takagi M. Cell processing engineering for ex-vivo expansion of hematopoietic cells. J Biosci Bioeng 2005;99:189–196.
32. Schmidt D, Mol A, Neuenschwander S, Breymann C, Gossi M, Zund G, Turina M, Hoerstrup SP. Living patches engineered from human umbilical cord derived fibroblasts and endothelial progenitor cells. Eur J Cardiothorac Surg 2005;27:795–800.
33. Wu X, Rabkin-Aikawa E, Guleserian KJ, Perry TE, Masuda Y, Sutherland FWH, Schoen FJ, Mayer JE, Bischoff J. Tissue-engineered microvessels on three-dimensional biodegradable scaffolds using human endothelial progenitor cells. Am J Physiol Heart Circ Physiol 2004;287:480–487.

34. Gang EJ, Jeong JA, Hong SH, Hwang SH, Kim SW, Yang IH, Ahn C, Han H, Kim H. Skeletal myogenic differentiation of mesenchymal stem cells isolated from human umbilical cord blood. Stem Cells 2004;22:617–624.
35. Heng BC, Cao T, Liu H, Phan TT. Directing stem cells into the keratinocyte lineage in vitro. Exp Dermatol 2005;14:1–16.
36. Valbonesi M, Giannini G, Migliori F, Dalla Costa R, Dejana AM. Cord blood (CB) stem cells for wound repair. Preliminary report of 2 cases. Transfus Apher Sci 2004;30:153–156.
37. Badiavas EV, Falanga V. Treatment of chronic wounds with bone marrow-derived cells. Arch Dermatol 2003;139:510–516.
38. Humpert PM, Bartsch U, Konrade I, Hammes HP, Morcos M, Kasper M, Bierhaus A, Nawroth PP. Locally applied mononuclear bone marrow cells restore angiogenesis and promote wound healing in a type 2 diabetic patient. Exp Clin Endocrinol Diabetes 2005;113:538–540.
39. Ayyappan T, Chadha A, Shaikh MF, Naik N, Desai I, Kadam, Shah C, Jain A, Baranwal P, Deepu NK, Patel V. Topically applied autologous bone marrow in healing of chronic non healing raw areas – a pilot study. Indian J Burns 2004;12:42–47.
40. Fathke C, Wilson L, Hutter J, Kapoor V, Smith A, Hocking A, Isik F. Contribution of bone marrow – derived cells to skin: collagen deposition and wound repair. Stem Cells 2004;22:812–822.
41. Han SK, Yoon TH, Lee DG, Lee MA, Kim WK. Potential of human bone marrow stromal cells to accelerate wound healing in vitro. Ann Plast Surg 2005;55:414–419.
42. Ichioka S, Kouraba S, Sekiya N, Ohura N, Nakatsuka T. Bone marrow-impregnated collagen matrix for wound healing: experimental evaluation in a microcirculatory model of angiogenesis, and clinical experience. Br J Plast Surg 2005;58:1124–1130.
43. Rasulov MF, Vasilchenkov AV, Onishchenko NA, Krasheninnikov ME, Kravchenko VI, Gorshenin TL, Pidtsan RE, Potapov IV. First experience of the use bone marrow mesenchymal stem cells for the treatment of a patient with deep skin burns. Bull Exp Boil Med 2005;139:141–144.

Chapter 13
Umbilical Cord Blood Transfusion – A Clinical Overview

Himansu Kumar Basu

Introduction

Fetal blood from the umbilical cord and placenta is a commodity which is wasted and disposed of after birth. Placental vessels at term contain an average of 150 ml of blood [1].

Umbilical cord blood is a convenient source of hematopoietic stem cells and can be used as an alternative to bone marrow or peripheral stem cells for transplantation in the treatment of malignant and non-malignant conditions in children and also in adults. Such transfusion or transplantation of hematopoietic stem cells has several advantages, including ready availability, decreased risk of transmission of viral infections and graft-versus-host disease (GVHD) in both human leukocyte antigen (HLA)-matched and HLA-mismatched transplants. Collection of blood is convenient with minimum risk to the mother or newborn.

Children who develop cancers such as leukemia and lymphoma often need bone marrow transplants following attempts to eradicate the cancer with strong chemotherapy and radiotherapy.

If matching bone marrow cannot be obtained from a relative, then the search for a match can be lengthy and often fruitless.

But stem cell from the subject's cord blood which had been collected and stored will always be a perfect match, and can be thawed out and delivered in an autologous blood transfusion.

Recently, there has been considerable interest in the use of cord blood as an alternative stem cell source to treat cancer and genetic diseases. An estimated 20,000 cord blood transplantations of matched and partly matched blood have been reported in the world literature.

Practical techniques have developed for collection, scrutiny, and storage of cord blood. Indications for umbilical cord blood (UCB) transfusion/transplantation are also expanding.

H.K. Basu (✉)
Consultant Gynaecologist, Shorne, Kent DA12 3HH, England

N. Bhattacharya, P. Stubblefield (eds.), *Frontiers of Cord Blood Science*,
DOI 10.1007/978-1-84800-167-1_13, © Springer-Verlag London Limited 2009

Characteristics of Umbilical Cord Blood

The yield of the cord blood varies from vol. 67–134 ml (mean 88 ± 14 ml SD) and mean hemoglobin 17.6 gm percent [2]. This blood has a much higher hemoglobin (mostly fetal hemoglobin), platelet and, leukocyte content than adult whole blood. Additionally, it has a high concentration of cytokine/growth factors in its plasma, which eventually helps in the gene-switching mechanism after the birth of the baby.

This blood has a much higher oxygen-carrying capacity than that of adult whole blood, and hence, the transfusion of fetal hemoglobin-rich cord blood has the potential for better tissue perfusion of oxygen (v/v) to the recipient's tissue than an identical volume of adult whole blood.

Compared with bone marrow cells, CD34+/CD3− cord blood cells proliferate more rapidly and generate larger numbers of progeny cells. Cultures of cord blood CD34+ cells increase in cell number every 7–10 days, several hundred-fold greater than the increase in cultures of similar cells from adult bone marrow.

Cord blood contains a high proportion of T cells expressing the CD45RA+/ CD45RO−, CD62L+ "naive" phenotype [3].

Some studies show that cord blood cells produce increased amounts of the anti-inflammatory cytokine and interleukin-10, which may down modulate GVHD [4].

Indications for Cord Blood Transfusion

There are two basic reasons for collection and transfusion of cord blood:

a. As a source of hematopoietic progenitors for allogenic stem cell transplantation in cases of leukemia or bone marrow aplasia. The treatment has been undertaken in children and less commonly in adults. However, new strategies are now being explored to address the obstacles of reduced cell dose on engraftment, risk of transplant-related complications and mortality [5].
b. As a source of hemoglobin in cases of anemia for transfusion in sickle cell disease, HIV, thalassemia. It has also been suggested as a source for possible peri-operative blood transfusion.

Indeed, it is possible to transfuse umbilical cord whole blood to older men and women after removing the stem cell content (0.01% of the nucleated cells of the cord blood), to combat anemia and raise immunity [2].

Umbilical Cord Blood Transfusion for Anemia

Clinical indications which are expanding, currently include cases of severe anemia, renal or hepatic dysfunction, and other conditions of diminished cardio-respiratory reserve or tissue hypoxic conditions, in any age group.

Hassall and colleagues [6] lowered mortality of children with severe anemia in sub-Saharan Africa by transfusing umbilical cord blood with a mean volume of 85 ml (SD 28.0). This amount of blood is sufficient to raise the hemoglobin concentrations in 28 (21%) of 131 children requiring transfusions in the same hospital, by 30 g/l.

Bhattacharya and colleagues [2] reported on the use of cord blood for transfusion in adults. They have transfused more than 350 units of freshly collected umbilical cord whole blood in different indications of adult blood transfusion, without encountering any immunological or non-immunological reactions.

Umbilical cord blood transfusion has also been suggested in cases of thalassemia, HIV infection with anemia, and leprosy with anemia [7].

Elderly Patients

Umbilical cord blood transfusion had been carried out in elderly patients after removing the stem cell content (0.01% of the nucleated cells of the cord blood), to combat anemia. This cord blood is rich in fetal hemoglobin (which carries 60% more oxygen than adult hemoglobin), growth factors and cytokines, etc., and therefore has a potential growth-promoting role. In the light of recent developments in molecular biology, it has been suggested that fetal stem cells and germ line cells, which express telomerase reverse transcriptase, can divide indefinitely and thus have the potential to increase cell numbers in a failing organ in the elderly after fetal cell transplantation and its homing effect on the hosts' organ [8].

Umbilical Cord Blood Stem Cell Transplantation

The indications are expanding. These can be considered under three headings:

a. Children with malignant disease – Umbilical cord blood had been used successfully in related transplants or with minor mismatch (with one or two loci unmatched) for both malignant and non-malignant diseases. There is a low but definite incidence of GVHD (10–15%). Cord blood, with low content of T cells is suitable for non-malignant diseases as there is no requirement for graft-versus-leukemia effect. Engraftment occurs in over 80% of cases. The event-free survival at 24 months is about 30–40% [9].
b. Metabolic disorders – Cord blood transplantation has also been shown to be effective in metabolic storage diseases. There were 20 children with Hurler syndrome, who received multiple chemotherapy followed by infusion of unrelated 1-, 2-, or 3-antigen-mismatched cord blood. With a median follow-up of 905 days, 17 of 20 children are alive with complete donor chimerism and normal peripheral blood alpha-1-iduronidase activity [10].

Cord blood transplantation can be successful, even if the patient and cord blood donor are mismatched at two antigen sites. GVHD is uncommon without a significant diminution of graft-versus-leukemia response.

c. Adult cord blood transplantation – Mismatched (unrelated) transplantation has been carried out in adults with leukemia, lymphoma, and myelo dysplasia along with a variety of conditioning and GVHD prophylaxis regimens. The results indicate high transplant-related early mortality mostly related to infection (47% death within 100 days) and 26% disease-free status at 22 months follow-up.

A comparison with unrelated but HLA-matched bone marrow transplants shows higher mortality, but lower GVHD in the cord blood group. Survival of around 20% was noted in recipients of unrelated cord blood and mismatched bone marrow. Indeed, studies suggest that outcomes are improved for patients receiving a matched unrelated bone marrow transplant.

Recipients of mismatched cord blood and 1-antigen-mismatched unrelated bone marrow had similar lower survival rates [11].

Although umbilical cord blood is often collected from unrelated donors, directed umbilical cord blood from sibling donors also provides an increasingly important source of UCB for transplantation. Blood is collected when an existing sibling suffers from a disease that may be treated by stem cell transplantation or a family history that could result in future birth of a sibling with a disease that could be treated by stem cell transplantation [12].

Improving Results of Cord Blood Transplantation in Adults

Mortality and disease-free survival in adult cord blood transfusion can be improved by:

a. pooled or sequential blood transfusion of a second partially matched cord blood unit,
b. cord blood expansion using mixtures of cytokines such as stem cell factor, G-CSF, and megakaryocyte growth factor, etc.,
c. combined cord blood and haploid identical CD34+ bone marrow transplants,
d. non-myeloablative or reduced strength conditioning regimens with one of the above.

Collection and Storage of Umbilical Cord Blood in Health

Blood from the maternal donor is tested for infectious disease markers, including tests for syphilis, human T-cell lymphotropic virus 1, HIV, hepatitis B, hepatitis C, and CMV.

The blood is taken from the placenta and umbilical cord just after birth and then frozen under liquid nitrogen at −180°C. This blood contains "stem cells," which can be harvested and kept in a frozen state.

Delayed cord clamping after birth appears to be beneficial for a term and particularly for a preterm fetus, equivalent to blood transfusion of an average of 21% of the neonate's blood volume.

For the purpose of in utero cord blood collection, too early cord blood clamping may deprive the fetus of this advantage and appears to be at variance with the recommended practice of delayed cord clamping [13].

The cord blood can be collected either in utero before the delivery of the placenta, or ex utero after delivery. In utero collections are usually performed by the obstetrician or nurse midwife attending the delivery, while trained personnel from the cord blood bank, who perform the collection outside the delivery room, more often perform ex utero collections.

Available evidence would favor collection of blood before the delivery of the placenta. There is a need to increase awareness and training among perinatal care providers who should be informed about the promising clinical potential of hematopoietic stem cells in umbilical cord blood and about current indications for its collection, storage, and use, based on sound scientific evidence. For detailed advice and recommendation, please see Armson [14] Of course it is important to recognize the primary importance of safety of the mother and child at all times, in relation to umbilical cord blood collection.

Potential Hazards

Recent research suggests that pre-cancerous cells can be found from birth onward, in children who go on to develop leukemia later on in life. If this is the case, returning umbilical blood to the same child may lead to renewed cancer a few years later – and by that time, the child may be at an age where chemotherapy is not so effective.

Of course, if a match can be found with another baby's umbilical cord blood, no such difficulties arise. Otherwise, a matched bone marrow transplant is preferable to autologous cord blood transplant.

Other risks are infection and transmission of damaged cells (please see below).

Blood Banking Issues

There are issues related to recruitment and screening of donors, consent of the mother, testing and processing after blood is collected, freezing, storage and distribution to recipients. For a review please see Ballen (2005) [9].

World's first public-private cord blood bank, the Virgin Health Bank has been established in the United Kingdom [15]. A number of potential conflicts, including the issue of safety of caring for the mother and the baby, and interest of cord blood collection, have been highlighted. The Royal College of Obstetricians and Gynaecologists has welcomed the public nature and international accountability of the Virgin Health Bank.

Future Trends

There is a trend toward utilizing cord blood instead of a matched unrelated donor, for example, in elderly patients with a high risk of GVHD. There appears to be a less risk of a GVHD. In this procedure, additional application in non-malignant diseases is likely to be introduced in the future.

Another intriguing application is in HIV disease which is a worldwide public health problem, in which the possibility of gene transfer to an hematopoietic stem cell reservoir may eventually be possible. An allogenic stem cell vaccine may replace hematopoietic stem cells infected with HIV with uninfected umbilical cord blood cells [16].

Another area of application could be autoimmune diseases, where there has been some success with autologous transplantation. The low risk of GVHD makes cord blood transplantation of positive benefit in comparison with bone marrow transplant.

Further future areas of cord blood transfusion may be other non-hematopoietic applications, such as the repair of damaged myocardium or neural tissue cord blood cells are a more primitive population than adult bone marrow, and have increased capacity for pluri-potential differentiation.

However, caution is needed in this line of research. There are unknown potential risks of transmission of malignant, autoimmune and infectious agents (prions) through blood transfusion. In many cases, screening tests do not exist and prevention of the passage of the harmful agent may not be possible [17]. Treatment should be carried out only in recognized centers with quality control.

An important future initiative is the practical possibility of collection of cord blood and transfusion in emergency situations, where an alternative source of blood may not be available [18]. If organisational problems can be overcome, this life saving method will have great potential, specially in areas or hospitals with high delivery rate.

References

1. Haselhorst G, Allmeling A. Die gwichtszunahme von neugeborenen infolge postnataler transfusion. *Z Geburtshilfe Perinatol* 1930;98:103.
2. Bhattacharya N. Umbilical cord whole blood transfusion: a suggested strategy to combat blood scarcity in Ireland. *BMJ* 2002;324:7330.
3. Szabolcs P, Park KD, Reese M, Marti L, Broad-water G, Kurtz berg. Coexistent naive phenotype and higher cycling rate of cord blood T cells as compared to adult peripheral blood. *J Exp Hematol* 2003;31:708–714.
4. Bacchetta R, Bigler M, Touraine JL, et al. High levels of interleukin 10 production in vivo are associated with tolerance in SCID patients transplanted with HLA mismatched haematopoietic stem cells. *J Exp Med* 1994;179:493.
5. Brunstein CG, Setubal DC, Wagner JE. Expanding the role of umbilical cord blood transplantation. *Br J Haematol.* 2007;137(1):20–35.
6. Hassall O, Bedu-Addo G, Adarkwa M, Danso K, Bates I. Umbilical-cord blood for transfusion in children with severe anaemia in under-resourced countries. *Lancet* 2003;361: 678–679.

7. Bhattacharya N. The safe use of placental umbilical cord whole blood transfusion in patients suffering from anaemia and thalassemia in under resourced regions of the world. *BMJ* 2004;328:7269.
8. Bhattacharya N. Immunization and fetal cell/tissue transplant: a new strategy for geriatric treatment. *BMJ* 2002;323:7320.
9. Ballen KK. New trends in umbilical cord blood transfusion. *Blood* 2005;105,10:3786.
10. Staba SL, Escolar ML, Poe M, et al. Cord-blood transplants from unrelated donors in patients with Hurler's syndrome. *N Engl J Med* 2004;350:1960–1969.
11. Laughlin MJ, Eapen M, Rubinstein P, et al. Outcomes after transplantation of cord blood or bone marrow from unrelated donors in adults with leukaemia. *N Engl J Med* 2004;351: 2265–2275.
12. Smythe J, Armitage S, McDonald D, et al. Directed sibling cord blood banking for transplantation: the 10-year experience in the national blood service in England. *Stem Cells* 2007;25(8):2087–2093.
13. Weeks A. Umbilical cord clamping after birth. *BMJ* 2007;385:312–313.
14. Armson B. Umbilical cord blood banking: implications for perinatal care providers. *J Obstet Gynaecol Can* 2005;27(3):263–290.
15. Mayor S. World's first public-private cord blood bank launched in UK by Richard Branson. *BMJ* 2007;334:277.
16. Goodwin HS, Bicknese AR, Chien SN, Bogucki BD, Quinn CO, Wall DA. Multilineage differentiation activity by cells isolated from umbilical cord blood: expression of bone, fat, and neural markers. *Biol Blood Marrow Transplant* 2001;7:581–588.
17. Braude P, Minger SL, Warwick RM. Stem cell therapy: hope or hype? *BMJ* 2005;330: 1159–1160.
18. Bhattacharya N. Placental umbilical cord whole blood transfusion: a safe and genuine blood substitute for patients of the under-resourced world at emergency. *J Am Coll Surg* 2005;200(4):557.

Section IV
Cord Blood Stem Cell Banking

Chapter 14
Establishment of the UK Stem Cell Bank and Its Role in Stem Cell Science

G.N. Stacey

Introduction

The United Kingdom has administered an in-depth and broad-ranging debate on the use of human embryos for research, stretching over at least two decades, which led to the Human Fertilisation and Embryology Act of 1990. The Human Fertilisation and Embryology Authority was established in 1991 to regulate and license all applications to work with human embryos in the United Kingdom. Following the publication of the first human embryonic stem (hES) cell lines [1], a Parliamentary House of Lords Select Committee was set up in 2001 to discuss the use of human embryos for research and the development of therapy as part of a broad public consultation. This process involved extensive dialogue between the public, politicians, and other professional stakeholders. Reporting in June 2002, the Select Committee recommended that there should be a bank established to provide stem cell researchers with ready access to embryonic stem cell lines of guaranteed purity and provenance from sources with appropriate ethical approval. In the same year, the Government endorsed the recommendations of the Select Committee report and announced that a National Stem Cell Bank would be established to curate and maintain stocks of somatic and embryonic stem cells, derived in the United Kingdom under the proposed regulation. Such cell lines would be prepared as quality-controlled cell banks, to enable ready access for researchers to reliable, high quality and ethically sourced stocks of these precious cells.

To establish the Bank, the Medical Research Council (MRC) coordinated competitive tenders from institutions with appropriate facilities and experience but not engaged in basic stem cell research. This selective process was important to ensure that the bank could operate as an independent custodian of the cells without the conflict of interest in using the cells that might occur in a center for stem cell research. Following a lengthy evaluation process, in January 2003, $2.6M was awarded to National Institute for Biological Standards and Control (NIBSC) for

G.N. Stacey (✉)
Director for the UK Stem Cell Bank, Head of the Cell Biology and Imaging Division, National Institute for Biological Standards and Control, Blanche Lane South Mimms, Herts, EN6 3QG, UK
e-mail: gstacey@nibsc.ac.uk

N. Bhattacharya, P. Stubblefield (eds.), *Frontiers of Cord Blood Science*,
DOI 10.1007/978-1-84800-167-1_14,

3 years from the MRC (75% of funds) and the Biotechnology and Biological Sciences Research Council (25% of funds).

Aims and Remit for the UK Stem Cell Bank

The primary remit of the Bank is to provide access to ethically sourced and well-characterized seed stocks of human stem cell lines of both somatic (adult and fetal) and embryonic origin. The Bank is also expected to work on an international collaborative basis with researchers and other banking centers. Stem cell lines will be provided for two types of use: first "research grade" banks will be prepared to promote basic research and second, "clinical grade" banks will provide seed stocks for clinical trials and the development of stem cell products.

Key Operational Principles for the UK Stem Cell Bank

The Bank is required to maintain transparent operational procedures including publication of the Code of Practice for the UK Stem Cell Bank (UKSCB; www.mrc.ac.uk) which describes how the bank can be expected to operate and interact with the stem cell community, and its responsibility to the Steering Committee for the UKSCB and the Use of Stem Cell Lines.

Given its unusual role as an independent "broker" in the stem cell community and to ensure that it cannot be accused of conflicts of interest, the Bank is prohibited from carrying out fundamental research on stem cell biology although it is permitted to develop and enhance methods for culture, preservation, characterization, and safety testing involved in the cell banking process. The Bank is also prohibited from engaging in commercial activities and specifically product development, although it is important that NIBSC and Bank staff are engaged with companies to support their work to enhance the safety and quality of stem cell products.

The Bank has also made extensive efforts to develop a strong and close liaison with the stem cell community. As a key part of NIBSCs work, there is close interaction with numerous regulatory bodies (approximately 80 world-wide) and this role is also developing for stem cell therapies as part of the Bank and general NIBSC activity. The Bank must be sensitive to the broad range of groups with interests in stem cells and their clinical potential, and also provides information for the press and media on the work of the Bank and its role in the stem cell community.

The high profile of the Bank means that it is focused on reliability of its outputs and achieved this thorough careful proofing of its procedures and trying to anticipate and explore the implications of potential future developments. This is achieved through building flexibility within staff and facilities and close interaction with lead research groups regulators and clinical groups.

Donating Cells to the Bank

Embryonic stem cell lines established in the United Kingdom are required, under the license for derivation from the Human Fertilisation and Embryology Authority, to be deposited in the UKSCB. Other groups working on the derivation of adult and non-UK hES cells are also very welcome to use the UKSCB facility. Donation of cell lines into the Bank is initiated by submission of information on the lines to the Bank's Steering Committee using the forms available on the Bank and Medical Research Council websites. Confirmation by the Steering Committee that the cells meet ethical requirements for the United Kingdom and other scientific and technical criteria then activates the depositing process with the Bank and establishment of the transfer agreements between depositor and the Bank. A generic agreement is also established to be put in place between depositor and any institution receiving cells from the Bank to protect the depositor's intellectual property in the cells.

Once a depositor's cell line is accepted by the Bank, then the depositor will hopefully begin to realize a series of technical, logistical, and other benefits that come with depositing cells in the UKSCB. These can include:

- Technical benefits
  - Detailed characterization and quality control of the cells.
  - Enhanced technical procedures for cell culture, preservation, and testing procedures.
- Resource benefits
  - The Bank takes on scale-up, quality control, and distribution.
  - The Bank provides an assured safe depository.
- Potential economic benefits
  - Added value in having cell banks that meet international quality standards thus aiding development for both clinical and testing applications of the cells.
  - Safety testing regimes for clinical grade cell banks.
  - Promote wider use of depositors' cells for research whilst protecting Intellectual Property Rights (IPR) under a Materials Transfer Agreement established by the depositor.
  - For the purposes of filing stem cell patents, the Bank can also provide patent deposit facility (see next).

Stem cell lines released from the UKSCB must be used only in projects that have appropriate ethical review and approval. Requests to obtain cell lines from the Bank must be submitted to the Bank's Steering Committee using the forms available on the Bank and Medical Research Council websites. This is a straightforward process of submitting a summary of the scientific and ethical information associated with the intended use of the cells to the UK Steering Committee. Early contact with the Bank is recommended to assist applications.

What is a Cell Bank?

The term "cell bank" has been applied generically to describe what is in fact a very broad range of entities. There are a wide variety of "tissue banks" established for cell and tissue transplantation for a range of tissues requiring different approaches and procedures. Whilst they all have a common need for donor consent and the need for donor medical histories and screening for viral markers, these requirements will differ between countries. Public service culture collections (see www.eccosite.org and www.wfcc.info) provide cell banks but are customer-focused and provide immortalized cell lines with fundamental quality control for a very broad range of uses in research and industry. Moving to another level pharmaceutical grade, cell banking facilities are required to comply with Good Manufacturing Practices [2] and intensive quality control and safety testing where cells are used for product manufacture. The UKSCB for stem cell lines must combine all of these activities in its role as a public service collection for research and as a source of seed stocks for clinical trials.

Principle of Cell Banking

An important principle of banking for any microorganism including cell lines is that there should be an early passage stock of viable cryopreserved cells that provide a primary source of material as an archive of the original material for future reference. This stock may be referred to as the Master Cell Bank and samples from this bank should be fully quality controlled and characterized. Ampoules from the master bank are recovered to produce expanded cultures at slightly higher passage level that can be cryopreserved as Working Cell Banks that may be used for R&D, production, or clinical therapy. If prepared correctly, this tiered master/working bank system (Fig. 14.1) can provide reproducible and reliable supplies of identical cultures for many decades.

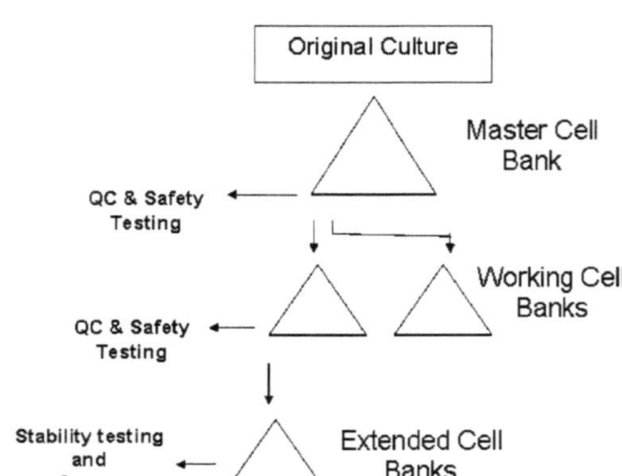

Fig. 14.1 Schema for preparation of master and working banks

Fundamental Criteria for Assurance of Quality of Cell Lines

There are three fundamental characteristics of a cell line required to promote good quality and valid cell culture work:

- Purity: absence of microorganisms
- Authenticity: correct identity and absence of "other" cells
- Stability: passage *in vitro* and storage

In general, most rigorous testing is performed on the Master Cell Bank, but for both master and working stocks it is important to have a combination of quality control tests for all these features whilst for extended cell banks of stem cell lines the main focus would be on the genetic/phenotypic stability of the cells in the undifferentiated state and their sustained ability to differentiate reproducibly [3].

In Europe, regulation of tissue engineering has begun to develop and in the United Kingdom guidance in this area has been in place for some time as Codes of Practice to provide guidance for tissue banks [4], manufacturers of human tissue products [5], and for the banking of stem cell lines (www.ukstemcellbank.org).

The general risk from endogenous contaminants of the cells or the original tissue of origin may be assessed from their tissue and species of origin. Trypsin and serum can be tested for likely contaminants or treated by irradiation, and there are also alternatives such as materials of plant or crustacean origin that may be used in place of animal proteins such as trypsin. In addition, serum-free growth media can be used to avoid the risks of virus and mycoplasma contamination. However, it is important to recognize that some cells may not be amenable to the use of these alternatives and that their use may introduce new complexities or contaminants to the *in vitro* culture environment and, moreover, may alter certain characteristics of the cell lines.

Viral contamination may arise from the original tissue used to derive a cell line or from materials of animal origin used in the cell line derivation process as already indicated, and it is important to evaluate these risks. Important sources of information that promote safety of cell therapy products include: donor screening for viral markers, and risk assessment of material of animal origin. However, additional risk factors include contamination from cell culture operators, and endogenous viruses that may emerge from the host genome.

Embryonic Stem Cells *in vitro:* Control and Standardization for Research and Therapy

Stem cells cultured *in vitro* are potentially unstable and highly sensitive to environmental variables with much of their cell biology yet to be determined. Nevertheless, if work with these cells is to progress, there is a clear need for reliable and reproducible supplies of cells that perform consistently. At the UKSCB, we aim to address this by: (1) attempting to minimize variation in culture environment, (2) establishment of a framework of controls and well-defined culture reagents, procedures, and quality control tests, and (3) attempting to characterize the residual variation in the cultures.

Maintaining accurate measurement and control of the temperature and gaseous environment provided for cell culture is vital to these aims, as will be the use of reagents and media that are closely specified for their composition, purity, and batch-to-batch reproducibility. Culture protocols will also be carefully captured from the laboratory of origin that will also be engaged in an ongoing interaction to ensure that scientific and technical best practice are maintained as methods are improved. Further definition of the culture environment may be achieved as serum-free and feeder cell-free methods are developed. Such approaches have significant benefits in reducing the media variation and the risk of certain types of viral contamination from culture reagents. However, the effect of such conditions on the performance of the cells must also be carefully monitored.

Stem Cell Lines for Clinical Use: Three Translational Phases

UKSCB provides a translational role taking research developments and attempting to translate these into starting materials (cell banks) that are appropriately qualified for use in clinical trials. The first phase is to capture a set of methodologies and protocols from the research environment that will give laboratory workers support in achieving technical proficiency. This role will also be very important for the development of protocols that can be used reliably in the product development and production settings for initiation of clinical trails.

In the next phase, the Bank must establish robust and reliable banking procedures that may vary for different cell lines depending on their growth characteristics. A core quality control and safety testing regime will be applied to each bank and for each line a specification is produced to describe and quantify, wherever possible, the key characteristics to be maintained. This specification is used to assess the certificate of analysis compiled for each new cell bank of that line and to assess if the bank is of the appropriate standard for release.

In the final phase, cell bank vials are transferred to researchers or clinical trials. In the former case, obtaining feedback on the performance of the cells will be vital to maintaining the standards of the Bank and responding to customer difficulties. It is anticipated that with cells released for clinical trial there will be a period of iteration for the bank and the recipients to discuss the testing protocol appropriate for the clinical trial, for the specific cell line. In addition, mechanisms will have to be established for recall procedures due to post-donation disease in donors and adverse event reporting from patients in the clinical trial.

Progress in Establishing the UK Stem Cell Bank

The establishment of the Bank has been a high-profile activity due to the associated ethical concerns and high expectations of the public for stem cell research.

Accordingly, the Steering Committee for the Bank has taken a very careful approach to setting up its framework and the Bank has reflected this in developing a robust and thoughtful approach to its establishment and operation. Appropriate time has been allocated to these activities and to the physical construction of the Bank. In 2003, four new core staff were recruited, facilities for research grade cells were established, a GMP-compliant facility was constructed, and a Code of Practice describing how the Bank should operate was published on the Medical Research Council website.

In 2004, the Bank achieved accreditation to provide cells for clinical use from the Medical and Healthcare products Regulatory Authority (MHRA). The Steering Committee approved the first lines for the Bank in May 2004 (the first two hES cell lines derived in the United Kingdom at Kings College and Newcastle Centre for Life) and in December a further 22 hES cell lines from the United Kingdom, the United States, and Australia were approved. The Bank also achieved patent depositary status in 2004 which is recognized by the World Intellectual Property Organisation. Currently, the staff comprises a total of nine scientists including four PhDs and a quality manager with Qualified Person experience for release of medical products. Since 2003, the Bank has also been involved in training activities for culture of hES cells with Professors Harry Moore and Peter Andrews at the University of Sheffield and more recently with a number of other organizations worldwide. During 2004–2005, the Bank provided the hub for the International Stem Cell Initiative (see next) and is now banking the remaining cell lines approved by the Steering Committee.

UK Stem Cell Bank/NIBSC Interactions with the Stem Cell Community

The staff at NIBSC have been engaged with the transplantation community for many years and have coordinated a liaison group on hematopoietic stem cells for a number of years (see http://www.nibsc.ac.uk/aboutus/ukscbliason.html). The Bank has engaged directly with stem cell biologists in many countries and has presented at scientific conferences on stem cells and regenerative medicine conferences around the world. The Bank has also provided the hub for the Medical Research Council led project called the International Stem Cell Initiative. This project headed by Professor Peter Andrews of Sheffield University aims, through a carefully standardized process, to compare the characteristics of around 70 hES cell lines in 17 expert research centers around the world [6]. Details of this activity can be found at http://www.stemcellforum.org/ and the results of the whole project will be published in 2006.

Conclusions

Whilst stem cell lines have the potential to deliver an exciting new range of therapies, there are still important issues to address to establish safe and efficacious cell therapy products. There is still considerable research to be performed on the basic culture and differentiation processes required for the development of therapeutic applications. The UKSCB aims to support the stem cell community at various levels: providing banking facilities and collaboration on technical, safety issues, and training. The NIBSC, the host institution for the UK Bank, has a background and long-standing experience in the field of biological medicines, which enables it to provide an advisory role free of conflicts of interest. The Bank is therefore well placed to help setting standards for safe and reliable stem cell therapies as they are developed and provide a valuable advisory role in the stem cell field.

References

1. Thomson, J., Itskovitz-Eldor, J., Shapiro, S., et al., (1998) Embryonic stem cell lines derived from human blastocysts. Science. 282, 1145–7.
2. MCA (MHRA) (2002) Rules and Guidance for Pharmaceutical Manufacturers and Distributors 2002. TSO, London.
3. Stacey, G. (2005). Human Stem Cell Lines: The Role of Cell Banks in Assuring Quality for Research and Clinical Development in Cell Therapy. European Biopharmaceutical Review. Winter Edn., 112–5.
4. DH (2001). A code of practice for tissue banks-providing tissues of human origin for therapeutic purposes. Department of Health, London. www.dh.gov.uk/Publications
5. DH (2002). A code of practice for the production of human derived therapeutic products. Department of Health., London. www.mhra.gov.uk/home (see "How We Regulate – Tissue Engineered Products").
6. Andrews, P.W., Benvenisty, N., Mckay, R., Pera, M.F., Rossant, J., Semb, H. and Stacey, G.N. (2005) The International Stem Cell Initiative: toward bench marks for human embryonic stem cell research. Nature Biotechnology, 23, 795–7.

Chapter 15
Cord Blood Allogeneic and Autologous Banking

Carolyn Troeger and Wolfgang Holzgreve

After delivery of the infant, its umbilical cord blood (UCB) has been found to contain sufficient numbers of hematopoietic stem cells (HSC) to be used for stem cell transplantation (CBT) in children and to a certain extent in adults. The first successful allogeneic-related CBT has been performed in 1988 in a boy affected by Fanconi's anemia from the CB of the HLA-identical newborn sister [1]. Since then, more than 6,000 unrelated allogeneic CBT have been performed worldwide. It has become a widely used alternative source for HSC to transplant patients suffering from several different diseases, such as malignancies of the hematopoietic system, bone marrow failure syndromes, inborn errors of metabolism, hemoglobinopathies, and others [2]. Survival rates after CBT are comparable to bone marrow transplantation (40–80% according to the indication); related allogeneic CBT leads to survival rates as high as 75–90%. These comparable results have led to the establishment of public allogeneic UCB banks where more than 165,000 UCB units are stored frozen and HLA typed [3, 4, 5]. In contrast to these allogeneic UCB banks, autologous UCB banks have been established by private companies. These so-called private UCB banks market properties of primitive progenitors found in UCB for regenerative purposes. Although numerous UCB units are stored in these private UCB banks, only few of these units have been used for transplantation, more in related allogeneic than in autologous settings [6].

Advantages and Disadvantages of HSC from UCB

The major aim of a public UCB bank is to store UCB units with a great HLA diversity to deliver matched transplants to patients in need, that otherwise would not find a HLA-matched donor in registries for bone marrow or peripheral blood-derived stem cells [7]. The analysis of the Swiss cord blood inventory with 1,441 CB units revealed that even between the two UCB banks within Switzerland (Basel and Geneva) certain HLA types are significantly different, being most stringent for HLA-DR*0101, 0701, and 1501. Furthermore, rare alleles (defined as

C. Troeger (✉)
University Women's Hospital Basel, Spitalstrasse 21, CH-4031 Basel, Switzerland

N. Bhattacharya, P. Stubblefield (eds.), *Frontiers of Cord Blood Science*,
DOI 10.1007/978-1-84800-167-1_15, © Springer-Verlag London Limited 2009

less than 1/500 in the normal population) had been identified, such as A*0202, HLA DR1*1304, and DR1*0302 (mainly abundant in Africans) and HLA-A*0211 (frequent in American Indians) [8]. Since the units are stored frozen and already at least low-resolution HLA-typed, the time interval between a search and the transplantation procedure is very short (see Table 15.1) [9]. UCB is collected under sterile condition right after delivery of the infant, which had not been exposed to bacteria or viruses. This leads to a very low risk of transmission of infectious agents that are acquired later in life (e.g., cytomegalievirus, Epstein-Barr virus etc.). On the other hand, the UCB sampling immediately after delivery has the problem that certain genetic diseases, such as M. Recklinghausen or Philadelphia chromosome-positive leukemia, are not evident at that early time in infant's life and follow-up information is difficult to gain. This risk is minimized by the application of very strict exclusion criteria in the donor selection process. The stem cell collection early in donor's life has also an influence on the behavior of the progenitors in that they have a higher proliferative capacity; this leads to comparable long-term engraftment levels although transplanted cell numbers are lower than in bone marrow transplantation [10, 11]. The immaturity of the co-transplanted leukocytes leads to less graft-versus-host disease, but on the other hand to a decreased graft-versus-leukemia effect, which is important for the success rate in the treatment of malignant disorders [12]. Since the UCB is collected after the cord has been clamped and therewith separated from the newborn infant, the sampling can be performed without pain and risk for the donor. The timing of the cord clamping should be influenced only by the common obstetrical practice, but not by the planned UCB sampling. A very early cord clamping would increase the volume of the blood that is left in the placenta and umbilical cord, but therewith would decrease the blood volume in the infant's circulation, leading to anemia [13].

One major drawback of UCB is the limited volume and number of progenitors. On average, 50–200 ml UCB can be collected [14]. The minimum HSC number of UCB units considered for an allogeneic UCB bank is defined at 80×10^7 nucleated cells. Since these units for allogeneic, unrelated transplantation are stored

Table 15.1 Advantages and disadvantages of transplants derived from bone marrow compared to UCB

	Cord blood	Bone marrow
Median search time	<1 Month	3–6 Months
Donor not available	<1%	30%
Rare HLA types present	29%	2%
Limiting factors for use	Cell dose $>8 \times 10^8$ NC, HLA match 4/6	HLA match 6/6
Possibility of booster or donor lymphocyte injection	Only in related allogeneic UCBT	Yes
Risk of viral transmission	No	Yes
Risk for unknown congenital diseases	Yes	No
Risk for donor	No	Yes

anonymously, any booster transplantation to enhance engraftment derived from the same donor is excluded [2]. For a successful transplantation, at least 1–2 × 10^7 nucleated cells per kg are needed, thus most units if applied as single transplants are available mainly for children [15, 16]. In contrast, adults can be transplanted with UCB only under certain circumstances, e.g., low body weight, absence of alternative matched donors, or in double transplantations, where two UCB units are transplanted to the same recipient [17, 18]. It has been shown that only one of the two grafts is detected in long term. A co-transplantation of third-party mesenchymal stem cells alleviates single-donor predominance and increases the engraftment level of the HSC from CB [19].

Factors that Influence the Number of Progenitors in UCB

Umbilical cord blood contains relatively high numbers of HSC and other progenitors representing 1–3% of the nucleated cell population [20]. Compared to adult peripheral blood numbers of CD34+ and CD34+CD38− cells are tenfold increased, being comparable to adult bone marrow [9, 21]. Since fetal hematopoiesis switches from liver and spleen to bone marrow in the 3rd trimester of pregnancy, levels of HSC are increased in the peripheral blood of the fetus and therewith also in UCB after delivery. Due to this fact, levels of the above-mentioned stem cell populations are significantly elevated in late 2nd and early trimester compared to term (CD34+: 2.51% vs. 0.88%; CD34+CD38−: 0.65 vs. 0.13%) [22, 23]. But not only preterm delivery is associated with elevated levels of HSC, but also chronic fetal stress like in pre-eclampsia and intrauterine growth retardation has an influence on the content of UCB after delivery. Certain obstetrical factors that are also associated with acute and chronic fetal distress such as vaginal-operative and operative deliveries (vacuum or forceps extraction, cesarean section) compared to normal deliveries, prolonged labor, and low pH values in UCB lead to increased numbers of HSC in UCB [24, 25, 26]. It can be speculated that an elevated secretion of pro-inflammatory cytokines, such as IL-1β and IL-6 as well as stress hormones, such as cortisol and adrenalin results in mobilization of progenitors to the periphery [27]. This is in accordance with the fact that elevated numbers of HSC are found in secondary cesarean sections that are performed due to fetal distress, compared to those performed for failure to progress or primary planned cesarean sections. In this study, we found that although the collected volumes of UCB were similar, the content of nucleated cells and CD34+ in UCB was significantly elevated if the cesarean section was indicated because of fetal distress (see Fig. 15.1) [28 Although it has been shown that UCB volume does not necessarily correlates with the number of HSC, higher UCB volumes are associated with higher numbers of HSC. Similarly, a big placenta with long umbilical cord contains more stem cells, as well as an infant with higher birth weight is associated with higher numbers of stem cells. Recently, it has been shown that certain HSC populations, e.g., CD34+CD61+ are increased in UCB collected from male infants. Significant differences in the lymphocyte and CD34+ subsets exist between different ethnic subset, for instance CD34+CD38− cells are

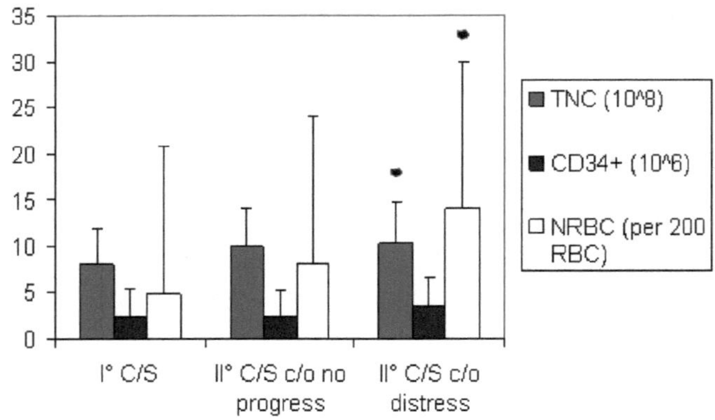

Fig. 15.1 Analyzed hematopoietic parameters in comparison between primary (group 1) and secondary cesarean section for failure to progress in labor (group 2) and fetal distress (group 3). *Indicates significant differences between groups 1 and 3, whereas there is no difference between groups 1 and 2

significantly lower in African American and Asian compared to Caucasian and Hispanic population. Whether this different distribution has an impact on engraftment kinetics and levels is currently under investigation [29, 30].

UCB Collection, Processing, and Quality Management

Realizing the great therapeutic potential of allogeneic UCB stem cell transplantation in children and adults has led to the establishment of allogeneic UCB banks in nearly all countries worldwide. The first institution was founded in 1993 in New York (New York Blood Center, NYBC) and has now the longest experiences in processing and long-term storage and de-freezing of cryopreserved UCB units [7].

Umbilical cord blood collection has become a routine service in many obstetrical units though adequate donor selection and clean UCB sampling, quick processing and precise documentation of the whole process is a serious issue. It has been shown recently that quality issues (quality control, medical history, labeling, and documentation) affect more than half of UCB units stored in recent UCB inventories [31]. But also in the pre-sampling period, it is important to accurately select the donor because due to the strict exclusion criteria for stem cell donation, UCB sampling and processing would be very ineffective if many units have to be excluded after processing [32].

Routinely, healthy pregnant women with unremarkable course of pregnancy as well as unremarkable family and personal medical history can be recruited for allogeneic UCB donation. This consent procedure should optimally take place before women come into the labor ward. It is feasible to obtain written informed consent after delivery of the infant and UCB collection if the pregnant woman has given oral informed consent before labor. An UCB collection from an expulsed placenta in a separate room before any informed consent had been obtained is ethically not correct [33].

The UCB sampling is best performed with the placenta still in utero after the umbilical cord had been clamped. To not deprave the infant because of UCB collection, cord clamping should be performed not earlier than 20 seconds after delivery of the baby. On the other hand, early cord clamping is an issue in preventing severe postpartum hemorrhage [34].

Units that contain more than 80×10^7 nucleated cells are further processed if all JACIE/FACT guidelines (Joint Accreditation committee ISCT and EBMT/ Foundation for the Accreditation of Cellular Therapy) have been followed and the delivery was unremarkable, e.g., any chorioamnionitis, severe maternal hemorrhage, and fetal malformations had been excluded (see Fig. 15.2) [35].

As stated above, the numbers of HSC in UCB is a critical factor for the success of the transplantation in terms of speed of recovery, transplant-related events and long-term survival rates. Because nowadays the UCB transplantation is more and more performed in adult patients, the required cell doses has increased since the beginning of UCB banking from 2.1×10^8 to 10×10^8 nucleated cells. These increased requirements parallel with a relatively high deferral rate of UCB samples due to so-called low cell count. In a study performed at our institution recently, we could show that half of the collected samples were deferred because of low volume or low cell count. Other logistic problems (UCB sampling during cesarean section, weekend, patients in labor, no consent and obstetrical work load) and obstetrical conditions (very preterm delivery, twins) were the reason not to collect UCB in 88 of 131 eligible patients (67%). All these factors result in a relatively low banking rate, being 10% of all deliveries at our institution and even as low as 1% in others [35, 36].

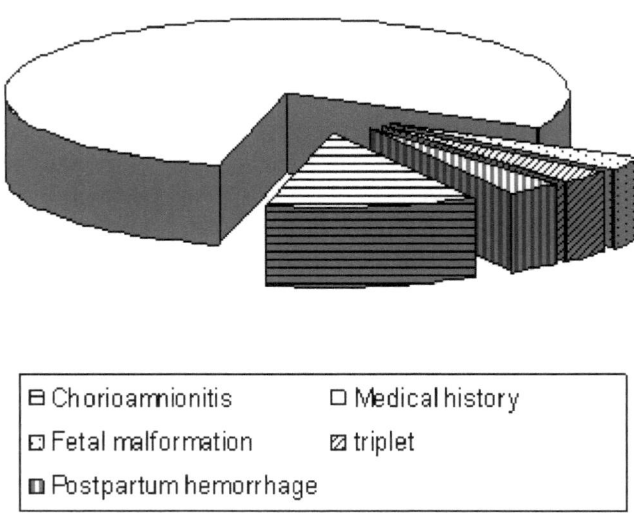

Fig. 15.2 Exclusion criteria for allogeneic UCB donation

Further processing of the UCB has to be started within 24 hours. It has been shown that storage of UCB units longer than 24 hours would decrease the yield of nucleated cells and CD34+ cells. A volume reduction is usually performed to decrease the space that is needed for storage in liquid nitrogen. Different procedures are used such as different filter systems, hydroxyethyl starch sedimentation, and automated centrifugation (Sepax®). It has been shown recently that the automated Sepax method results in higher total nucleated cell and CD34+ cell recoveries compared to other methods [37]. After cell separation, the fraction containing the HSC is supplemented with DMSO and controlled-rate frozen. Finally, UCB units are stored in liquid nitrogen containers at −180°C until use. Although one major aim of an UCB bank is to have a constant turnover of UCB units with a delivery rate of about 1% of the units per year, long-term cryopreservation cannot be excluded. To test the potential of HSC stored for 15 years, Broxmeyer et al. could show that immature UCB-derived primitive progenitors with high proliferative, replating, ex vivo expansion and engrafting capacities can be retrieved with high efficiency [38].

Controversies Between Public and Private UCB Banking

Pregnant women have the option to store their UCB within a private UCB bank for possible use by the child or other family members, or to donate it to a public bank for later anonymous use within an allogeneic UCB transplantation. As stated above, public UCB banks are well-established worldwide and store about 200,000 units usually for allogeneic, mostly unrelated transplantation. Public UCB banks do not charge the parents for collection and processing of the UCB unit. Costs to establish the bank are often covered by philantrophic or tax payer's money. Stored UCB units are registered at a stem cell donor registry such as "Bone marrow donors worldwide" (www.bmdw.org), where 165,000 HLA-type UCB units are registered. If an UCB unit is requested and used for HSC transplantation, the unit is delivered from the UCB bank to the transplantation center and paid by the institution, respectively, the health insurance of the recipient. If the turnover of UCB units exceeds a certain level (about 1%), costs for processing new units equal the costs that are charged for the delivered units [39]. Most public banks offer both unrelated and related allogeneic UCB units to be used for HSC transplantation in patients with leukemia or genetic diseases. In related allogeneic UCB transplantation, a sibling with its UCB serves as a donor for a family member that has a disease that can be treated by HSC transplantation. If the UCB bank targets on a great HLA diversity, it might provide HSC also for ethnic minorities that are under-represented in the common bone marrow registries.

In contrast to the public UCB banks, private companies offer their service in processing and storage of UCB units for future use by the donor itself or a family member who hypothesize that they would be once affected by a disease that can be cured by HSC transplantation. The number of stored UCB units in private inventories is not published, but will most probably exceed the number stored in public UCB banks. However, the rate of transplantation of privately stored UCB units is extremely low. In the literature, only single cases are reported since the probability of ever suffering from a disease that requires HSC transplantation is estimated at 1:2,700 to 1:20,000 [40, 41]. In some cases, UCB units stored in private banks have been used for related allogeneic HSC transplantation, a service that is also offered by the public UCB banks. Here, the probability of HLA match is 25%. An autologous HSC transplantation with UCB from private UCB banks is hardly ever used. In this case, it has to be excluded that the defect leading to some hematopoietic diseases or leukemias is not already found in the UCB-derived stem cells [6]. The rate of relapse is known to be higher after an autologous UCB transplantation. Recent indications for an autologous UCB transplantation are solid tumors, lymphomas, and auto-immune diseases. Again, the probability for these conditions is extremely low. Since data on the quality of the UCB units stored in private companies are not available, it can only be speculated whether cell numbers are sufficient for use in adults. Although stem cells derived from UCB have a higher seeding and proliferative capacity than stem cells from adult sources, it would be possible to harvest autologous progenitors from peripheral blood or bone marrow of the patient if needed.

These facts lead to the major criticism of many scientific and public societies, such as American Academy of Pediatrics, American College of Obstetrics and Gynecology, Royal College of Obstetricians and Gynaecologists, French National Consultative Ethics Committee for Health and Life Sciences and European Union do not recommend private UCB banking in a low-risk population, because the cost-to-benefit ratio is very high [42, 43, 44, 45]. Private UCB banks charge their customers between $1000 and $1500 for UCB collection and $100 per year for storage. They market their service especially with promising data on stem cells used for regenerative purposes. If pregnant women, however, were asked, whether UCB stem cells have ever been successfully used for diseases, like Alzheimer's or Parkinson's disease, only a quarter of them knew correctly that it had not [46].

In summary, it needs to be discussed who should cover the costs of UCB stem cell collection for future use in regenerative medicine. Private UCB banks need to advertise correctly about the probabilities of ever needing an autologous UCB transplantation for both, current and future treatment options.

References

1. Gluckman E, Broxmeyer HE, Auerbach AD et al. (1989) Hematopoietic reconstitution in a patient with Fanconi's anemia by means of umbilical-cord blood from an HLA-identical sibling. N Engl J Med 321: 1174–1178.
2. Gluckman E, Rocha V (2004) Cord blood transplant: strategy of alternative donor search. Springer Seminars in Immunopathology 25: Epublication ahead of print. DOI: 10.1007/s00281-004-0157-3.
3. Barker JN, Davies SM, DeFor T et al. (2001) Survival after transplantation of unrelated donor umbilical cord blood is comparable to that of human leukocyte antigen-matched unrelated donor bone marrow: results of a matched-pair analysis. Blood 97: 2957–2961.
4. Locatelli F, Rocha V, Reed W et al. (2003) Related umbilical cord blood transplantation in patients with thalassemia and sickle cell disease. Blood 101: 2137–2143.
5. www.bmdw.org

6. Hayani A, Lampeter E, Viswanatha D et al. (2007) First report of autologous cord blood transplantation in the treatment of a child with leukaemia. Pediatrics 119: e296–e300.
7. Rubinstein P (2006) Why cord blood? Hum Immunol 67: 398–404.
8. Meyer-Monard S, Roosnek E, Troeger C et al. (2007) Public cord blood banks in Switzerland recruit rare and diverse HLA alleles. (Submitted to Bone Marrow Transplantation).
9. Broxmeyer H, Douglas G, Hangoc G et al. (1989) Human umbilical cord blood as a potential source of transplantable hematopoietic stem/progenitor cells. Proc Natl Acad Sci USA 86: 3828–3832.
10. Gluckman E, Rocha V, Boyer-Chammard A et al. (1997) Outcome of cord-blood transplantation from related and unrelated donors. N Engl J Med 337: 373–381
11. Lu L, Xiao M, Shen R-N et al. (1993) Enrichment, characterization, and responsiveness of single primitive CD34 human umbilical cord blood hematopoietic progenitors with high proliferative and replating potential. Blood 81: 41–48.
12. Rocha V, Wagner JE, Sobocinski KA et al. (2000) Graft-versus-host disease in children who have received a cord-blood or bone marrow transplant from an HLA-identical sibling. N Engl J Med 342: 1846–1854.
13. Yao Moinian M, Lind J (1969) Distribution of blood between infant and placenta after birth. Lancet 2 (7626): 871–873.
14. Surbek DV, Schönfeld B, Tichelli A, Gratwohl A, Holzgreve W (1998) Optimising umbilical cord blood mononuclear cell yield for hematopoietic stem cell transplantation. Bone Marrow Transplant 22: 311–312.
15. Laughlin MJ, Barker J, Bambach B et al. (2001) Hematopoietic engraftment and survival in adult recipients of umbilical-cord blood from unrelated donors. N Engl J Med 344: 1815–1822.
16. Sanz GF, Saavedra S, Planelles D et al. (2001) Standardized, unrelated donor cord blood transplantation in adults with hematologic malignancies. Blood 98: 2332–2338.
17. Almeida-Porada G, Porada CD et al. (2000) Cotransplantation of human stromal cell progenitors into preimmune fetal sheep results in early appearance of human donor cells in circulation and boosts cell levels in bone marrow at later time points after transplantation. Blood 95: 3620–3627.
18. Zou HY, Li Z, Deng ZH et al. (2004) Experimental study on quantitative monitoring engraftment of an adult with mixed umbilical cord blood transplantation. Zhongguo Shi Yan Xue Za Zhi 2: 179–184.
19. Kim D-W, Chung Y-J, Kim T-G et al. (2004) Cotransplantation of third-party mesenchymal stromal cells can alleviate single-donor predominance and increase engraftment from double cord transplantation. Blood 103: 1941–1948.
20. Knudtzon S (1974) In vitro growth of granulocytic colonies from circulating cells in human cord blood. Blood 43: 357–361.
21. Hao Q-L, Shah A, Thielmann F et al. (1995) A functional comparison of CD34+ CD38− cells in cord blood and bone marrow. Blood 86: 3745–3753.
22. Surbek DV, Holzgreve W, Jansen W et al. (1998) Quantitative immunophenotypic characterization, cryopreservation, and enrichment of second and third trimester human fetal cord blood hematopoietic stem cells (progenitor cells) Am J Obstet Gynecol 179: 1228–1233.
23. Wyrsch A, dalle Carbonare V, Jansen W et al. (1999) Umbilical cord blood from preterm human fetuses is rich in committed and primitive hematopoietic progenitors with high proliferative and self-renewal capacity. Exp Hematol 27: 1338–1345.
24. Ballen KK, Wilson M, Wuu J et al. (2001) Bigger is better: maternal and neonatal predictors of hematopoietic potential of umbilical cord blood units. Bone Marrow Transplant 27: 7–14.
25. Aufderhaar U, Holzgreve W, Danzer E et al. (2003) The impact of intrapartum factors on umbilical cord blood stem cell banking. J Perinat Med 31: 317–322.
26. Donaldson C, Armitage WJ, Laundry V et al. (1999) Impact of obstetric factors on cord blood donation for transplantation. Br J Hematol 106: 128–132.

27. Zandaro V, Solda G, Trevisanuto D (2006) Elective cesarean section and fetal immune-endocrine response. Int J Gynaecol Obstet 95: 52–53.
28. Manegold G, Meyer-Monard S, Tichelli A et al. (2007) Cesarean section due to fetal distress increases the number of stem cells in umbilical cord blood. Transfusion 48: 871–876.
29. Cairo MS, Wagner EL, Fraser J et al. (2005) Characterization of banked umbilical cord blood hematopoietic progenitor cells and lymphocyte subsets and correlation with ethnicity, birth weight, sex, and type of delivery: a cord blood transplantation (COLBT) study report. Transfusion 45: 856–866.
30. Aroviita P, Teramo K, Hiilesmaa V, Kekomaki R (2005) Cord blood hematopoietic progenitor cell concentration and infant sex. Transfusion 45: 613–621.
31. McCullough J, McKenna D, Kadidlo D et al. (2005) Issues in the quality of umbilical cord blood stem cells for transplantation. Transfusion 45: 832–841.
32. Jefferies LC, Albertus M, Morgan MA et al. (1999) High deferral rate form maternal-neonatal donor pairs for allogeneic umbilical cord blood bank. Transfusion 39: 415–419.
33. Vawter DE, Rogers-Chrysler G, Clay M et al. (2002) A phased consent policy for cord blood donation. Transfusion 42: 1268–1274.
34. Winter C, MacFarlane A, Deneux-Tharaux C et al. (2007) Variations in policies for management of third stage of labour and the immediate management of postpartum haemorrhage in Europe. BJOG 114: 845–854.
35. Troeger C, Meyer-Monard S, Tichelli A et al. (2007) Problems in umbilical cord blood collection. Transfus Med Hemother 34: 95–98.
36. McCullough J, Clay M (2000) Reasons for deferral of potential umbilical cord blood donors. Transfusion 40: 124–125.
37. Lapierre V, Pellegrini N, Bardey I et al. (2007) Cord blood volume reduction using an automated system (Sepax) vs. semi-automated system (Optipress II) and a manual method (hydroxyethyl starch sedimentation) for routine cord blood banking: a comparative study. Cytotherapy 9: 165–169.
38. Broxmeyer HE, Srour EF, Hangoc G et al. (2003) High-efficiency recovery of functional hematopoietic progenitor and stem cells from human cord blood cryopreserved for 15 years. PNAS 100: 645–650.
39. Sirchia G, Rebulla P, Tibaldi S et al. (1999) Cost of umbilical cord blood units released for transplantation. Transfusion 39: 645–650.
40. Ecker JL, Greene MF (2005) The case against private umbilical cord blood banking. Obstet Gynecol 105: 1282–1284.
41. Steinbroock R (2004) The cord-blood-bank controversies. NEJM 351: 2255–2257.
42. FIGO Committee for the Ethical Aspects of Human Reproduction and Women's Health (2006) Ethical guidelines regarding the procedure of collection of cord blood (Cairo, 1998). London, FIGO, pp. 67 (http://www.figo.org/docs/Ethics%20 Guidelines.pdf).
43. WMDA Policy Statement on the Utility of Autologous or Family Cord Blood Unit Storage (2006) The WMDA Board adopted this policy on 25th of May 2006. (http://www.worldmarrow.org/fileadmin/WorkingGroups_Subcommittees/DRWG/Cord_Blood˙Registries/WMDA_Policy_Statement_Final_02062006.pdf).
44. Rosell PP, Virt G (2004) Ethical aspects of umbilical cord blood banking: Opinion of the European Group on Ethics in Science and New Technologies to the European Commission. No. 19. (http://ec.europa.eu/european˙group˙ethics/docs/avis19˙en.pdf).
45. Royal College of Obstetricians and Gynaecologists (2006) Umbilical cord blood banking: Scientific Advisory Committee Opinion Paper 2. (http://www.rcog.org.uk/resources/Public/pdf/umbilical_cord_blood_banking_sac2a.pdf).
46. Fox NS, Stevens C, Ciubotariu R et al. (2007) Umbilical cord blood collection: do patients really understand? J Perinat Med 35: 314–321.

Section V
Potential Engineering Application of Cord Blood

Chapter 16
Possibilities of Using Cord Blood for Improving the Biocompatibility of Implants

K. Kaladhar and Chandra P. Sharma

Cord blood is a rich source of stem cells, growth factors and immune suppressing cytokines. We have reviewed its potential for enhancing material integration in the case of implants. We have reviewed the problems with the current degenerative therapy, future outlook and also the potential of using cord blood to mimic the biological way of, delivery of active molecules, immune suppression and tissue regeneration.

Introduction

Degenerative disease affecting different organs like kidney, liver, heart etc., often end up in loss of tissue or organ function. The current therapy of most of these diseases is by using medical devices or using tissue, from different sources for the partial recovery of their functions. These treatment methodologies are often assisted with drug therapy to improve the patency of the implants. The continuous monitoring and assisting drug therapy often seems to be costly and cumbersome. The synthetic medical devices reduce this problem to certain extent because of its improved durability as compared to its tissue counterparts. However, substitution of synthetic implants seems to be impossible at certain regions where correction is needed than replacement of the organs; for example, urinary bladder, heart tissue, etc.

The major problem associated with the medical devices inside the body is performance failure due to biological reactions, regulated by the adsorbed proteins and the pathological cells on the material surface. Usually the surface of the material is being modified to make the material biocompatible. Introducing specific surface groups, immobilizing proteins with certain conformations, or by immobilizing certain cell lines, often do this. Strategies have also been adopted to modify the material/biology interphase. Basically, this type of cell-mediated therapy is being done to improve the device integration by augmenting the tissue regeneration.

K. Kaladhar (✉)
Biosurface Technology Division, Biomedical Technology Wing, Sree Chitra Tirunal Institute for Medical Science and Technology, Poojappura, Thiruvananthapuram, 695 012, Kerala, India

N. Bhattacharya, P. Stubblefield (eds.), *Frontiers of Cord Blood Science*,
DOI 10.1007/978-1-84800-167-1_16,

For example, endothelialization of the vascular grafts to improve the blood compatibility [1]; utilizing platelet-rich plasma for improving the tissue regeneration in periodontitis [2]; etc.

However, the lessons from the organ morphgenesis, and wound healing suggests that specific chemokines are being sequentially released during the tissue regeneration. The tissue regeneration and wound healing are the important events after any tissue damage, whether it is due to trauma or implanting a medical device. Here, the difference is that when a medical implant is placed in the surgical wound the implant surface along with the adjuvant medication seems to regulate the normal wound healing process. Surface modification of the devices for improved biocompatibility by varying techniques both by mimicking the biology and by understanding the biological processes is in extensive research today. The cells are migrated from the neighboring environment for the wound healing. Alternative methods by making biofriendly surfaces with, endothelialization [1] and immobilization of the extracellular matrix (ECM) proteins [3], looks promising. However, immune rejection cannot be neglected in this case. Stem cells are an alternative choice for this problem, as human leukocyte antigen (HLA)-matched stem cells are less prone to immune rejection [4].

Cord blood is a rich source of growth factors, immunosuppressant chemokines, and stem cells. Here, we have reviewed the possibilities of using cord blood as a "cocktail" of stem cells, growth factors, and immunosuppressant cytokines for the integration of implant to the biological environment.

Degenerative Diseases and the Current Treatment Methodology

Many of the degenerative diseases affecting various vital organs leads to functional loss of that tissue or organ. In the case of organs that are performing mechanical functions like heart, blood vessels, bone, etc., artificial implants of synthetic origin is being used. However, in the case of organs that are performing synthesis of hormones, e.g., pancreas or partial loss of organ function like heart valve the synthetic implants seems inferior to allogenic or xenogenic tissue implants [5]. However, tissue engineering looks to be an alternative approach in all these cases. Table 16.1 gives the current strategy and future promises in the treatment of degenerative diseases affecting vital organs. The current tissue engineering strategies are either partial functional restoration as in the case of artificial pancreas or surface modification using endothelialization. Immune reaction to the xenogenic tissue seems to be an important problem in these cases. Despite these allogenic or immune protected in vitro cultured tissue grafts, attempts have also been made for tissue regeneration at the site of injury. This has been achieved with chimeric-morphoneogenesis with the help of porous scaffolds and bioactive molecules [6]. Here, the number of allogenic cells at the wound site is important for tissue regeneration, wound healing, and integration of the material into the body. This is to avoid the overgrowth of the other cells that may get migrated to the site.

Table 16.1 Different degenerative diseases and treatment methodologies (current and future perspectives)

Organ	Disease	Current treatment	Problems to be resolved	Future trends based on biomimicry	References
Blood vessel	Aneurysmal disease, abdominal aortic aneurysm, popliteal aneurysm, advanced artherosclerosis, traumatic injury	Surgical intervention and replacing the vascular grafts of both the biological and synthetic origin (e.g., cephanous vein and PTFE grafts)	Pseudointimal hyperplasia, early thrombosis	Tissue engineering of vascular grafts and endothelialization	[7, 8]
Heart valves	Symtomatic valvular heart disease	Surgical intervension and Mechanical devices and Prosthesis (both allogenic and synthetic vascular grafts)	Lesser half life for the tissue based vascular grafts as compared to the synthetic one	Tissue engineering of vascular tissue and grafts	[5, 9]
Liver	Hepatic encephalopathy	Total liver transplantation	Scarcity of the liver source	Liver assist device with liver tissue regeneration	[10, 11]
Kidney	Chronic renal failure	Kidney transplatation, Hemodialysis, Chronic ambulatory peritoneal dialysis	–	Tissue regeneration of the kidney tissues	[12, 13]
Pancreas	Diabetes mellitus	Drug therapy to increase the synthesis or utilization of the insulin or direct administration of insulin	“Tolerance” on prolonged drug therapy leads to the associated events in other organs like kidney or liver	Tissue regeneration of the islets of langehans of the pancreas	[14, 15]

Stem Cells – Cells with High Plasticity

Stem cells being totipotent and compatible with all the cell lineages could be used as an alternative strategy for this purpose. They have the capacity to self renew and give rise to differentiated progeny. These stem cells are present in virtually all parts of the human body such as liver, muscle, brain, blood, bone, and even in teeth. The introductory chapters have given a detailed introduction about the plasticity of stem cell plasticity; here, we are discussing about the potentialities relevant to in vivo tissue engineering required for the surface modification of biomaterials, with the help of cord blood.

The hematopoietic stem cells and the adult stem cells present in the stem cell niches of various tissue help in renewal and regeneration of the tissue under damage [16]. The specific signal molecules called growth and differentiation factors stimulate the differentiation of these stem cells, first to transit amplifying cells and then to terminally differentiated cell lineages. The stem cells can be switched to differentiate into various cell lineages and also could be trans-differentiated or dedifferentiate back, in an altered environment [17]. The plasticity to cross the different cell lineage boundaries invoked significant scientific attention, and invited research in understanding the molecular mechanism governing differentiation. This would possibly have therapeutic impact in future in the area of degenerative diseases. Cord blood is a rich source of stem cells is being extensively explored for bone marrow transplantation (BMT) [18]. Cord blood stem cells (CBSC), different from other stem cell sources like embryonic stem cells and bone marrow stem cell, have demonstrated rapid colony inducing ability [19] and less immune reaction.

However, the stem cells are to be differentiated to the corresponding cell lineages prior to its application. The teratoma formation due to undifferentiated stem cells has been identified [20]. Various growth and differentiation factors have been proposed to improve the proliferation as well as the differentiation of these stem cells.

Inductive Factors in Cell Proliferation and Differentiation – Biomimicry in Drug Delivery

Professor Hans spenman, one of the pioneers in developmental biology, who won the nobel prize in 1935, demonstrated that the inductive signals generated in embryonic tissue can regulate the differentiation in neighboring tissues. [21, 22]. This invited a lot of scientific interest in understanding the inductive stimuli and their role in governing the molecular mechanism of the morphogenesis. The present understanding is that the inductive chemical stimuli can be in the soluble form like growth factor, cytokines, etc. or in the insoluble form like the peptide sequences of the ECM proteins or adhesion proteins like fibronectin or vitreonectin. Both kinds of the inductive stimuli seem to do transmembrane signaling by binding to specific receptors. These receptors are G protein coupled will act on to different types of effector enzymes like adenylate cyclase, phosphodiesterase, and phospholipase C and through the secondary messengers like cAMP acts on to specific phosphatases and protein kinases. This will initiate the different cytoskeletal and nuclear cell activation processes leading to the different cellular effects including differentiation and proliferation [23].

There are evidences that the collaboration of the inductive stimuli (growth factor and matrix mediated) in cell proliferation [24].

In a wound the thrombus formed acts as a scaffold for the cells to migrate and grow, in addition to stopping the loss of blood. Here, the bioactive molecules are immediately delivered to the site by the platelets and from the damaged cells [25]. After the initial cleansing of the wound site by the neutrophils macrophages are invited to the site to remove the particulate matter and synthesis of growth factors. They further invite fibroblasts to synthesize the collagen, which form the basic structural unit of the ECM. All these cell–cell communications happens sequentially regulated by specific inductive signals (cytokines and growth factors) in normal wound healing and will be altered under infection or in the presence of a xenobiotic [26]. However, the combination as well as exact mechanism of action of these inductive signals is far from understood.

To simulate the biological mode of delivering these soluble active molecules, various techniques have been adopted at different fields for tissue culture. Co-culturing of two different cell lines has been proposed and is being successfully utilized in tissue engineering [27]. Otherwise this is the basic principle of using serum for tissue culture [28]. Combination of specialized differentiation factors and serum has been proposed for tissue engineering as well as stem cell differentiation [29]. This is an alternative successful approach for co-culture systems. Development of cocktails for specific tissue regeneration using this various bioactive molecules seems to have large market potential and invites a lot of research. For example, hematopoietic growth factors such as human recombinant erythropoietin, GM-CSF and G-CSF are commonly used in allogenic and autologous stem cell transplantation [30].

Cord blood is a rich source of this bioactive molecules and stem cells [31]. Apart from that under in vivo conditions they form the interface between the mother and the fetus, which also appears that it can possibly regulate the growth of neighboring cell lineages without inducing an immune reaction. However, its potential for generating a bioactive interface for implant is not being explored (Table 16.2).

Apart from this soluble inductive signals, the insoluble signals (i.e., the peptide sequences from the precipitated protein of the ECM) also have to be found to generate the transmembrane signal for the cell growth and differentiation (Table 16.3).

These soluble and the insoluble cues direct the cell migration and proliferation at the wound site. Evidences also suggest that there is a signal correlation inside the cell after receptor activation [63, 64]. As Prof. Vacanty foresees one of the next breakthrough, research will be circumventing the immune response of this tissue engineered materials [65], here is an example of tissue integration for specified duration regulated by humoral response. Attempts in this direction may help in reducing the immune rejection of implant material also.

Table 16.2 Family of growth and differentiation factors tried for stem cell differentiation

Growth factor	Tissue	References
Self-renewal of stem cells while suppressing differentiation		
Leukocyte inhibitory factor (LIF)	Suppresses differentiation by activating transcription of pluripotent gene Oct-4	[32, 33]
Differentiation factors		
Transforming growth factor â	Growth and proliferation	[34, 35]
Bone morphogenic protein (BMP)	BMP's is used for chondrogenic differentiation, and cartilage formation	[36, 37]
Fibroblast growth factor (FGF)	Growth and proliferation	[38, 39]
Hedghog, Notch, and WnT	Growth and proliferation	[16, 40]
Platelet-derived growth factor	Growth and proliferation	[41, 42]
Insulin-like growth factor	Growth and proliferation	[43, 44]
Epidermal growth factor	Growth and proliferation	[45, 46]

Table 16.3 Insoluble inductive signals from extra cellular matrix

Peptide sequences	Parent protein	References
RGD	Fibronectin, collagen, fibrinogen, laminin, vitronectin, Von Willebrands factor, entactin, tenascin, thrombospondin	[47, 48]
YIGSR	Laminin	[49, 50]
IKVAV	Laminin	[51, 52]
LRE	Laminin	[53, 54]
REDV	Fibronectin	[55, 56]
DGEA	Collagen	[57, 58]
GXG	Thrombospondin	[59, 60]
VGVAPG	Elastin	[61, 62]

Immune Reaction to the Implant – A Lesson from Fetal Survival

The fertilized egg (embryos) seeks nutrients from mother by forming contact through the placenta. The reason for tolerance of the embryos by the maternal immune system despite the presence of paternal MHC histocompatibility antigens has invited a lot of research. The local immune response at the site of contact is suppressed by the anti immune cytokines produced locally at the site of contact.

There is also clear evidence that the maternal immune system during pregnancy can enhance or inhibit the development of fetoplacental unit. Recent data support that some cytokines produced by both T cells and non-T cells (IL-3, GM-CSF, TGF-â, IL-4, and IL-10) favor fetal survival and growth. In contrast, other cytokines, such as IFN-ã, TNF-â, and TNF-á, can rather compromise pregnancy. They have classified the human lymphocyte CD4+ T-helper cells into two classes – T helper 1 (Th1) and T helper 2 (Th2) – based upon these cytokine secretion profiles. The Th1 cells produces IFN-ã and TNF-â, whereas the second type, Th2 cells produces IL-4 and IL-5, and a third type (Th0) is also observed, that produce both Th1 and Th2 cytokines. They concluded that the cytokine network maintaining the fetal survival mainly belongs to the Th2 pathway, whereas the failure of pregnancy is associated with the dominance by Th1-type cytokines. In vitro studies suggest that progesterone enhances the preferential development of Th2-like cells and enhances transient IL-4 production [66], while relaxin another corpous-luteum-derived hormone mainly promotes the development of Th1-like cells [67]. Further during the development of the umbilical cord this principle is maintained and the cord blood contains more Th2 cytokines rather than the proimmune cytokines. At situations like urinary infection and associated abortion of the fetus the shift in paradigm of increased production of Th1 cytokines have been observed. This clearly demonstrates the endocrine immune relationship in maintaining the pregnancy.

Here is an equivalent situation when an implant, whether tissue or artificial implant, is placed in a wound (implant site). When the body identifies the implant as a xenobiotic, it first try to destroy the implant, if not possible isolate with the help of a fibrous capsule. If the inflammatory reaction persists due to variety of reasons like leachables, abration of the implant, infection at the implant site etc., lead to the immune response against the implant. This can be type I–IV depending upon the solubility, size, and surface chemistry of the xenobiotic formed from the implant. Most of the materials using for developing the implants are tested for each class of immune reaction preclinically, and qualifies for the implantation [68]. However, taking care of the difference in pathogenesis of various microorganisms, between the animals (using for preclinical studies) and human, certain clinical evaluation protocols are also to be followed to avoid any hyper sensitivity cascades during implantation [69]. Both the humoral immunity due to the formation of antibodies against the soluble leachables and cell-mediated immune reactions against the particulate material due affect the biomaterials. In that, the cell-mediated immunity due to the surface identification of the biomaterials invites chronic inflammatory responses which will complementarily activate the humoral immune system and further decides the fate of implant. The nature of the lymphocytes at the implant site and their cytokine responses regulate the cell–cell signaling during chronic inflammatory response. Here also the Th1 cell response is higher lead to excessive secretion of the IL-1, IFN-ã, TNF-â, and TNF-á at the implant site [70, 71]. These lymphokines are proinflammatory in nature, as said earlier.

The comparison between the fetus and the implant illustrate, the implant exposes to a big area, and so more amount of proinflammatory agents are released, and with time the environment at the implant site decides, the paradigm shifts toward tissue integration or immune rejection. The lymphocytes at the implant site through different cytokine profiles regulate the "paradigm shift," which is similar to the maintenance of fetomaternal system. Different from the fetus, in the case of implant, if it is not identified as a xenobiotic they tend to integrate with the tissue, otherwise it will be isolated with a fibrous capsule. In this case, the long-term chronic inflammatory responses may lead to performance failure of the implant. The current developments are toward integrating the implant to the body [72]. Various surface modification techniques have been adopted to look the surface more natural. However, least attempts have been made to manipulate the interphase. Few of the current techniques include endothelialization, coating the surface with adhesive proteins or peptides etc., are attempts in that direction. Again here the possibilities of immune rejection cannot be totally neglected. As the restoration of complete homeostasis is required for proper integration of the implant, it needs not to be two-way like in the case of fetus, but it should be able to form full circuit with the circulatory system. Porous matrix approach compounded by proper engineering principles to relax the applied stress, found to be the most promising approach toward achieving this goal in all the fields, right from vascular grafts to hip replacement. The tissue integration is regained in these porous structures, but at a slow pace.

The ability of the cord blood to reduce the immune reaction selects it as a good candidate for modifying the interface. The higher concentration of the Th2 cytokines may be the reason for the reduced activation of cord blood lymphocytes [73]. This is observed as a reduced immune response in BMT using CBSC [74]. This inefficiency could be used for modifying the interfacial immune reactions at an implant site, provided all the precautions are taken care off, as in BMT [75]. The tolerogenic potential of the cord blood could be further improved by redirecting the cytokine profile with the help of specific bioactive signals., e.g., macrophage colony stimulating factor (CSF) [76]. This is because cord blood contains every primary requirement like growth factors, stem cells, and immune suppressing chemokines for tissue regeneration.

Conclusion

We have reviewed the possibilities of using cord blood as a "cocktail" for modifying the interface of material–biology interaction for the fast integration of the implants with the neighboring tissue. There is interesting correlation in immune profiles of fetomaternal system and implant in host environment. The role of Th2 cytokines in regulating the maintenance of fetomaternal system could be mimicked using cord blood for implant integration. The tissue integration should sufficiently supported with sufficient blood vessels at the implant site (with proper homeostasis), as in the fetomaternal system to avoid any necrosis and chronic inflammation. The growth factors present in the cord blood could be able to sufficiently enhance the angiogenesis at the implant site along with growth and integration of the neighboring tissue. The stem cells can be differentiated to any cell lineages according to the inductive stimuli at the implant site once the tissue regeneration is induced. The current strategy of implant-tissue integration in biomaterials is by utilizing the acute inflammatory reactions favorable, by modifying the surface properties of the implant. However, using cord blood, the implant site could be introduced to a new environment of cocktail containing growth hormones, anti-immune cytokines, and stem cells for fast and effective regeneration and integration of the implant with the tissue.

References

1. Pawlowski KJ, Rittgers SE, Schmidt SP, Bowlin GL. Endothelial cell seeding of polymeric vascular grafts. Front Biosci. 2004;9:1412–21.
2. Grageda E. Platelet-rich plasma and bone graft materials: a review and a standardized research protocol. Implant Dent. 2004;13:301–9.

3. Lutolf MP, Hubbell JA. Synthetic biomaterials as instructive extracellular microenvironments for morphogenesis in tissue engineering. Nat Biotechnol. 2005;23:47–55.
4. Elsner HA, Blasczyk R. Immunogenetics of HLA null alleles: implications for blood stem cell transplantation. Tissue Antigens. 2004;64:687–95.
5. Love WJ. Cardiac prosthesis. In: *Principles of Tissue Engineering* ed. Lanza RP, Langar R, Chick WL. Academic Press, San Diego, CA, USA 1997;365–80.
6. Langer R, Vacanti JP. Tissue engineering. Science. 1993;260:920–6.
7. Kakisis JD, Liapis CD, Breuer C, Sumpio BE. Artificial blood vessel: the Holy Grail of peripheral vascular surgery. J Vasc Surg. 2005;41:349–54.
8. Daly CD, Campbell GR, Walker PJ, Campbell JH. In vivo engineering of blood vessels. Front Biosci. 2004;9:1915–24.
9. Hopkins RA. Tissue engineering of heart valves: decellularized valve scaffolds. Circulation. 2005;111:2712–4.
10. Vacanti JP, Langer R. Tissue engineering: the design and fabrication of living replacement devices for surgical reconstruction and transplantation. Lancet. 1999;354 (Suppl. 1): SI32–4.
11. Chan C, Berthiaume F, Nath BD, Tilles AW, Toner M, Yarmush ML. Hepatic tissue engineering for adjunct and temporary liver support: critical technologies. Liver Transpl. 2004;10:1331–42.
12. Mooney DJ, Kim BS, Vacanty JP, Langer R, Atula A. An overview of the pathology and approaches to tissue engineering. In Principles of Tissue Engineering, Eby Lanza RP, Langar R, Chick WL. Academic Press, San Diego, CA, USA 1997;591–600.
13. Tiranathanagul K, Eiam-Ong S, Humes HD. The future of renal support: high-flux dialysis to bioartificial kidneys. Crit Care Clin. 2005;21:379–94.
14. Lanza RP, Chick WT. Endocrinology: pancreas. In Principles of Tissue Engineering, Eby Lanza RP, Langar R, Chick WL. Academic Press, San Diego, CA, USA 1997;405–25.
15. Miyamoto M. Current progress and perspectives in cell therapy for diabetes mellitus. Hum Cell. 2001;14:293–300.
16. Tsai RY, Kittappa R, McKay RD. Plasticity, niches, and the use of stem cells. Dev Cell. 2002;2:707–12.
17. Odelberg SJ. Inducing cellular dedifferentiation: a potential method for enhancing endogenous regeneration in mammals. Semin Cell Dev Biol. 2002;13:335–43.
18. Cohen Y, Nagler A. Umbilical cord blood transplantation – how, when and for whom? Blood Rev. 2004;18:167–79.
19. Broxmeyer, HE. Stem and progenitor cells isolated from cord blood. In Hand Book of Stem Cells, Lanza R, Weissman I, Thomson J, Pedersen R, Hogan B, Gearhart J, Blau H, Melton D, Moore M, Verfaillie C, Thomas ED, West M. Volume 2. Academic press. 2004, Elsevier, pp. 760–99.
20. Heng BC, Cao T, Lee EH. Directing stem cell differentiation into the chondrogenic lineage in vitro. Stem Cells. 2004;22:1152–67.
21. Gilbert SF. Developmental Biology, 6th edition. Sinauer Associates, Sunderland, MA, 2000.
22. West LJ. Wound healing. In Frontiers in Tissue Engineering, Eby Patrick CW, Mikos AG Jr, McIntire L. Pergamon Press, New York, 1998.
23. Miyamoto S, Katz B-Z, Latrenie R, Yamada KM. Fibronectin and integrin in cell adhesion, signaling, and morphogenesis, in morphogenesis: cellular interations. Ann N Y Acad Sci. 1998;857:143–154.
24. Mcnamee HP, Ingber DE, Shwartz MA. Adhesion to fibronectin stimulates inositol lipid synthesis and enhances PDGE – induced inositol lipid breakdown. J Cell Biol. 1993 May; 121(3):673–678.
25. Tozum TF, Demiralp B. Platelet-rich plasma: a promising innovation in dentistry. J Can Dent Assoc. 2003;69:664.
26. Denel TF. Polypeptide growth factors: role in normal and abnormal cell growth. Annu Rev Cell Biol. 1987;3:443–492.

27. Vacanti JP, Vacanti CA. The challenges of tissue engineering. In Principles of Tissue engineering, Eby Lanza RP, Langar R, Chick WL. Academic Press, San Diego, CA, USA 1997; 344–86.
28. Ang LP, Tan DT, Seah CJ, Beuerman RW. The use of human serum in supporting the in vitro and in vivo proliferation of human conjunctival epithelial cells. Br J Ophthalmol. 2005;89:748–52.
29. Heath JK, Smith AG. Regulatory factors of embryonic stem cells. J Cell Sci Suppl. 1988;10:257–66.
30. Jansen J, Hanks S, Thompson JM, Dugan MJ, Akard LP. Transplantation of hematopoietic stem cells from the peripheral blood. J Cell Mol Med. 2005;9:37–50.
31. Almici C, Carlo-Stella C, Wagner JE, Rizzoli V. Umbilical cord blood as a source of hematopoietic stem cells: from research to clinical application. Haematologica. 1995;80:473–9.
32. Chambers I, Smith A. Self-renewal of teratocarcinoma and embryonic stem cells. Oncogene. 2004;23:7150–60.
33. Zandstra PW, Le HV, Daley GQ, Griffith LG, Lauffenburger DA. Leukemia inhibitory factor (LIF) concentration modulates embryonic stem cell self-renewal and differentiation independently of proliferation. Biotechnol Bioeng. 2000;69:607–17.
34. Chang H, Brown CW, Matzuk MM. Genetic analysis of the mammalian transforming growth factor-beta superfamily. Endocr Rev. 2002;23:787–823.
35. Chen Y, Lebrun JJ, Vale W. Regulation of transforming growth factor beta- and activin-induced transcription by mammalian Mad proteins. Proc Natl Acad Sci USA 1996;93:12992–7.
36. Nieden Z. Embryonic Stem Cell Therapy for osteodegenerative diseases. Biotech Int. 2005;17:2.
37. Chen D, Zhao M, Harris SE, Mi Z. Signal transduction and biological functions of bone morphogenetic proteins. Front Biosci. 2004;9:349–58.
38. Kashiwakura I, Takahashi TA. Fibroblast growth factor and ex vivo expansion of hematopoietic progenitor cells. Leuk Lymphoma. 2005;46:329–33.
39. Moroni E, Dell'Era P, Rusnati M, Presta M. Fibroblast growth factors and their receptors in hematopoiesis and hematological tumors. J Hematother Stem Cell Res. 2002;11:19–32.
40. Watt FM. Unexpected Hedgehog-Wnt interactions in epithelial differentiation. Trends Mol Med. 2004;10:577–80.
41. Lee SJ. Cytokine delivery and tissue engineering. Yonsei Med J. 2000;41:704–19.
42. Giannobile WV. Periodontal tissue engineering by growth factors. Bone. 1996;19 (Suppl. 1):23S–37S.
43. Yakar S, Pennisi P, Wu Y, Zhao H, LeRoith D. Clinical relevance of systemic and local IGF-I. Endocr Dev. 2005;9:11–6.
44. Cheng CL, Gao TQ, Wang Z, Li DD. Role of insulin/insulin-like growth factor 1 signaling pathway in longevity. World J Gastroenterol. 2005;11:1891–5.
45. Hayashi M, Tomita M, Yoshizato K. Production of EGF-collagen chimeric protein which shows the mitogenic activity. Biochim Biophys Acta. 2001;1528:187–95.
46. Kanematsu A, Yamamoto S, Ozeki M, Noguchi T, Kanatani I, Ogawa O, Tabata Y. Collagenous matrices as release carriers of exogenous growth factors. Biomaterials. 2004;25: 4513–20.
47. Takagi J. Structural basis for ligand recognition by RGD (Arg-Gly-Asp)-dependent integrins. Biochem Soc Trans. 2004;32(Pt3):403–6.
48. Meinhart JG, Schense JC, Schima H, Gorlitzer M, Hubbell JA, Deutsch M, Zilla P. Enhanced endothelial cell retention on shear-stressed synthetic vascular grafts precoated with RGD-cross-linked fibrin. Tissue Eng. 2005;11:887–95.
49. Itoh S, Matsuda A, Kobayashi H, Ichinose S, Shinomiya K, Tanaka J. Effects of a laminin peptide (YIGSR) immobilized on crab-tendon chitosan tubes on nerve regeneration. J Biomed Mater Res B Appl Biomater. 2005;73:375–82.
50. Genove E, Shen C, Zhang S, Semino CE. The effect of functionalized self-assembling peptide scaffolds on human aortic endothelial cell function. Biomaterials. 2005;26:3341–51.

51. Matsuda A, Kobayashi H, Itoh S, Kataoka K, Tanaka J. Immobilization of laminin peptide in molecularly aligned chitosan by covalent bonding. Biomaterials. 2005;26:2273–9.
52. Adams DN, Kao EY, Hypolite CL, Distefano MD, Hu WS, Letourneau PC. Growth cones turn and migrate up an immobilized gradient of the laminin IKVAV peptide. J Neurobiol. 2005;62:134–47.
53. Hunter DD, Cashman N, Morris-Valero R, Bulock JW, Adams SP, Sanes JR. An LRE (leucine-arginine-glutamate)-dependent mechanism for adhesion of neurons to S-laminin. J Neurosci. 1991;11:3960–71.
54. Hunter DD, Porter BE, Bulock JW, Adams SP, Merlie JP, Sanes JR. Primary sequence of a motor neuron-selective adhesive site in the synaptic basal lamina protein S-laminin. Cell. 1989;59:905–13.
55. Girotti A, Reguera J, Rodriguez-Cabello JC, Arias FJ, Alonso M, Matestera A. Design and bioproduction of a recombinant multi(bio)functional elastin-like protein polymer containing cell adhesion sequences for tissue engineering purposes. J Mater Sci Mater Med. 2004;15:479–84.
56. Sasabe T, Suwa Y, Kiritoshi A, Doi M, Yuasa T, Kishida K. Differential effects of fibronectin-derived oligopeptides on the attachment of rabbit lens epithelial cells in vitro. Ophthalmic Res. 1996;28:201–8.
57. Mizuno M, Fujisawa R, Kuboki Y. Type I collagen-induced osteoblastic differentiation of bone-marrow cells mediated by collagen-alpha2beta1 integrin interaction. J Cell Physiol. 2000;184:207–13.
58. Luzak B, Golanski J, Rozalski M, Boncler and MA, Watala C. Inhibition of collagen-induced platelet reactivity by DGEA peptide. Acta Biochim Pol. 2003;50:1119–28.
59. Maeda T, Oyama R, Titani K, Sekiguchi K. Engineering of artificial cell-adhesive proteins by grafting EILDVPST sequence derived from fibronectin. Biochem (Tokyo). 1993;113: 29–35.
60. Komoriya A, Green LJ, Mervic M, Yamada SS, Yamada KM, Humphries MJ. The minimal essential sequence for a major cell type-specific adhesion site (CS1) within the alternatively spliced type III connecting segment domain of fibronectin is leucine-aspartic acid-valine. J Biol Chem. 1991;266:15075–9.
61. Floquet N, Hery-Huynh S, Dauchez M, Derreumaux P, Tamburro AM, Alix AJ. Structural characterization of VGVAPG, an elastin-derived peptide. Biopolymers. 2004;76:266–80.
62. Senior RM, Griffin GL, Mecham RP, Wrenn DS, Prasad KU, Urry DW. Val-Gly-Val-Ala-Pro-Gly, a repeating peptide in elastin, is chemotactic for fibroblasts and monocytes. J Cell Biol. 1984;99:870–4.
63. Dedhar S, Williams B, Hannigan G. Integrin-linked kinase (ILK): a regulator of integrin and growth-factor signalling. Trends Cell Biol. 1999;9:319–23.
64. Takahashi MO, Takahashi Y, Iida K, Okimura Y, Kaji H, Abe H, Chihara K. Growth hormone stimulates tyrosine phosphorylation of focal adhesion kinase (p125(FAK)) and actin stress fiber formation in human osteoblast-like cells, Saos2. Biochem Biophys Res Commun. 1999;263:100–6.
65. Mikos AG, McIntire LV, Anderson JM, Babensee JE. Host response to tissue engineered devices. Adv Drug Deliv Rev. 1998;33:111–39.
66. Joachim R, Zenclussen AC, Polgar B, Douglas AJ, Fest S, Knackstedt M, Klapp BF, Arck PC. The progesterone derivative dydrogesterone abrogates murine stress-triggered abortion by inducing a Th2 biased local immune response. Steroids. 2003;68:931–40.
67. Piccinni MP, Bani D, Beloni L, Manuelli C, Mavilia C, Vocioni F, Bigazzi M, Sacchi TB, Romagnani S, Maggi E. Relaxin favors the development of activated human T cells into Th1-like effectors. Eur J Immunol. 1999;29:2241–7.
68. Park JC, Lee DH, Suh H. Preclinical evaluation of prototype products. Yonsei Med J. 1999;40:530–5.
69. Leuschner J, Rimpler M. Preclinical safety testing of plastic products intended for use in man. Biomed Tech (Berl). 1990;35:44–7.

70. Mohanty M. Cellular basis for failure of joint prosthesis. Biomed Mater Eng. 1996;6:165–72.
71. Shanbhag AS, Jacobs JJ, Black J, Galante JO, Glant TT. Cellular mediators secreted by interfacial membranes obtained at revision total hip arthroplasty. J Arthroplasty. 1995;10: 498–506.
72. Meffert RM. Do implant surfaces make a difference? Curr Opin Periodontol. 1997;4:104–8.
73. Cohen SB, Perez-Cruz I, Fallen P, Gluckman E, Madrigal JA. Analysis of the cytokine production by cord and adult blood. Hum Immunol. 1999;60:331–6.
74. Nomura A, Takada H, Jin CH, Tanaka T, Ohga S, Hara T. Functional analyses of cord blood natural killer cells and T cells: a distinctive interleukin-18 response. Exp Hematol. 2001;29:1169–76.
75. Rocha V, Sanz G, Gluckman E. Eurocord and European Blood and Marrow Transplant Group. Umbilical cord blood transplantation. Curr Opin Hematol. 2004;11:375–85.
76. Li G, Kim YJ, Broxmeyer HE. Macrophage colony-stimulating factor drives cord blood monocyte differentiation into IL-10(high)IL-12absent dendritic cells with tolerogenic potential. J Immunol. 2005;174:4706–17.

Chapter 17
Potential of Stem Cell to Tailor the Bone-Ceramic Interface for Better Fixation of Orthopedic Implants

Jui Chakraborty and Debabrata Basu

The main cause of premature failure of an orthopedic implant in vivo is due to various biological reactions with the surrounding tissues/environment. Therefore, to combat this situation, continuous efforts have been concentrated to improve biocompatibility of the implant material by adopting different strategies. Extensive study is being made to modify the implants by plasma-spraying bioactive materials, introducing specific surface groups, immobilizing proteins with certain conformations, or by immobilizing certain cell lines. In addition, investigations are in progress to modify the implant/biology interface and study its influence on long-term stability of the material to improve the integration by augmenting the tissue regeneration. Such modification of the devices for enhanced biocompatibility following varying techniques is a subject of extensive research today. In last few decades, though the innovative use of long-lasting bioceramic-based implants have revolutionized the treatment procedure, it is strongly felt that the implant integration/fixation with the surrounding tissue improvement can be obtained by developing a more biofriendly interface through reconstructive surgery. Thus, the implant integration with the damaged/diseased tissue needs a biofriendly interface. For this purpose, bioactive ceramics in the form of scaffold, powder, or granule is used more extensively to fill the space of the damaged hard tissue or bioactive coating plasma sprayed on the surface of the implant cement-less fixation. Recently, for reconstruction surgery, ceramic scaffolds are manufactured from the computer tomography (CT) scan data of the patient by adopting rapid prototyping method that, however, needs to be stably fixed to the operation site, although this may not be applicable in case of load-bearing implants. Human leukocyte antigen (HLA)-matched stem cells, which are less prone to immune rejection and capable of self-renewal and has compatibility to all cell lineages, are being considered to be an effective alternative to address this problem in future.

With growing age, the hard tissues in our systems that are natural living composites of calcium phosphate-based ceramics and collagen are especially vulnerable to fracture as the osteoblasts (bone-growing cells) become less productive and lead

---

J. Chakraborty (✉)
Bio-ceramics and Coating Division, Central Glass and Ceramic Research Institute, 196, Raja S.C. Mullick Road, Kolkatta 700032, India

N. Bhattacharya, P. Stubblefield (eds.), *Frontiers of Cord Blood Science*,
DOI 10.1007/978-1-84800-167-1_17, © Springer-Verlag London Limited 2009

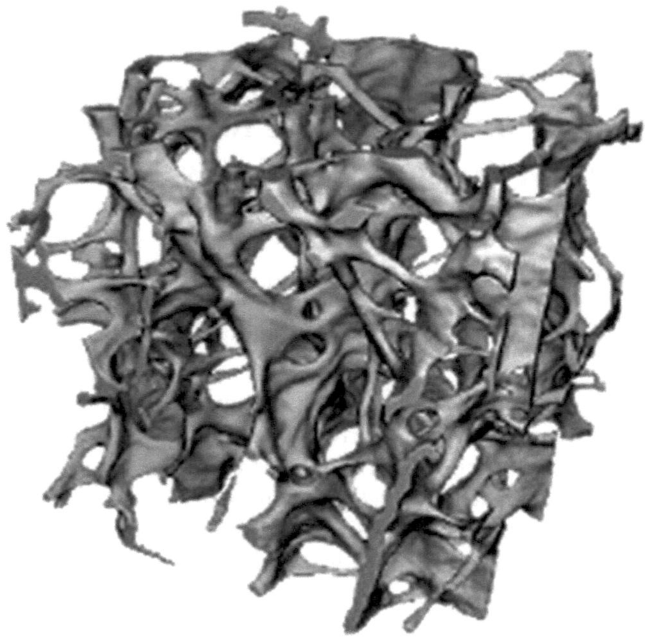

Fig. 17.1 A 5.5 mm cube of trabecular bone taken from a human lumbar vertebrae that has a volume fraction of approximately 7%

to reduction of bone density and strength [1]. In this stage, the strength of trabecular/cancellous bones of vertebrae is greatly deteriorated, which are even otherwise very porous and fragile (Fig. 17.1). This leads to fracture of the hip, knee joints, collapse, and compression fracture of vertebrae/spine, which need to be repaired immediately to restore the normal function of the limb. To address the need for intervention in these cases, implants/scaffolds of different materials are currently in use, which include natural autografts (tissue harvested from the same patient), allografts (tissue harvested from a similar species) as well as a variety of biomaterials based on ceramics, metals, polymers, and a host of composites. The use of allografts is limited by the possibility of an immunological response and risk of disease transmission, whereas autografts are restricted by a limited number of donor sites and are associated with an additional trauma resulting from the collection of the bone tissue. In this scenario, manmade materials stand out as potential solution, being easily available, processed, and modified to suit the needs of a given application, although many problems persist as a result of the inability to match exactly to the natural tissue [2]. Also, high chemical inertness, absence of adverse effects on the surrounding tissue, long-term life expectancy, and fatigue strength are some other criteria, summarized under the term 'biocompatibility', which need to be studied in detail prior to inserting these materials into the living system. The clinical success of bioceramics (a specially designed ceramics for reconstruction of diseased/damaged parts of the body, e.g., hips, knees, wrists, spines, jaws, long-bones as well as maxillofacial periodontal diseases) in these application areas triggered extensive activities to develop suitable stable interface with connective tissue and a match of mechanical behavior of the implant with the tissues to be replaced. In this regard, various techniques have been attempted using bioactive glass/ceramic coating on inert metal/ceramic implant surfaces to tailor the hard tissue–implant interface for their cement-less fixation at the damaged tissue site. Preliminary research results indicate that the development of bioactive hydroxyapatite (microporous) coating on the metal implant surface renders fast osseointegration kinetics and enhances the strength of the interface, although it is still far from ideal. So far, these bioceramic coatings on porous metal surfaces for fixation of orthopedic prostheses in the osseous surrounding achieved by various means [3, 4, 5] have become popular, of which plasma-sprayed ones are generally preferred [6]. Another emerging technique, called biomimetic coating, is being explored extensively at present by various research groups [7, 8, 9, 10]. Since, apparently, replacement of a damaged organ by transplantation of tissues is hindered by many factors, such as immune rejection, limited supply, and morbidity of the donor site, the limitations of these techniques (either using artificial implants or transplantation of living tissues) in restoration of the function of a damaged organ/tissue in vivo triggered a new area to be explored with an innovative insight. Here, the general principle of tissue engineering offers a promising solution. A potential idea involves the combination of living cells with natural or synthetic support (scaffold) to produce a three-dimensional analog of the damaged organ. There are a number of different sources of living cells that can be used for tissue repair and regeneration, but not all are suited to serve the purpose. The mature cells isolated from tissue biopsies can effectively be used for re-implantation into the same donor, although they suffer from few intrinsic limitations. For them, the generation of sufficient number of cells for complete tissue repair is not possible, and they are already committed to a particular cell lineage, which is restricted to the type of tissue from which they are harvested. Hence, there lies the demand for 'immature' or 'undifferentiated' cells – the stem cells that can overcome the drawbacks of living cells harvested from various sources.

Scope of Bioceramics as Implant Materials

With rapid economic globalization, people are compelled to adopt a faster life style, which in turn increases the number of accidents and trauma in an alarming rate. In addition, the increasing rate of average life expectancy has significantly increased the need for replacement of old/damaged bones. The success of bioceramics in hard tissue replacement primarily depends on the fact that our natural bone is a supportive living tissue composed of a carbonate containing calcium apatite ($\sim$60 wt%) in type I collagen ($\sim$30 wt%) matrix. It also contains $\sim$10 wt% water. The mineral component of bone is a form of calcium phosphate/calcium apatite known as hydroxyapatite (HAp). Stoichiometric HAp has a molecular formula $Ca_{10}(PO_4)_6(OH)_2$, whereas the bone mineral contains many substitutions like magnesium, sodium, potassium, fluoride, chloride, and carbonate ions This apatitic mineral is closely

Table 17.1 Classification of bioceramics

S. No.	Type of bio-ceramics	Mechanism of attachment	Type of attachment	Example
A	Bioinert	Bone growth occurs into the surface irregularities by cementing/press-fitting into a defect	Morphological fixation	Al_2O_3/ZrO_2
B	Bioactive	Attach directly by chemical bonding at the surface	Bioactive fixation	Bioactive glasses/glass-ceramics/dense HAp
C	Resorbable	Slowly replaced by bone	–	Calcium sulphate, tricalcium phosphate, some bioactive glasses

associated with collagen fibers (highly aligned, anisotropic structure) to yield flat, plate-like nanocrystals ($40 \times 10\,nm^2$). The organic matrix renders the tensile strength whereas the mineral component gives rise to compressive strength of the bone. Cross-sectionally dissected view of a bone exhibits two types of tissues – the dense cortical outer layer that has ~90% solid bone tissue, and the softer inner layer of trabecular bone that is spongy and contains 80% marrow filled with voids. Bone is a dynamic tissue subject to constant deposition by osteoblast activity and subsequent resorption by osteoclasts. When a new surface is introduced into the bone tissue, a sequence of complex interactions is triggered [11]. Based on the host tissue response that varies with the bulk/surface properties of the particular prostheses when implanted in vivo, the bioceramic implant/prostheses materials are classified as shown in Table 17.1.

In addition, in some cases, if the bioinert/bioactive bioceramic is porous, bone in-growth may occur, which mechanically attaches the bone to the material. This type of attachment may be termed as *biological fixation* at the site of the damaged tissue.

Bioinert Ceramics

At present, every year, globally, about 600,000 of hip replacement surgeries take place, while in India alone the number is around 50,000. Women of 55–60-year age group, who after menopause usually suffer from severe osteoporosis that ultimately results in the breakage of neck femur bone, specifically need these prostheses to serve for more than 25 years of their life span. Conventional hip joints made out of stainless steel/Co–Cr alloy/Ti–6Al–4 V alloy last only for 10–15 years, and therefore need to be replaced several times, which involves risk and enormous

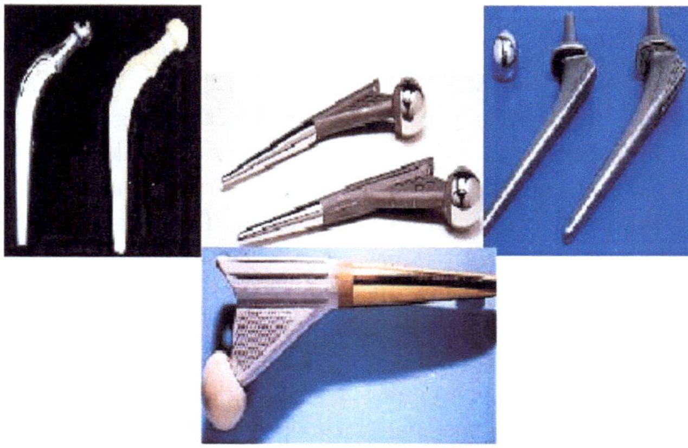

Fig. 17.2 Stem and acetabular cup of hip implants: Charnley's, Freeman's Cobalt Chrome, Johnson & Johnson's Titanium and Hybrid implant

expenditure. For this purpose, mainly with an expectation to provide longer trouble-free life, bioinert ceramics are replacing metals, particularly for femoral head applications; at present, globally, about 10% of the femoral components of total hip joints are made out of ceramics. Two of the three components of these joints, i.e., the stem and the acetabular cup (Fig. 17.2), need to be fixed with the surrounding bony tissue, and for this purpose, poly(methyl methacrylate (PMMA)-based bone cement is generally used. The major long-term problem with cemented hip replacement is the loosening of the bond between the implant and the bone, which often needs a second surgery to fix it once again. This has led to the development of cement-less hip-replacement in which the surface of the metal part is porous. The most remarkable evolution has been in the area of porous coating along the stem and number of porous layers. Initially, it was a full-length coating with two to three layers, while the current trend is to give a single-layer coating towards proximal end. Only a few years ago, bone in-growth fixation was considered to be most desirable, while currently more importance is given to tissue stabilization at the interface. Judging from the multiple interrelated factors of fixation and durability, it is believed that the ideal prosthesis would have a tight fitting that stabilizes itself and achieves equilibrium. Since fibrous interposition is an inevitable biological consequence under dynamic load against implant material, the crucial issue is how one can make the fibrous tissue remain stable, thin, and inactive. The absence of macro-motion of the implant is expected to play a vital role. Thus, if the design of the implant follows the anatomic shape and size of recipient bone, the interference fit is possible to result in a pain-free joint, which would serve for a long time. These materials are potential candidates for development of other articulating surfaces of many joints, such as knee, shoulder, elbow, wrist, etc., although, for their maximum utilization, a more efficient fixation system need to be developed. Other clinical applications of this class of ceramics include dental implants, bone screws, alveolar ridge and maxillofacial reconstruction, ossicular bone substitution, keratoprostheses, segmental bone replacements, etc. All these are due to a combination of a range of structural properties – corrosion resistance, biocompatibility, wear resistance, low friction, and high strength [3, 12, 13]. Medical grade bioinert ceramics offer two main advantages over other materials, e.g., metals/polymers – (1) low wear rates generate much lower concentration of wear debris in the surrounding tissue, and (2) high corrosion resistance (rate of corrosion 10^{-4} g cm^{-2}/day corresponding to a maximum corrosion rate of 1 mm in 10 years) ensures trouble-free service.

Superior tribological properties of high-density, small-grain-size ceramics (<4 μm, having a very narrow size distribution) (Fig. 17.3) result in exceptionally low coefficient of friction and minimal wear rates [3, 14], and this has established the credential of the material as the articulating surface in different load-bearing joints. Extensive characterization of the material to predict its suitability for long-time usage under typical biological conditions points out that it offers excellent resistance to dynamic/impact fatigue and to sub-critical crack growth [14, 15]. Detailed gate analysis of the human hip has pointed out [16] that, when walking, the maximum load encountered by the hip of a 100-kg weighing person is about 4.3 kN (Fig. 17.4a). To assess the trouble-free service life of these prostheses, the ceramic-based hip joint balls were exposed to 10^8 walking cycles (which is equivalent to 20 years of walking) of the persons with varied body weights up to 400 kg, and it was observed that the balls could withstand the test parameters (Fig. 17.4b). The study concluded that the balls with uniform and sub-micron average grain size would improve the fatigue properties of these balls even further, and eventually fatigue life of the prostheses would be longer.

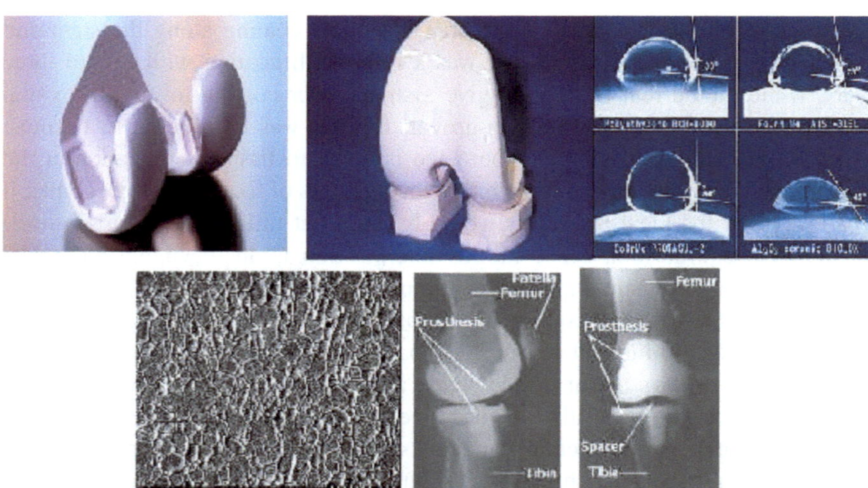

Fig. 17.3 Total knee-joint prosthesis showing (clockwise from left) femoral components, XRD of the prosthesis, side view and rear view, SEM of surgical grade aluminad

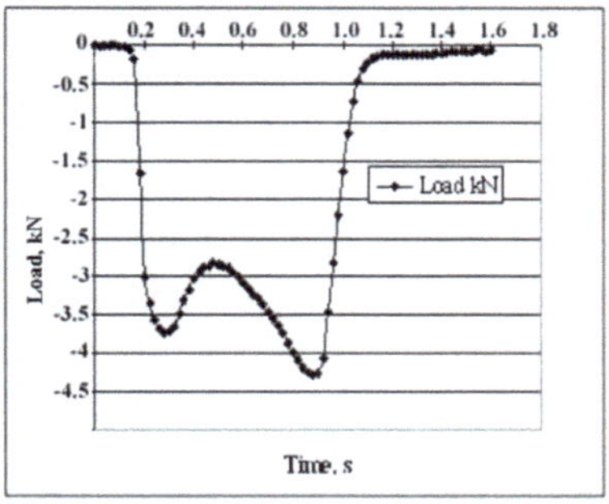

(a)

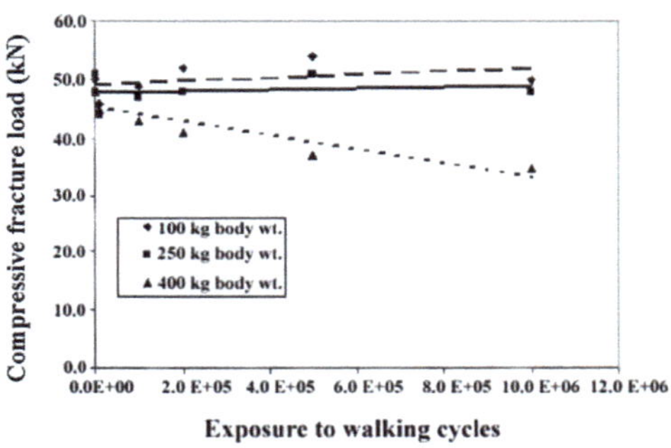

(b)

ACTIVITY	MAXIMUM LOAD ON HIP JOINT (Multiples of body weight)
SLOW WALKING	4.3
NORMAL WALKING	4.3
FAST WALKING	7.6
CLIMBING UPSTAIRS	7.2
CLIMBING DOWNSTAIRS	7.1
RUNNING	8.9
HIGH JUMPING	10 – 12
UP RAMP	5.9
DOWN RAMP	5.1

Fig. 17.4 (A) Typical stress pattern experienced by a human hip during walking (body weight of the person has been assumed to be 100 kg; (B) fracture strength of the ceramic heads after being exposed to walking cycles of varied conditions

Bioactive and Resorbable Ceramics

Calcium Phosphate Ceramics

Calcium phosphate ceramics is a well-known inorganic constituent of normal (bones, teeth, fish enamel, and some species of shells) and pathological (dental and urinary calculus, stones, and atherosclerotic lesions) calcifications. In bone, they occur mainly in the form of poorly crystallized non-stoichiometric sodium-, magnesium-, and carbonate-containing HAp (termed as ‘biological apatite’ or dahllite). There are a number of biologically relevant calcium phosphate ceramics in normal human calcified tissues [11]. At body temperature, in a body fluid, the stable phase of calcium phosphate is $CaHPO_4.2\,H_2O$ (brushite, at pH < 4.2), whereas at pH > 4.2, the stable phase is $Ca_{10}(PO4)_6(OH)_2$ (HAp). At a higher temperature, other phases, e.g., $Ca_3(PO_4)_2$ (β-tricalcium phosphate, whitlockite) and $Ca_4P_2O_9$(tetracalcium phosphate), are formed. These anhydrous, high-temperature calcium phosphate phases interact with water and body fluids at optimum temperature (37°C) to form

HAp. The importance of Ca:P ratios in determining the solubility and tendency for resorption in body have been discussed by De Groot [4], Williams [17], and Le Geros et al. [18]. It has been observed that the presence of micropores in the sintered material increases the solubility of these phases [5, 19, 20, 21]. The induction time to form crystallized carbonated apatite increases as follows: Ca-deficient HAp (CDHA) < poorly crystallized HAp (pcHA) < crystallized HAp (cHA) < coralline HAp (I-HAp) < β-tricalcium phosphate (β-TCP) < calcium carbonate marine coral (I-CC) < β-calcium pyrophosphate (I-β-CP). Among these, β-TCP and HAp are the two ceramics used widely for clinical applications.

Among the different phases of calcium phosphates discussed so far, hydroxyapatite is the main mineral constituent of the bone and, therefore, is biocompatible, exhibits only limited degree of surface reaction with bone tissues, and is integrated within the system. It is used as an implant material in various forms: as a solid body with little porosity, as granular particles, as porous structure, or as coating on metallic implants. There are different forms of porous HAp, which have undergone major clinical trials in maxillofacial and orthopedic surgery. These porous HAp blocks are also extensively used in long-bone reconstructions that are often stabilized with plate and screw fixation systems particularly in case of some traumatic defects like road accident/gunshot injury. In restorative surgery, granules of the material are used in treating parodontopathy (local and generalized, moderate and acute parodontitis, and idiopathic parodontopathy accompanying insulin-independent diabetes mellitus) and periodontal, follicular, and residual maxillary cysts. In implantable drug delivery systems, the presence of a large number of small interconnected pores in porous HAp granular matrix and the small diffusion coefficient of the drug to the capillary action [22] lead to the stabilization of the drug concentration at the desired level for a targeted time period. In the 21st century, CAD/CAM (computer-aided design/computer-aided manufacturing) is also emerging as a potential development process of porous HAp blocks in cases where medical interventions favor the application of an anatomic patient-specific, custom-made implant. The anatomic shapes of degenerated/damaged human bone system (marrow cavity, etc.) can be interpreted and identified on the basis of CT data, which can be digitized and transferred to a CAD/CAM model. This possibility allows the surgeons to perform a mock operation to perfect the process prior to the actual operation and take the final decision on the selection of prosthesis from a standard set. Further, by adopting rapid proto-typing route through selective laser sintering, efforts are being made to develop bioactive, patient-specific porous prosthesis as per the surgeon's need, which would decrease the operation time and, in turn, the risk in operation. However, for easy and better fixation as well as restoration of the functionality of the operated zone, efforts are being made to incorporate protein and stem cells into the scaffold.

To produce implants capable of withstanding mechanical loads, it is reasonable to use densely sintered ceramics, which surpass porous ceramics in strength. For load-bearing applications, ceramics should consist of fine grains because, according to the well-known Hall-Petch formula [23], mechanical strength increases with decreasing grain size. Dense ceramics can be produced by pressing or slip-casting followed by pressure-less sintering or hot uniaxial or isostatic pressing [24, 25, 26, 27, 28]. In this, the density of the ceramics is ~3.16 g/cm [3, 29]. An addition of 5% Na_3PO_4 was shown to reduce the sintering temperature necessary for the preparation of dense HAp ceramics by about 50°C. The use of bioglass (2.6 mol% P_2O_5, 26.9 mol% CaO, 24.0 mol% Na_2O, 46.1 mol% SiO_2) as a sintering aid made it possible not only to improve the mechanical properties of HAp ceramics but also their behavior in biological environments [30].

In surgery, both dense and porous HAp ceramics are used depending on the need for strength-bearing of the implants. The various dental and medical applications of dense HAp (39.68 wt% Ca, 18.45 wt% P, Ca:P weight ratio 2.151, Ca:P molar ratio 1.667) are mainly for (a) repair of bony defects in dental and orthopedic applications [31], (b) immediate tooth root replacement [32], (c) adjuvant to the placement of metal implants [21], (d) enhancement of guided tissue regeneration, etc. [33]. Porous ceramics have low strength and, therefore, are suitable for implantation into tissues that experience no substantial stresses (middle ear base for plastic surgery, coatings on metallic/ceramic/polymer-based implants and some maxillofacial applications, and local drug delivery). Pores in implants are necessary for osteointegration, a process that depends on the pore size, volume, and interconnectivity. The minimum pore size for bone in-growth into the implants is 100–135 μm; to ensure blood supply to the contact surfaces and tissue in-growth and fixation [34, 35, 36], smaller pores favor protein adsorption and adhesion of osteogenic cells, and therefore a bimodal pore-size distribution in porous ceramics is considered to be necessary for fixation and quick wound-healing of the operation site. These ceramic materials were examined for their efficacy as bone substitutes in filling traumatic or pathological bone defects in tumor/fracture, and were found to have satisfactory progress in the fracture union/healing of trauma with increase in radiographic density at the ceramic implant sites. There were no toxic effects, and evidence of bone formation around HAp granules with good incorporation into the host bone was noticed [37, 38].

In addition, porous synthetic hydroxyapatite was started to be used widely as integrated ocular implants in the field of ophthalmology, which is generally introduced to fill up the void in the orbital socket after the removal of an infected/diseased eye through evisceration or enucleation surgery. However, HAp-based artificial eyeball was designed and developed with the purpose of not only filling the orbital cavity volume to prevent deformation of the eye but also to provide movement of the fellow eye to improve cosmetic rehabilitation of the patient [39]. Figure 17.5 depicts the design of the actual implant along with one such patient inserted with the implant. Presently, clinical trials with these implants in 40 human patients in various medical institutions revealed no side-effects, and in all the cases they provided adequate motility and mimicked the other eye for both horizontal and vertical movements [11]. Periodic MRI after 4, 6, and 8 months of the surgery showed that the implants maintained their exact location with adequate degree of fibrovascularization. The images of gadolinium contrast exhibited that early peripheral activities start within 4 months, whereas 70% of fibro-vascularization is completed within 6–8 months in centrally located implants.

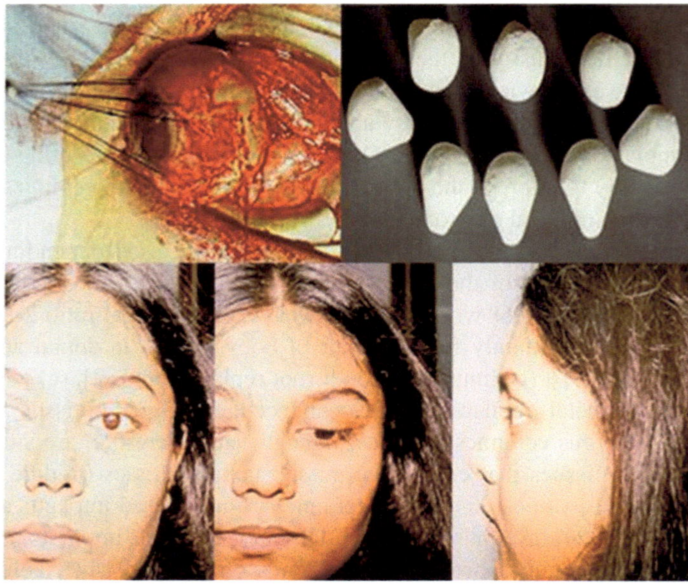

Fig. 17.5 Design of hydroxyapatite-based integrated orbital implant developed at CGCRI along with one such patient inserted with the implant showing the movement of her artificial eye

Hydroxyapatite coatings for cement-less fixation of orthopedic implants are osteo-conductive in nature, increase the kinetics of tissue in-growth, and enhance the strength of the interface. Hydroxyapatite (HA)-coated stems have been shown to have less micro-motion and subsidence than porous-coated and cemented stems. Concerns with regard to HAp delamination and third-body wear have not materialized with thin, dense plasma-sprayed coatings. The results demonstrate excellent lasting fixation to a grit-blasted, tapered titanium stem with dense, highly crystalline, pure-proximal HAp coating. These stems have performed well in young and active patient population, and have already become popular with orthopedic surgeons.

However, there are some potential problems associated with these plasma-coated prosthesis for bone in-growth fixation, which are as follows:

- According to Wolff's law of bone remodeling, load is concentrated at the area of rigid fixation and would bypass a large area resulting in stress-shielded bone resorption.
- During revision surgery, the removal of such a stem without destruction of bone would be difficult.
- Varying degrees of heat treatment required for sintering porous surfaces substantially reduce the fatigue strength of the implant due to various microstructural as well as other transformations. In addition, the porous layer substantially increases the surface area of the metal, resulting in the acceleration of the corrosion process, which may lead to prosthesis-loosening and metal ion-releasing. Accumulated metal ion may cause adverse systemic effects.

Therefore, at present, biomimetic coating has emerged as a promising technique that overcomes some of the intrinsic drawbacks of the plasma-spraying method. It elaborates a 30–50 μm uniform and homogeneous hydroxyapatite coating with tailored porosity on metal substrates at room temperature. For this purpose, bioactive metal implants (Ti metal, Ti metal alloys, stainless steel, Co–Cr alloys) are soaked into a solution called simulated body fluid (SBF) at physiological pH (7.4) and room temperature (37°C) [10]. Under such experimental conditions, it is possible to coat heat-sensible metals, e.g., porous implants. Also, this technique can successfully be employed to cover implants with new Ca–P phases [8, 40], which is otherwise not possible to obtain at high temperatures. Depending on the crystal size of the precipitating phase, biomimetic coating has different structures, dissolution behavior, and phase composition [9]. These specific characteristics of the method could be highly beneficial for bone formation as compared with the HAp plasma-sprayed coating. The time consumption factor in this process is shortened or overcome by chemical treatment of the substrate or by increasing the concentration of the SBF solution. A preliminary result of this study is summarized in Fig. 17.6 [41].

Another widely used bioceramics is β-TCP, which has a nominal chemical composition of $Ca_3(PO_4)_2$ and a Ca:P ratio of 1.5. Due in part to its crystalline structure, the biodegradation rate of TCP is much faster than that of HAp. Although the exact mechanism of biodegradation is not clear, it has been reported [1] that β-TCP dissolves in situ in acidic environment and undergoes cellular breakdown by macrophages among the osteoclast-like cells attached to the implanted TCP. Consequently, the function of these totally biodegradable (resorbable) biomaterials is merely to serve as a scaffolding/filler of space, thereby permitting tissue infiltration and replacement. This leads to the elimination of a second surgical procedure as is evident in autologous bone grafts, although there is a serious reduction in strength that occurs during the resorption process. The chemical interaction of the implanted TCP with the body fluid to form HAp may be given as:

$$4Ca_3(PO_4)_2(s) + 2\,H_2O \rightarrow Ca_{10}(PO_4)_6(OH)_2(\text{surface}) + 2Ca^{2+} + 2HPO_4^{2-}. \quad (17.1)$$

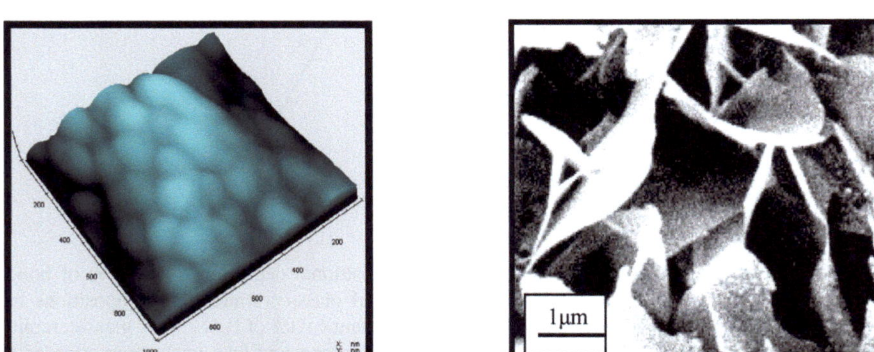

Fig. 17.6 The AFM and SEM microstructures of biomolecular template-induced biomimetic coating of hydroxyapatite (HAp) on Ti-6Al-4 V substrate, developed at CGCRI, Kolkata

This reaction decreases the pH of the solution adjacent to the implant, which in turn increases the solubility of TCP. Therefore, after implantation, TCP progressively degrades and is slowly replaced with natural tissues. It is important to note that it leads to the regeneration of tissues instead of their replacement, and thus renders good interfacial stability. Although an ideal implant material, some limitations restrict further extensive use of TCP in clinical applications [11, 42].

Bioactive Glasses and Glass-Ceramics

Bioactive glasses are manufactured by conventional glass manufacturing methods [1]. The choice of raw materials here can affect the properties of glass, which can be tailored according to the application area. Basically, the most well-studied composition of these materials is 45 wt% SiO_2, 24.5 wt% Na_2O, 24.5 wt% CaO, and a constant 6 wt% of P_2O_5. Bioglasses are known to form stable bonding (chemical bonding of hydroxyapatite, embedding collagen fibers and bone cells) to the bone when implanted in vivo for repair and reconstruction of diseased and damaged tissues, especially hard tissues. The ternary SiO_2-Na_2O-CaO diagram (Fig. 17.7) represents the bioactive bonding-boundary compositions. At the center, composition A is most suitable for the rapid formation of apatite and hence termed as 'bioactive region', whereas the composition at region B is 'bioinert' as it is SiO_2-rich and leads

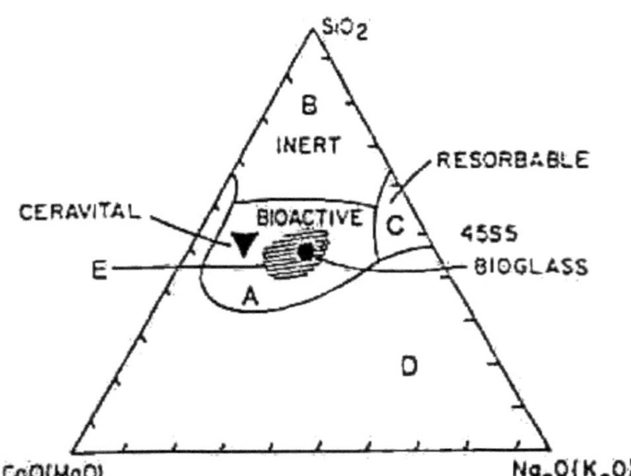

Fig. 17.7 The ternary SiO_2-Na_2O-CaO diagram: compositional dependence (in wt%) of bone bonding and soft tissue bonding of bioactive glasses and glass-ceramics. All compositions in region A are bioactive and bind to bone. They have a constant 6 wt% of P_2O_5. A/W glass-ceramic has higher P_2O_5 content. Compositions in region B are bioinert and lead to the formation of a non-adherent fibrous capsule. Compositions in region C are resorbable. Region D is restricted by technical factors. Region E (soft tissue bonding) is inside the dashed line where the index of bioactivity, IB, is >8[5]

to the formation of a non-adherent fibrous capsule. Region C with poor CaO content comprises the resorbable glass/glass-ceramics. Earlier, it was believed that P_2O_5 is an essential constituent of glass to make it bioactive, although it has been shown presently that the minimal melt-derived glass compositional system for bioactivity is CaO-SiO_2 (compositional limit 60 mole%) (Kokubo et al.), and for gel-derived glasses, it is SiO_2-Na_2O-CaO (compositional limit 85 mole%). The role of phosphate in glass is to aid in the nucleation of calcium phosphate phase on the surface of the glass substrate.

In all known bioactive implants, including bioactive glass and glass ceramics, it is essential that a layer of biologically active hydroxycarbonate apatite (HCA) must develop on the surface to form a bond with the surrounding tissue. A sequence of chemical reactions including leaching, dissolution followed by precipitation of an amorphous calcium phosphate-rich layer on the surface later crystallizes to a HCA structure slowly by incorporating carbonate ions from the body fluid [43]. Rapid growth of HCA agglomerates incorporates collagen, monopolysaccharides, and glycoproteins consequently into the active surface layer forming an organic–inorganic composite [44]. Within a week, the mineralizing bone appears at the interface of more reactive bioactive glass substrate, and by 4 weeks, the interface is completely bonded to the bone without any intervening fibrous tissues. Studies on bone bonding to bioactive glasses and glass-ceramics exhibited very high interfacial strength values using different mechanical test methods. Bioglass implants in rat tibia ($4 \times 4 \times 1\,mm^3$) exhibited a pull-out strength of $\sim$30 N within 30 days after implantation, while the control implants of stainless steel and alumina showed much lower pull-out strength of less than 10 N. So, it is evident that the bonding ability and bond strength of bioactive glasses to both hard and soft tissues of the musculoskeletal system are distinctly higher than other bioactive implants that do not bond to soft tissues.

Some of the important characteristics of bioactive glasses are as follows:

1. exhibits a rapid rate of surface reaction that leads to fast tissue-bonding in vivo
2. has a low elastic modulus of 30–35 GPa, which is close to that of a cortical bone
3. mechanical weakness and low fracture toughness due to amorphous two-dimensional glass network
4. low tensile bending strength (40–60 MPa)

The latter two properties make them unsuitable for load-bearing applications, although they can be used as coating, buried implants, or low-loaded/compressively loaded devices in the form of powders/bioactive phase in composites. The strength of bioglasses can be increased by preparing a fine-grained apatite containing glass ceramic, comprising 10–15 wt% P_2O_5 in high-SiO_2 and high-CaO glass, termed as Ceravital [45]. Another bioactive glass ceramic, termed as A/W (Apatite, Wollastonite) consists of 38 wt% apatite, 34 wt% wollastonite, and 28 wt% residual glassy phase (MgO 16.6 wt%, CaO 24.2 wt%, and SiO_2 59.2 wt%), has an especially important load-bearing clinical application in the replacement of vertebrae (Kokubo et al., 1982) [46, 47, 48, 49, 50]. Previously, autograft or allograft in combination with metals, PMMA bone cement, or Al_2O_3 ceramics were attempted for the

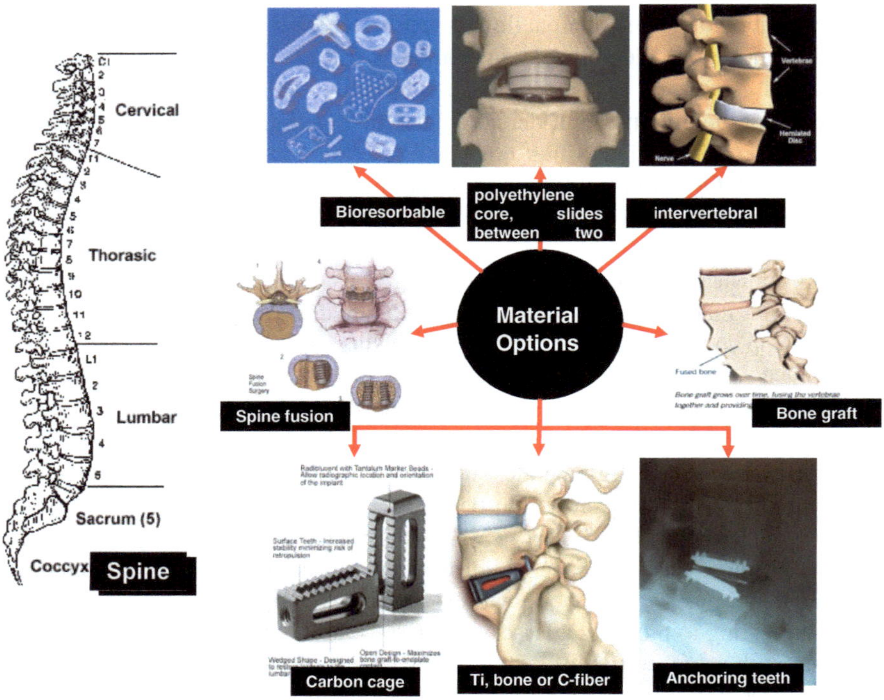

Fig. 17.8 Glass ceramic and composite materials used as vertebral implants

reconstruction of extensively damaged vertebral column (Fig. 17.8). All these were often unsatisfactory because of limited availability/non-bonding, resulting in loosening and dislocation of the implant during use [51, 52]. However, pore/crack-free, dense, homogeneous glass-ceramic prepared by densifying 5 μm glass powders with oxyfluorapatite ($Ca_{10}(PO_4)_6(O,F_2)$) and wollastonite ($CaO\text{-}SiO_2$) phases exhibited high compressive/bending strength (1080 MPa, 215 MPa) and fracture toughness (2.0 $MPa^{1/2}$) [1], and interfacial bond strength to bone showed great promise for in vivo experiments to replace surgically removed vertebrae.

Vast advances in fusion techniques and instrumentation have markedly facilitated the treatment of various spinal disorders. Discs are cartilages that lie between the bony vertebral bodies of the spine, and are the most vulnerable component of a human vertebra. Since motion occurs in this area, these are considered joints, and in aging process, discs lose their water content and are degenerated. Tear occurs in the outer lining of the disc (annulus), causing degenerative disc disease (DDD), which requires artificial disc replacement. The implant is designed with polyethylene core (Fig. 17.8) slides between two metal end plates that are attached to the vertebral body with anchoring teeth built along the rim of the end plates. This replaces the injured disc, and the polyethylene core allows movement of the spine unlike fusion that prevents normal movement.

When a disc ruptures, it is not able to support the body weight, the space between the vertebra narrows, the nerves are pinched, and slowly the facet joints become arthritic, get larger, develop bone spurs resulting in spondylolisis, which leads one vertebra to slip on the other. This is a dynamic process and the disc is to be removed (by laminectomy/disectomy) to relieve pressure on the nerve. During the process, a titanium-based BAK (Bagby and Kuslich) cage is inserted, which allows spinal fusion to relieve pain and keep the vertebra from slipping. The device is a hollow threaded cylinder with holes that are filled with bones taken from the lamina/bioactive ceramics. Bone grows through the holes to fuse the vertebra from above and below. On the other hand, a carbon fiber cage is a composite of long carbon fibers and a polymer matrix (polyether ether ketone) designed in the shape of a trapezoidal hollow box (Fig. 17.8). As in the previous case, the upper and the lower surfaces of the cage are open to allow packing with bone graft/bioceramics and to provide a wide area of contact between the graft and the adjacent vertebra [53].

The use of bioabsorbable implants, e.g., alpha-polyesters, in the current development of spinal instrumentation and surgery is widespread. Polylactide and polyglycolide, whose breakdown products are lactic and glycolic acids, are familiar to the physiological milieu of the body. With its gradual resorptive properties, bioresorbable implants gradually decrease the stress shielding effect that is common with rigid metallic implants, stabilize motion segments, allow a greater transfer of load to the host spine during resorption, and minimize junctional degeneration [54].

In another approach, hydroxyapatite–collagen composites having a bone-like nanostructure was synthesized and shaped as an implant. This study was to develop artificial vertebra using this novel implant for anterior fusion of the cervical spine. Histological and radiographical analyses after initial studies on beagle dogs suggested that the composite material adsorbing rhBMP-2 may be a suitable replacement for the existing ceramics in anterior inter body fusion of the cervical spine [55].

In an intermediate stage, after extraction of teeth and prior to fitting of dentures, the preservation of jaw-bone of patients is essential and is done by endosseous ridge maintenance implant (ERMI; Stanley et al.) [56, 57]. Another clinical problem called 'conductive hearing loss' [58, 59, 60, 61] caused by chronic infection of the ossicles (small bones of the middle ear) is met by 'ossicular prosthesis' using bioactive glass-ceramic-based implant (Fig. 17.9). Here, the bioglasses bond both to the collagen of the eardrum and to the bones of the stapes footplate, thereby anchoring the implant firmly on both ends. This prevents extrusion possibility and micro-motion of the implant–tissue interface, which occurs when bioinert implants are used. Also, there is no growth of fibrous tissue to impair sound transmission, and so the sound conduction was excellent in a patient [61]. Because of disadvantages of autograft materials and homograft implants, alloplastic materials (biocompatible, bioinert, or bioactive) have replaced the former in ossicular prostheses. It was found that, among the introduced materials like stainless steel, titanium, gold, and alumina, the latter one used for ossicular reconstruction does not release any detectable trace substances and, therefore, became popular in Germany and Japan, and the developed implant was fixed to the undersurface of the tympanic membrane without cartilage coverage. The high surface energy and extremely low surface

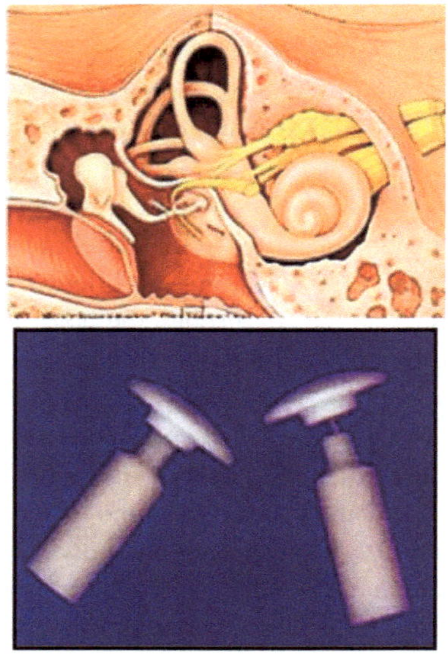

Fig. 17.9 Middle ear prosthesis using hydroxyapatite. (Article: Hydroxyapatite composite biomaterials: evolution and application, Fig. 3, Source: Materials World, Vol. 5, no. 1, pp. 18–20, January 1997, Courtesy: http://www.azom.com/details.asp?ArticleID=1718)

roughness result in fast and strong adsorption of biological molecules in alumina. These adsorbed molecules limit the direct contact of the articulating solid surface, resulting in hindrance in the transmission of sound [62], although it showed better performance in comparison to polymeric components. Bioactive implants (HAp, bioglass) react favorably with the body tissues to promote soft tissue attachment. It is a direct chemical bond to the surface of the material unlike the mechanical attachment that occurs with bioinert and biocompatible materials, and as a consequence, it is expected to offer better property and longer life.

New-Age Innovation in Bioceramic Implants

Composites

These comprise a notable example of the innovation of a second-generation biomaterial, provided by a hydroxyapatite-reinforced polyethylene composite, for use as a bone analog pioneered by Bonfield et al. [63]. Modeled on the structure of cortical bone as a natural composite of collagen fibers and apatite, the material was tailor-made to provide matching deformation characteristics and superior fracture toughness to cortical bone, so as to produce bone apposition rather than bone resorption at an implant surface. The concept was developed with incremental testing and processing to produce an optimized composite, which entered clinical trial as a suborbital floor implant [64]. It was established that the material could be trimmed readily by the surgeon to fit precisely the skeletal defect and promote bone bonding without the need for cement. The material became very popular in UK and USA for application as a trimmable shaft in a middle ear implant (replacing partially or totally damaged or diseased bones that transmit sound from the diaphragm to the inner ear) and achieved immediate clinical success with its advantages of trimmability, providing a precise fit to the individually varying middle ear space, and of bonding to the residual bony base. Clinical follow-up has indicated very satisfactory restoration of hearing [65], and this has triggered to develop altogether 22 different designs of middle ear implant, with benefits already to about 60,000 patients. From this base, other implants for bone replacement or augmentation became possible, with commercial potential for a range of minor and major load-bearing applications, including maxillofacial reconstruction, spinal prostheses, and revision hip prostheses.

Tissue Engineering

Recently, in the third generation of biomedical implants, the developed knowledge-base of other allied fields, e.g., tissue engineering, nanoscience and technology, etc., is amalgamated to design more efficient implants/devices/new tissues/organs. Synthetic biomaterials and stem cells are two important tools that tissue engineering utilizes as building blocks for new tissues that incorporate living cells. More precisely, it is the application of principles and methods of engineering and life sciences toward fundamental understanding of structure–function relationships in normal and pathological mammalian tissues and development of biological substitutes (for replacements as opposed to the use of inert implants) to restore, maintain, or improve tissue function. The modern-day 'tissue engineering' aims to manufacture complete tissues outside the body ready for future transplant of skin, cartilage, regeneration of bone, and other connective structural substitutes. These replacements may consist of cells in suspension, cells implanted on a scaffold such as collagen, and replacements that entirely consist of cells and their extracellular products. The three general strategies identified for the creation of new tissues involve the use of (1) isolated cells or cell substitutes, (2) tissue-inducing substances, or (3) cells placed on or within matrices.

In this case, the product consists of individuals' own cells; therefore, transplantation of engineered tissues or organs resides in the immunological acceptance, and it is not expected to evoke rejection. On the other hand, differentiated donor cells from another individual would likely have one or more surface markers that would be incompatible to the host. Since the availability of individual's own cells at the time of need is unlikely, cost-effective universal donor cell lines that are non-immunogenic are needed. Preliminary data suggest that tissue-engineered composites can be designed to cross the blood-brain barrier, and thus have the potential to correct deficits associated with brain tissues such as those found in Alzheimer's disease and Parkinson's disease.

A multitude of applications for engineered tissues and organs exist in human health arena. Examples include whole organ replacements in life-threatening situations associated with liver, pancreas, heart, or kidney failure and replacement of lost skin-covering due to massive burns or chronic ulcers. Other applications include repair of defective or missing supportive structures, such as long bones, cartilage, connective tissue, and intervertebral discs; replacement of worn out and poorly functioning tissues as exemplified by aged muscle or cornea; replacement of damaged blood vessels; and restoration of cells to produce necessary enzymes, hormones, and other metabolites.

In addition, tissue-engineered composites will be useful to establish safety and efficacy of potential new drugs, and may contribute to the development of understanding of genetic or environmental factors that may be responsible for the onset of diseases.

Orthopedic Tissue Engineering

Bioactive composites for bone substitutes provide an approach to skeletal regeneration in which the implant surface provides a favorable site for the recruitment of cells from the surrounding biological environment, with the subsequent cellular processes leading to the expression of matrix and tissue formation. In cellular or tissue engineering, such cells are cultured outside the body to develop tissues that can be used subsequently for tissue repair. The primary advantage of a tissue substitute obtained by this route is that some or all of the biological growth factors would be immediately available, rather than needing to be recruited. Such an approach has particular appeal, for example, in the potential repair of regions of healthy cartilage damaged by injury, as a more conservative treatment than that of total joint replacement. There are enormous intrinsic challenges in the production of tissues ex vivo in a bioreactor as compared (in terms of composition and properties) to normal natural tissues. Other key challenges are to develop a source of cartilage cells (chondrocytes) with a favorable immune response, to design an approach method of fixation, and to provide effective storage. The pioneering work of Langer [66] to develop prototype cartilage grafts by adapting this route has yielded the substitute with the composition and properties of the natural tissue (but not exactly equal), and this has triggered many new activities in this area.

For bone tissue engineering, there is a direct link from the research on porous hydroxyapatite, which could provide a suitable matrix delivery system for osteoblasts or precursor stem cells. In the former case, such an approach would provide an autograft equivalent to bone grafting, without the need for a second operation. An exciting prospect in the latter case is the production of both bone and cartilage through cell differentiation locally directed by scaffolds and scaffold chemistries, so as to produce a mini-implant of cartilage already in place on bone, e.g., a replacement acetabulum of bone complete with its cartilage lining, which would eliminate the considerable difficulty of fixing cartilage to bone in vivo. A complementary approach is to stimulate osteoblast recruitment, e.g., by local delivery of parathyroid receptor agonists through prior transfection of the PTH gene into local fibroblasts.

During the last decade, considerable attention has been directed toward the use of implants with bioactive fixation. This is defined as interfacial bonding of an implant to tissue by means of formation of a biologically active hydroxyapatite layer on the implant surface [67, 68]. Hence, the bioactive bond formed at the implant-bone interface has strength equal to or greater than that of bone. The level of bioactivity of a specific material can be related to the time taken for more than 50% of the interface to bond to bone ($t_{0.5bb}$):

Bioactivity index, $I_B = 100/t_{0.5bb}$

In this, materials that exhibit an I_B value greater than 8, e.g., 45S5 Bioglass, will bond to both soft and hard tissues, whereas materials that have I_B value less than 8 but greater than 0, e.g., synthetic hydroxyapatite, will bond only to hard tissue [26]. Also, a bioactive glass undergoes surface dissolution in a physical environment in order to form a hydroxycarbonate apatite (HCA) layer [69]. The larger the solubility of the bioactive glass, the more pronounced the effect on the bone-tissue growth [70].

Three-dimensional porous scaffolds promote new tissue formation by providing a surface and void volume that promotes the attachment, migration, proliferation, and desired differentiation of connective tissue progenitors throughout the region where new tissue is needed. Critical variables in scaffold design and function include the bulk material or materials from which it is made, the three-dimensional architecture, the surface chemistry, the mechanical properties, the initial environment in the area of the scaffold, and the late scaffold environment, which is often determined by degradation characteristics.

The stem cells, the immature/undifferentiated cells capable of producing an identical daughter cell that may perpetuate over many generations resulting in considerable amplification of their numbers (when subjected to the right biochemical signal), are the key elements to conceive the idea of developing a complete implant consisting of bone and cartilages. Depending on their respective decrease in potency, stem cells can be totipotent (e.g., the fertilized egg or zygote), pluripotent [e.g., embryonic (ES) and germ (EG) cells], or multipotent (bone marrow, stromal or mesenchymal stem cells). The characteristics that make stem cells an attractive proposition for tissue repair and regeneration have been outlined [71] below, and there are specified mechanisms that activate stem cells or progenitor cells to replace the damaged cells:

(1) generation of adequate number of cells and tissues to fill the defect or complete the repair
(2) differentiation of the cells toward the correct phenotype and maintenance of this
(3) ensuring that the cells of tissues adopt the appropriate three-dimensional organization and produce the extracellular matrix. This may require provision of structural support in the shape of resorbable scaffold
(4) production of cells or tissues that are structurally and mechanically compliant with the normal demands of the native tissue
(5) achievement of full integration with the local tissue with vascularization, if required
(6) overcoming the risk of immunological rejection

The three major components of the acellular structure of bone are collagen, which is flexible but very tough; hydroxycarbonate apatite, which is the reinforcing phase of the composite; and bone matrix or the ground substance, which performs various cellular support functions – all are organized into a three-dimensional system that has maximum strength and toughness along the lines of applied stress. Two of the various types of bones that are of most concern in bioceramics are the cancellous bone and the cortical bone. The cancellous bone that occurs across the end of the long bones has lower modulus of elasticity and higher strain to failure than that of the cortical bone. The difference in elastic moduli between various types of soft connective tissues, e.g., tendons and ligaments, renders a smooth gradient in mechanical stress across a bone, between bones, and between muscles and bones.

Bone at the interface with an implant is often structurally weak because of disease or aging, and there is progressive loss of volume of bone with age that can deteriorate even further due to the presence of the implant or the method of fixation.

Another problem, called stress shielding, occurs when the implant prevents the bone from being properly loaded. The higher modulus of elasticity of the implant results in its carrying nearly all the load. The elastic modulus of the anisotropic cortical bone ranges between 7 and 25 GPa, depending upon age, location of the bone, and direction of measurement. This is 10–50 times lower than that of alumina, while the value for cancellous bone is several hundred times less than that of alumina. Stress-shielding weakens bone in the region where the applied load is lowest or in compression. Bone that is unloaded or is loaded in compression will undergo a biological change that leads to bone resorption. The interface between a stress-shielded bone and an implant deteriorates as the bone weakens, resulting in the loosening of the implant or fracture of the bone at the interface. Moreover, the presence of wear debris associated with the synthetic hip and knee joint prostheses accelerates the weakening of stress-shielded bone, because of increased cellular activity involved in the removal of foreign wear particles. Such combination of stress shielding, wear debris, and motion at an interface damages and leads to the failure of the implant.

The challenge in the current bone-tissue engineering is the design of a matrix that is capable of mimicking the natural properties of bone while providing a temporary scaffold for tissue regeneration [72]. This involves the combination of cells with synthetic biodegradable or biocompatible scaffold architecture that supports vascular cell in-growth through neovascularization and osteogenesis. It has been observed that a certain size of pore geometry supports osteoblastic activities related to vascularization, and pore dimension and interconnectivity are the key factors in structural design that ensure tissue attachment and osteoid formation.

Mesenchymal stem cells are one of the adult stem cell types that can be made to develop a limited number of different kinds of tissues, with bone, cartilage, muscle and skin being the most important types (Figs. 17.10 and 17.11). They are found primarily in bone marrow, but also elsewhere in the body, such as in umbilical blood or fatty tissue.

One possible application of these versatile cells is to aid in the production of optimized materials for bone implants, such as those used in artificial hip joints.

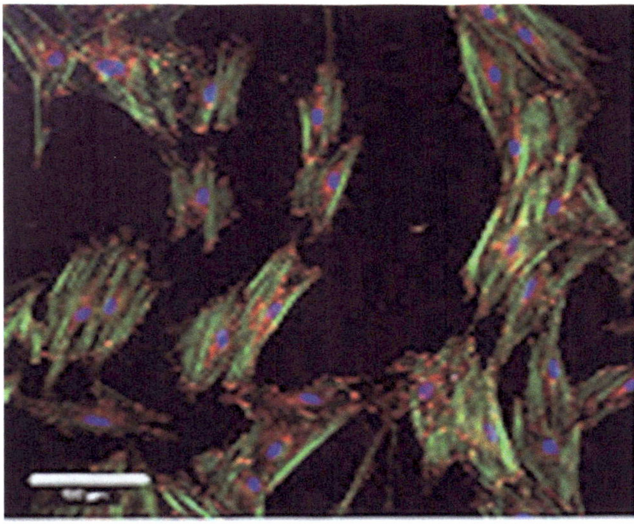

Fig. 17.10 Human mesenchymal cells: To improve visibility, the three cellular proteins have been stained: blue, core; green, F-Actin; red, Vinculin. (Article: 'All rounder helps to heal damage bones', of 'International Workshop: Stem Cells and Medical Materials', published by Empa, a Research Institute of the ETH domain, dated Nov. 10th, 2005, Courtesy: http://www.empa.ch/plugin/template/empa/*/44348/---/l=2)

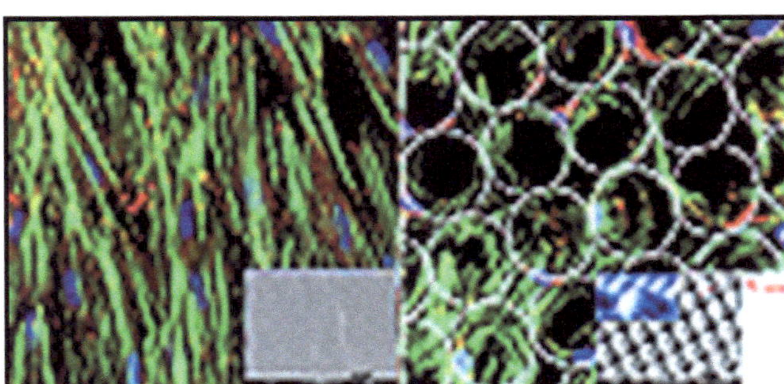

Fig. 17.11 Human mesenchymal cells on structured surfaces: left, unstructured; right, hemispheres. (Article: 'All rounder helps to heal damage bones', of 'International Workshop: Stem Cells and Medical Materials', published by Empa, a Research Institute of the ETH domain, dated Nov. 10th, 2005, Courtesy: http://www.empa.ch/plugin/template/empa/*/44348/---/l=2)

Beyond this, it might one day be possible to grow bone replacement material using the patient's own bone marrow. Given the huge number of hip replacement operations and the currently unsatisfactory healing rate of bone disorders, it is clear that the mesenchymal stem cells show a great promise – not least for commercial reasons.

An attempt to make biocompatible bone has been initiated at the University of Central Florida, Orlando. In this, combining coatings, nanotechnology and stem cell

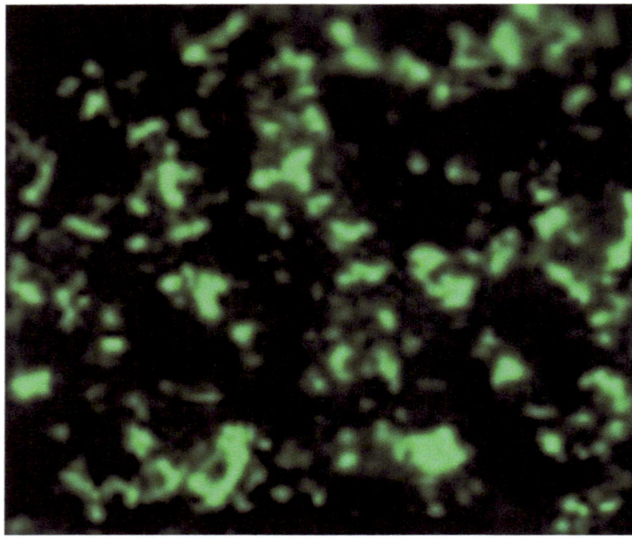

Fig. 17.12 Biocompatible bone

technology have been combined to create a better transplanted bone. As said above, the bone is coated with the patient's own stem cells with a hope that this bone will incorporate into the patient's own tissue much faster than the artificial bone – and that will help build new bone marrow tissue (Figs. 17.12 and 17.13).

Recently, Ito et al. [73] of Hiroshima University used hydroxyapatite-based scaffold with interconnected porous structure on which mesenchymal stem cells harvested from the bone marrow of green rats containing green fluorescent protein were cultured, and finally these hybrids were implanted into the tibias of Sprague–Dawley rats. The hybridized feeler showed that the stem cells were differentiated into osteoblast-like cells within 8 weeks, resulting in excellent bone formation through osteoconduction, and is expected to have extensive clinical applications. Harris et al. studied the influence of local environment established by scaffold

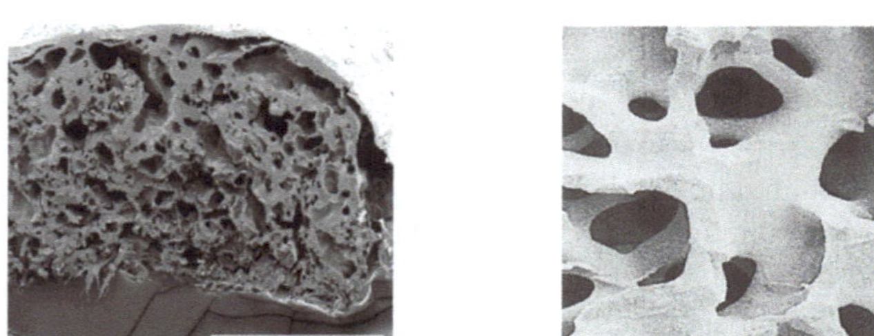

Fig. 17.13 SEM displaying the cross-section of a composite disk, which had been seeded with cultured bone marrow stromal cells

chemistry/architecture on the potency of the human bone marrow-derived mesenchymal stem cells, which were culture-expanded on different scaffold and finally placed into the dorsum of SCID mice for 5 weeks. It was reported that scaffolds made of hydroxyapatite and β-TCP were the best ones to exhibit 8.8% and 13.8% bone formation. Bo et al. [74] reported that bone marrow-derived mesenchymal stem cells when expanded in vitro, implanted to β-TCP-based pre-molded scaffolds and finally implanted into the cranial defect of New Zealand rabbits, showed excellent bone formation on the surface and along the cross-section of the scaffold within first 6 weeks. The study pointed out that transplantation of mesenchymal stem cells from rat with β-TCP could serve as an example of a cell-based treatment for bone regeneration in skeletal defects. Yamada et al. [75] explanted mesenchymal stem cells from rat femur, cultured in vitro, fragmented, and mixed with fibrin glue and β-TCP admixtures, and finally injected into the subcutaneous space on the dorsum of a rat to study the effect of fibrin glue and β-TCP mixture on new bone formation at heterotrophic sites in the rat with plasticity. The results revealed that, within 8 weeks, newly formed bone structure with pearly opalescence and firm consistency appeared at the injected site, and the study pointed out that this technique holds the promise of a minimally invasive means of generating autogenous bone to reconstruct bony defects.

Arinzeh et al. [76] studied the influence of calcium phosphate-based scaffolds on the performance of human mesenchymal stem cells to induce bone formation in large, long bone defects. For this purpose, bone marrow was collected from two healthy human donors, which was further treated to isolate the mesenchymal cells. These cells were culture-expanded in Dulbecco's modified eagle's medium containing 10% fetal bovine serum and 1% antibiotic/antimycotic. Thawed cells were then loaded onto ceramic scaffolds at 5×10^6 cells/mL using a vacuum-based technique. Ceramic scaffolds of varied hydroxyapatite/β-TCP content with 60–70% total porosity, pore size range 60–70%, and grain size 0.5–1.5 μm were prepared separately, and the cells were allowed to attach to the ceramics for 2 h at 37°C prior to implantation. The kinetics of bone formation was studied in vivo by introducing these implants subcutaneously in the back of 24 SCIP mice and harvesting them for 6 and 12 weeks to study the formation of osteoblasts at the interface. The study revealed that the scaffold with 20:80 HA:TCP showed the highest new bone formation with higher abase activity, which was evident even within 28 days after implantation. In India, Basu et al. [77] have started a fresh activity to develop porous hydroxyapatite/TCP layer-based scaffold by adopting a biomimetic technique in which a protein-based layer is developed at first within the simulated body fluid medium. The nanosized holes within the protein molecules were utilized to synthesize hydroxyapatite/TCP nanocrystals. Mesenchymal stem cells extracted from New Zealand rabbits were culture-expanded separately and attached to the surface of porous scaffold layers of protein and hydroxyapatite. The hybridized implants when put back to the tibia of rabbits showed quick bone formation at the interface. The long-term immunogenic response of the surrounding tissues/organs is being studied at the moment. The initial results so far are highly encouraging.

Conclusions

Mechanical or chemical bonding of prosthesis to bone would enhance its stability, limiting the relative motion between the implant and the bone, thereby diminishing the risk of loosening. Without bonding, the prosthesis might migrate relative to the bone, and hence the risk of future loosening of the implant remains. The term osseointegration was coined by Brånemark in the 1970 s, in that a chemical bond may have been implied. Later, he suggested that chemical bonding of bone to the implant surface was a prerequisite for osseointegration, and so as to encourage faster bone growth to the implant surface, this may be done by coating titanium with a biocompatible and bioactive thin polymer film followed by the incorporation of bioactive substances like the protein BMP-2. Nevertheless, in this aspect, alongside the choice of implant material, three-dimensional design of scaffold is another important factor, as 3D structures not only permit the tuning of chemical and mechanical properties but also copy the outer form of the required bone or cartilaginous structures. Recently, a vast area has opened up to explore the application of mesenchymal cells as a source of bone-cartilage forming cells upon seeding within resorbable polymeric scaffolds in the presence of bioactive growth factors. The pluripotent nature of these progenitor cells is consistent with their involvement in developmental and biological repair processes, such as embryonic skeletal formation and fracture-healing leading to faster implant fixation.

References

1. Hench LL and Wilson J. An Introduction to Bioceramics. London: World Scientific; 1993.
2. Lawson AC and Czernuska JT. Collagen-Calcium Phosphate Composites. Proc. Inst. Mech. Eng. H. 1998; 212: 413–25.
3. Hulbert SF, Bokros JC, Hench LL et al. Ceramics in Clinical Applications: Past, Present and Future. In: Vincenzini P, editor. High Tech Ceramics. Amsterdam, the Netherlands: Elsevier; 1987. p. 189–213.
4. de Groot K. Bioceramics of Calcium Phosphate. Boca Raton, FL: CRC Press; 1983.
5. de Groot K, Klein CPAT, Wolke JGC et al. Chemistry of Calcium Phosphate Bioceramics. In: Yamamuro T, Hench LL and Wilson J, editors. Handbook of Bioactive Ceramics, Vol. II. Boca Raton, FL: C.R.C Press; 1990. p. 3–15.
6. Klein CPAT, Wolke JGC and de Groot K. Stability of Calcium Phosphate Ceramics and Plasma Sprayed Coating. In: Hench LL and Wilson J, editors. An Introduction to Bioceramics. London, UK: World Scientific; 1993. p. 199–21.
7. De Groot K. Calcium Phosphate Bioceramics: Their Future in Clinical Practice. Rev. Eur. Tech. Biomed. 1991; 13: 88–91.
8. Barre F, Laryrolle P, van Bitterswijk CA et al. Biomimetic Coatings on Titanium: A Crystal Growth Study of Octacalcium Phosphate. J. Mater. Sci. Mater. Med. 2001; 12: 529–34.
9. Barre F, Stigter M, Layrolle P et al. In Vitro Dissolution of Various Calcium Phosphate Coatings on Ti-6Al-4 V. Bioceramics 2001; 13: 67–70.
10. Kokubo T, Kushitani H, Sakka S et al. Solutions able to Reproduce *In Vivo* Surface Structure Changes in Bioactive Glass-Ceramics A/W. J. Biomed. Mater. Res. 1990; 24: 721–34.
11. Kundu B and Basu D. Ceramics for Biomedical Applications-An Insight. Sci. Cult. 2005; 71[5–6]: 144–58.

12. Hench LL and Ethridge EC. Biomaterials: An Interfacial Approach. New York, USA: Academic Press; 1982.
13. Black J and Hastings G. Handbook of Biomaterial Properties. London, UK: Chapman and Hall; 1998.
14. Willmann G. Ceramic Components for Total Hip Arthropasty. Orthop. Int. Ed. 1997; 5[4]: 110–15.
15. Dorre E and Dawihl W. Ceramic Hip Endoprotheses. In: Hastings GW and Williams DF, editors. Mechanical Properties of Biomaterials. New York: Wiley; 1980. p. 113–27.
16. Basu D. Fatigue Behaviour of Fine-Grained Alumina Hip-Joint Heads Under Normal Walking Conditions. Sadhana 2003; 28[3, 4]: 589–600.
17. Williams DF. The Biocompatibility and Clinical Uses of Calcium Phosphate Ceramics. In: Williams DF, editor. Biocompatibility of Tissue Analogs, Vol. II. Boca Raton, FL: CRC Press; 1985. p. 43–6.
18. Le Geros RF, Bone G and Le Geros RZ. Type of H_2O in Human Enamel and Precipitated Apatites. Calcif. Tissue Res. 1978; 26: 111–8.
19. de Groot K. Effect of Porosity and Physicochemical Properties on the Stability, Resorption and Strength of Calcium Phosphate Ceramics. In: Ducheyne P, Lemons J, editors. Bioceramics: Material Characteristics vs. *in vivo* Behaviour, Vol. 523. New York Academy of Science, New York, USA, 1988; p. 227–34.
20. de Groot K, Tencer A., Waite P., Nichols J., and Kay J. Significance of the porosity and physical chemistry of calcium phosphate ceramics. Dental and other head and neck uses, In: Ducheyne P., Lemons J., editors. Bioceramics: Material Characteristics vs. *in vivo* Behaviour Vol. 523., New York Academy of Sciences, New York, USA, 1988; p. 272–277.
21. Jarcho M. Calcium Phosphate Ceramics as the Hard Tissue Prosthetics. Clin. Orthop. Relat. Res. 1981; 157: 259–78.
22. Krajewski A, Ravaglioli A, Roncari E et al. Porous Ceramic Bodies for Drug Delivery. J. Mater. Sci. Mater. Med. 2000; 12: 763–71.
23. Kelly A. Strong Solids. London: Oxford University Press, 1971. Translated under the title. Vysokoprochnye Materialy. Moscow: Mir, 1976.
24. Suchanek W and Yoshimura M. Processing and Properties of HA-Based Biomaterials for Use as Hard Tissue Replacement Implants. J. Mater. Res. Soc. 1998; 13[1]: 94–103.
25. Hosoi K, Hashida T, Takashi T et al. New Processing Techniques for the hydroxyapatite Ceramics by the Hydrothermal Hot-Processing Method. J. Am. Ceram. Soc. 1996; 79: 2771–4.
26. Hench LL. Bioceramics: From Concept to Clinic. J. Am. Ceram. Soc. 1991; 75: 1487–510.
27. Le Geros RZ. Biodegradation and Bioresorption of Calcium Phosphate Ceramics. Clin. Mater. 1993; 14: 65–88.
28. De With G, Van Dijk HJA, Hattu N et al. Preparation, Microstructure and Mechanical Properties of Dense Polycrystalline Hydroxyapatite. J. Mater. Sci. 1981; 16: 1592–8.
29. Mizuno M, and Saito H, Preparation of Highly Pure Fine Mullite Powder. J. Am. Ceram. Soc., 1989; 72[3], 377–382.
30. Orlovskii VP, Komlev VS and Barinov SM. Hydroxyapatite and Hydroxyapatite-Based Ceramics. Inorg. Mater. 2002; 38: 973–84.
31. Ganeles J, Listgarten MA and Evian CI. Ultrastructure of Durapatite-Periodontal Tissue Interface in Human Intrabony Defects. J. Periodontol. 1986; 57: 133–40.
32. Denissen H, Mangano C and Cenini G. Hydroxylapatite Implants. India: Piccin Nuova Libraria, S.P.A, 1985.
33. Seibert J and Nyman S. Localised Ridge Augmentation in Dogs: A Pilot Study Using Membranes and Hydroxyapatite. J. Periodontol. 1990; 61: 157–65.
34. Hing KA, Best SM, Tanner KA et al. Quantification of Bone Ingrowth within Bone Derived Porous Hydroxyapatite Implants of Varying Density. J. Mater. Sci. Mater. Med. 1999; 10: 633–70.
35. Lu JX, Flautre B and Anselme K. Role of Interconnections in Porous Bioceramics on Bone Recolonization *In Vitro* and *In Vivo*. J. Mater. Sci. Mater. Med. 1999; 10: 111–20.

36. Yamamoto M, Tabata Y, Kawasakii H et al. Promotion of Fibrovascular Tissue Ingrowth into Porous Sponges by Basic Fibroblast Growth Factor. J. Mater. Sci. Mater. Med. 2000; 11: 213–8.
37. Sinha MK, Basu D and Sen PS. Porous Hydroxyapatite Ceramic and its Clinical Applications. Ceram. Asia 2000; 49: 102–4.
38. Shimizu T, Zerwekh JE, Videman T et al. Bone Ingrowth into Porous Calcium Phosphate Ceramics. Influence of Pulsing Electromagnetic Field. J. Orthop. Res. 1988; 6: 248–59.
39. Kundu B, Sinha MK and Basu D. Development of Bio-active Integrated Ocular Implant for Anophthalmic Human Patients. Trends in Biomaterials and Artificial Organs, 2002; 16: 1–4.
40. Barre F, Laryrolle P, van Bitterswijk CA et al. Biomimetic Ca-P Coating on Ti-6Al-4 V: Crystal Growth Study of Octacalcium Phosphate and Inhibition by Mg^{2+} and HCO^{-}_{3}. Bone 1999; 25: 107S–11S.
41. Chakraborty J, Sinha MK and Basu D, Biomolecular Template Induced Biomimetic Coating of Hydroxyapatite on SS 316 L Substrate. J. Am. Ceram. Soc., 2007; 90[4]: 1258–1261.
42. Sinha MK, Sen PS and Basu D. Synthesis, Sintering and Microstructure of Beta-Tricalcium Phosphate for Prosthetic Applications. J. Ind. Chem. Soc. 2001; 78[8]: 386 1/N388.
43. Hench LL, Bioceramics. J. Am. Ceram. Soc. 1998; 81: 1705–28.
44. Gosain AK, Bioactive Glass for Bone Replacement in Craniomaxillofacial Reconstruction. Plastic & Reconstructive Surgery. 2004; 114(2): 590–593.
45. Bromer H, Deutscher K, Blencke B et al. Properties of the Bioactive Implant Material 'Ceravital'. Sci. Ceram. 1977; 9: 219–25.
46. Kokubo T, Ito S, Sakka S et al. Formation of a high strength bioactive Glass-Ceramic in the System MgO-CaO- SiO_2- P_2O_5. J. Mater. Sci. 1986; 21: 536–40.
47. Kitsugi T, Yamamuro T and Kokubo T. Bonding Behaviour of a Glass-Ceramic Containing Apatite and Wollastonite in Segmental Replacement of Rabbit Tibia under Load Bearing Conditions. J. Bone Joint Surg. Am. 1989; 71A: 264–72.
48. Yoshii S, Kakutani Y, Yamamuro T et al. Strength of Bonding between A/W Glass Ceramic and the Surface of Bone Cortex. J. Biomed. Mater. Res. 1988; 22: 327–38.
49. Yamamuro T, Shikata J, Kakutani Y et al. Novel Methods for Clinical Applications of Bioactive Ceramics. In: Ducheyne P, Lemons D, editors. Bioceramics: Material Characteristics vs *in vivo* Behaviour, Vol. 523. New York, USA: Annals of New York Academy of Science; 1988; p. 107–114.
50. Yamamuro T, Hench LL and Wilson J, editors. Handbook on Biocative Ceramics: Bioactive Glasses and Glass-Ceramics, Vol. I. Boca Raton, FL: CRC Press; 1990.
51. Yamamuro T. Replacement of the Spine with Bioactive Glass-Ceramic Prostheses. In: Yamamuro T, Hench LL and Wilson J, editors. Handbook of Bioactive Ceramics: Bioactive Glasses and Glass Ceramics, Vol. I. Florida, Boca Raton, USA: CRC Press; 1990. p. 343–52.
52. Yamamuro T. A/W Glass –Ceramic: Clinical Applications. In: Hench LL and Wilson J, editors. An Introduction to Bioceramics. London, UK: World Scientific; 1993 p. 89–104.
53. Salame K, Quaknine G, Razon N et al. The Use of Carbon Fibre Cages in Anterior Cervical Interbody Fusion. Neurosurg. Focus 2002; 12: 1–5.
54. Robbins MM, Vaccaro AR and Madigan L. The Use of Bioabsorbable Implants in Spine Surgery. Neurosurg. Focus 2004; 16: 1–7.
55. Itoh S, Kikuchi M, Koyama Y et al. Development of an Artificial Vertebral Body Using a Novel Biomaterial, Hydroxyapatite/Collagen Composite. Biomaterials 2002; 23: 3919–26.
56. Stanley HR, Hall MB, Clark AE et al. Using 45S5 Bioglass Cones as Endosseous Ridge Maintenance Implants to prevent Alveolar Ridge Resorptions-A 5 Year Evaluation. Int. J. Oral Maxillofac. Implants 1997; 12: 95–105.
57. Stanley HR, Clark AE and Hench LL. Alveolar Ridge Maintenance Implants. In: Hench LL and Wilson J, editors. Clinical Performance of Skeletal Prostheses. London, UK: Chapman and Hall; 1996. p. 255–70.
58. Reck R, Storkel S and Meyer A. Bioactive Glass-Ceramics in Middle Year Surgery: an 8-Year Review. In: Ducheyne P, Lemons D, editors. Bioceramics: Material Characteristics vs *in vivo* Behaviour, Vol. 523. New York, USA: Annals of New York Academy of Science; 1988. p. 100.

59. Merwin E. Review of Bioactive Materials for Ottologic and Maxillofacial Applications. In: Yanamuro T, Hench LL and Wilson J, editors. Handbook of Bioactive Ceramics: Bioactive Glasses and Glass-Ceramics, Vol. I. Boca Raton, FL: USA; 1990. p. 323–8.
60. Wilson J, Douek E, Rust K et al. Bioglass Middle Ear Devices: Ten Year Clinical Results. In: Wilson J, Hench LL and Greenspan D, editors. Bioceramics, Vol. 8. Oxford, UK: Pergamon/Elsevier; 1995. p. 239–46.
61. Lobel K. Ossicular Replacement Prostheses. In: Hench LL and Wilson J, editors. Clinical Performance of Skeletal Prostheses. London, UK: Chapman and Hall, 1996. p. 214–36.
62. Pester D, Jahnke K. Ceramic Implants in Otologic Surgery. Am. J. Otol. 1981; 3: 104–8.
63. Bonfield W et al. Hydroxyapatite Reinforced Polyethylene – a Mechanically Compatible Implant Material for Bone Replacement. Biomaterials 1981; 2: 185–6.
64. Downs RN, Vardy S, Tanner KE et al. Hydroxyapatite–Polyethylene Composite in Orbital Surgery. Bioceramics. 1991; 4: 239–46.
65. Dornhoffer JL. Hearing Results with the Dornhoffer Ossicular Replacement Prostheses. Laryngoscope. 1991; 108: 531.
66. Langer R et al. Principles of Tissue Engineering. San Diego: Academic Press, 1997.
67. Cao W, Hench LL. Bioactive Materials. Ceram. Int. 1996; 22: 493–507.
68. Hench LL, West JK. Biological Application of Bioactive Glasses. Life Chem. Rep. 1996; 13: 187–241.
69. Wallace KE, Hill RG, Pembroke JT et al. Influence of Sodium Oxide Content on Bioactive Glass Properties. J. Mater. Sci. Mater. Med. 1999; 10: 697–701.
70. Ducheyne P, Qui Q. Bioactive Ceramics: The Effect of Surface Reactivity on Bone Formation and Bone Cell Function. Biomaterials 1999; 20: 2287–303.
71. Vats A, Tolley NS, Polak JM et al. Stem Cells: Sources and Applications. Clin. Otolaryngol. 2002; 27: 227–32.
72. Laurencin CT, Ambrosio AMA, Borden MD et al. Tissue Engineering: Orthopedic Applications. Annu. Rev. Biomed. Eng. 1999; 1: 19–46.
73. Ito Y, Tanaka N, Fujimoto Y et al. Bone Formation Using Novel Interconnected Porous Calcium Hydroxyapatite Ceramic Hybridized with Cultured Marrow Stromal Stem Cells Derived from Green Rat. J. Biomed. Mater. Res. A. 2004; 69: 454–61.
74. Bo B, Wang CY, Guo XM. Repair of Cranial Defects with Bone Marrow Derived Mesenchymal Stem Cells and β-TCP Scaffold in Rabbits. 1: Zhongguo Xiu Fu Chong, Jian Wai Ke Za Zhi, 2003; 17[4]: 335–8.
75. Yamada V, Boo JS, Ozawa R et al. Bone Regeneration following Injection of Mesenchymal Stem Cells and Fibrin Glue with a Biodegradable Scaffold. J. Craniomaxillofac. Surg. 2003; 31[1]: 27–33.
76. Arinzeh TL, Tran T, Mcalary J et al. A Comparative Study of Biphasic Calcium Phosphate Ceramics for Human Mesenchymal Stem Cell Induced Bone Formation. Biomaterials 2005; 26: 3631–8.

Section VI
Ethics

Chapter 18
Some Aspects of the Ethics of Stem Cell Research

Ranès C. Chakravorty

Ethics

Humans are guided by certain principles of behavior that relate to themselves, their relations to society (as an individual), and, if they belong to a specific group (e.g., professionals, caste, etc.) to that group. These principles are termed *ethics*. The Oxford English Dictionary defines "ethos" as "the characteristic spirit, prevalent tone of sentiment, of a people or community; the 'genius' of an institution or system" [1], "ethics" as "(3b) the moral principle by which a person is guided and (3c) the rules of conduct recognized in certain associations or departments of human life" [1]. Stedman's Medical Dictionary defines Medical ethics as – "The principles of proper professional conduct concerning the rights and duties of the physician himself, his patients and his fellow practitioners."

The Sanskrit term "*Dharma*" has some equivalence with "Ethics" in that Dharma implies those principles that "support" or guide an individual in the passage through life [2, 3].

For the individual then, the ethics of living depend upon personal rules of behavior, rules of behavior in his personal close society (family, relations, and friends), rules of behavior with society at large, and as a subset of this last, relationship with the group of people associated with her special interests such as livelihood. In most civilized societies, doing beneficial things to other members of the same society is a universal ethic.

People are constrained to behave ethically as such (ethical) behavior produces the least discomfort (internal) or punishment (external). In this paper, I propose to discuss my views (as mentioned above all ethics are finally individual) on the ethics of some aspects of stem-cell research.

I had been actively involved in the practice of surgery for half a century. As such, I have considerable personal knowledge of the suffering and the social consequences of chronic diseases. Though knowledge of and manipulation of genes have become possible for quite some time, human stem-cell research has a much shorter history.

R.C. Chakravorty (✉)
Department of Surgery, University of Virginia, Salem, Virginia, USA
e-mail: rchakrav@peoplepc.com

N. Bhattacharya, P. Stubblefield (eds.), *Frontiers of Cord Blood Science*,
DOI 10.1007/978-1-84800-167-1_18, © Springer-Verlag London Limited 2009

I have never been directly involved in human stem-cell research, hence I hope to be reasonably objective about its applications.

Stem-Cell Research

Stem-cell research is currently very much under discussion, amongst physicians, biologists, and even some religious groups [4]. Stem cells may some day provide the means of treating and possibly curing diseases such as diabetes, Parkinsonism, Alzheimer's etc., which can only be symptomatically palliated currently. The promise of stem-cell research products (medically and financially) is so great that in July 2005, the prestigious journal *Scientific American* had produced an entire section on stem-cell research in conjunction with the journal *Financial Times*.

A cursory Boolean search using the terms "stem-cell research" AND "ethics" in Google produced 383,000 hits [5] and 959 citations from 2000 to 2005 in Pubmed (National Library of Medicine) [6].

Modern Medical Ethics

As the practice of medicine becomes more complex and integrated with other scientific disciplines, the scope of medical ethics expands and diversifies. In the middle decades of the last century, medical ethics was a relatively simple set of principles. Since then, the great advances in medicine and allied sciences have given rise to ethical rules that relate to researchers and practitioners of specialized fields in medicine and the biological sciences. Today, we have ethics for transplant physicians, the trauma specialists, nurses in various specialties, researchers using animals in experiments, etc. Most of these are of course interrelated. Stem-cell research is closely associated with research in human and animal cloning, recombinant DNA, etc. I will try to limit myself to the ethical principles applicable to stem-cell research only.

A basic issue in scientific publications, in general, is veracity in publishing scientific papers. This has recently been highlighted by the revelation of false data in the publications of a previously noted Korean researcher in stem-cell research. However, that is not specific to stem-cell research, for similar scientific fraud has happened in other fields of research in the past.

General Principles of Medical Ethics

All medical ethical systems starting from the ancient Ayurvedic and Greek (Hippocratic) systems to the modern compilations of the American Medical Association (2001), the British Medical Association, the World Medical Organization (2003) etc. insist upon the following physician–patient relationships.

1. The patient should never be harmed (the implication is harmed intentionally, for unexpected harm might arise from the side-effects of drugs and vaccines and

complications from surgical operations). Some leeway is permitted in the process of treatment. For example, the effects of a surgical procedure could cause harm that would be offset by the ultimate benefit to the patient. Some medications, and most cancer chemotherapeutic agents cause significant, distressing and occasionally dangerous side-effects.

For some decades past, there has been an increasing stress on informed consent by the patient (and significant others) to the treatment(s) offered. This is to explain in as much detail as possible all possible ill effects of the proposed measures so that the patient can opt out before the measures can be applied.

2. In order to ensure that the patient has the best treatment available at the time, the physician has to be aware of the latest therapies as far as is possible. Hence the insistence (in many medical societies) on documented continuing medical education.

Stem-Cell Research

The improvement of the human condition without causing distress to others or degrading the environment is an accepted goal of most if not all ethical systems. The use of stem cells to combat disease is covered by the above ethical considerations. Stem cells are specially promising in that their use could possibly benefit some diseases such as Parkinsonism, diabetes etc., which currently cannot be cured though some symptomatic amelioration is possible. The potentialities are great though some current claims are manifestly exaggerated [7]. The major controversy is in obtaining the stem cells. Very early totipotent stem cell (from blastocysts) may produce cancers and that is an added concern.

The source and potentialities of human stem cells are not the subject of this essay. However, a short discussion is required to elucidate the major ethical questions.

Stem cells can be obtained from adult tissues (such as hematopoeitic stem cell from bone marrow – the patient's own, from a related human donor, from an unrelated human donor or from animals), from the cord blood or placenta (again mainly hematopoeitic stem cell) or from a human embryo/fetus at various stages of development. While adult-differentiated functioning cells have a built-in mechanism (apoptosis) for "death" after a certain number of self-replications, immature or stem or precursor cells do not have this inhibition (neither do cancer cells in general.) Besides, depending upon the degree of their differentiation, stem cells may be totipotent (i.e., capable of producing any type of functioning cell) or pluripotent (i.e., capable of producing multiple types though not all of functioning cells). The more immature the stem cell, the greater is its possible spectrum of differentiation.

There are many potential sources for stem cells. *Embryonic stem cells* are derived from the blastocyst (inner cell mass of a very early embryo) and are totipotent. *Embryonic germ cells* are collected from fetal tissue at a somewhat later stage of development (from a region called the *gonadal ridge*), they are pluripotent and the cell types that they can develop into may be slightly limited. *Adult stem cells* are derived from mature tissue.

In view of the theoretical potentialities of the benefits of treatment by stem cells, the use of this therapeutic modality is abundantly justified, provided appropriate (and supervised) informed consent is used. Early efforts with treatment by stem cells will undoubtedly produce adverse effects – however, that is inevitable, even with established methods of therapy.

Problems with stem-cell research arise mainly with the source of the cells. To a limited extent, stem cells can be obtained from an adult – the individual himself or another consenting immune-compatible individual. There are no ethical problems with this (except for the inherent problems of distress, failure to function and the possible complications of the techniques of harvesting). Unfortunately, such applications are limited – currently mainly to the transfer of bone-marrow hematopoeitic stem cells. More potent stem cells can only be obtained from embryos. Cord blood and placental tissue as stem cell source are usable – again, the potency of the cells obtained are limited. Cells from embryos or fetuses may be used though the ethical constraints may be more stringent (see below).

Historically, human embryonic tissue has been used for medical purposes in the past without any evident ethical conflicts at the time. Thus, tissue from human embryonic muscles was issued to culture poliomyelitis virus to prepare a vaccine. A promising present source is a fertilized ovum that is preserved in liquid nitrogen for later implantation in a contracted or gestational mother. Quite a few such ova are later destroyed when there is no further projected possibility of implantation. If the “owners” or “guardians” of such fertilized ova agree, there should be no ethical problems in using stem cells derived from such sources. Indeed, this should be the beneficial use of a non-replaceable resource that would otherwise be squandered. (See discussion on this further down.)

Whether procurement and fertilization of human ova specifically to obtain stem cells is another question. Where altruistic or compensated “surrogate” or “gestational” motherhood is accepted, there should be no hindrance. I do not know if surrogate motherhood is acceptable in South Korea, the donation of fertilized ova by some of the women associated with the stem-cell research of a now discredited Korean researcher have been considered unethical by the University where the research was conducted.

These constraints devolve around when the embryo can be considered to be a human (with a soul – whatever the soul is considered to be). If so, using embryonic tissues could be taken to be equivalent to destruction of a human. The issue is thus also equated with abortion, creating even more passion. The Catholic Church states that “At the very moment of conception a human being comes into existence. At any time after this the deprivation of life in this living matter, if done deliberately, is murder” [8]. Therefore, stem-cell research utilizing normal gestational and in vitro fertilization products is prohibited.

Totipotent stem cells are available from the human blastocyst, a very early stage of the fertilized human ovum. While the existence of a “soul” is accepted in many religions, the essence of human life is not so clear. Most medico-legal systems (including the American Medical Association and the American Bar Association) agree that the absence of any brain function is the equivalent of “death” [9].

The human brain develops from the primary brain vesicles and the cerebral hemispheres appear in the 5th week of embryogenesis – considerably after the blastocyst stage. The blastocyst, therefore, cannot under any circumstance be considered to be a "live human" [10].

The progression of a naturally fertilized human ovum to the delivery of a healthy child is in itself a hit or miss event. Under optimal conditions, 15% of oocytes do not fertilize, 10–15% start cleavage but fail to implant. Of the 70–75% that implant in the endometrium, 58% will survive until the 2nd week and 16% of these will be abnormal. When the first expected menstruation is missed, only 42% of eggs exposed to sperm are surviving. A number of these will be aborted during the subsequent weeks and some others will be abnormal at birth [11].

While the USA is a secular state, the US Congress under President George Bush has prohibited Federal Funding for establishing any new stem cell lines. A recent effort by the US Congress to permit such funding was vetoed by President George Bush. The US Congress brought together a body of experts whose interesting and informative deliberations are in the public domain [12]. A recent issue of the journal *Perspectives in Biology and Medicine* carried some further discussion on the ethical aspects of stem-cell research, which are well worth consulting [13]. Private funding is allowed and the state of California has reserved money specifically for stem-cell research. Similar efforts are being considered by other state legislatures while a number of States have individually permissive or restrictive guidelines. In states or countries where the willful destruction of human lives is permitted through judicial homicide and acts of war (or terror), governmental restriction of the use of human embryonic tissue (otherwise slated for destruction) for possible benefits to humanity seems confused at the best and hypocritical at worst.

Some Protestant Christian denominations also have taken a stance on stem cells. For example, a number of Baptist ministries are against the use of embryonic stem cells (not adult, cord blood or placental cells.) The 2003 General Convention of the Episcopal Church, considered and passed a resolution to support human embryonic stem-cell research.

Judaism holds that life-saving measures take priority and must be employed, even when conflicting with other laws. An embryo is not deemed a human being – life begins at birth, and Judaism favors life-that-is over life-that-can-be. At its 2003 General Assembly, the Union for Reform Judaism adopted a resolution supporting embryonic and adult stem-cell research as well as research using SCNT technology for therapeutic cloning, opposing efforts to restrict or penalize scientists, clinicians, or patients for participating in stem-cell research and SCNT technology for therapeutic purposes, and supporting efforts by the scientific community to develop regulations and monitor those using SCNT technology [14].

In Hinduism, physical existence is considered to be a transitory abode of the soul on its journey to be one with the Absolute. Death of the physical body is therefore considered to be irrelevant [15].

The Holy Qu'ran addresses the question of human embryonic development in Surahs 23:12–14. A translation is "We created man from an extract of clay. Then we made him as a drop in a place of settlement, firmly fixed..." The very early embryo thus does not seem to be infused with "human" life.

The official position of the US Government vis-à-vis stem-cell research has created considerable discussion, particularly as the US Government through the National Health Institute subsidizes and supports medical research abundantly. The American Association for the Advancement of Science (publishers of the prestigious journal Science) in a position paper stated that:

> "Existing federal regulatory and professional control mechanisms, combined with informed public dialogue, provide a sufficient framework for oversight of human stem-cell research.
>
> Federal funding for stem-cell research is necessary in order to promote investment in this promising line of research, to encourage sound public policy, and to foster public confidence in the conduct of such research.
>
> Public and private research on human stem cells derived from all sources (embryonic, fetal, and adult) should be conducted in order to contribute to the rapidly advancing and changing scientific understanding of the potential of human stem cells from these various sources.
>
> Embryonic stem cells should be obtained from embryos remaining from infertility procedures after the embryo's progenitors have made a decision that they do not wish to preserve them. This decision should be explicitly renewed prior to securing the progenitors' consent to use the embryos in ES cell research, and in order to allow persons who hold diverse moral positions on the status of the early embryo to participate in stem-cell research to the greatest degree possible without compromising their principles, and also to foster sound science, stem cells (and stem cell lines) should be identified with respect to their original source" [16].

Stem-cell research demands considerable complexity in its setup and is also expensive. Therefore, it is actively pursued in only a few countries, most of which already have ethical guidelines in place. The global pursuit of stem-cell research has been summarized in a map and listing available on the Internet [17]. Some countries, such as Brazil and Spain, have permissive laws for stem-cell research. Brazil has launched an ambitious program in stem-cell research, specially related to the use of stem cell in the treatment of heart disease. South Korea had a state-supported stem-cell research program, which has recently been tarnished by the revelation of false claims of success by the researchers. Singapore has abundantly welcomed stem-cell researchers who have faced problems in their countries and set up an excellent center for such pursuit.

India is a secular state and is active in stem-cell research. The Indian Council of Medical Research has published draft guidelines for stem-cell research though these have not yet been legislated into law [18]. As mentioned above, stem-cell research does not seem to have any prohibitions either in Hinduism or in Islam.

Epilogue

Curiosity and profit are two of the most potent driving forces for humans. As mentioned already, stem-cell research is expensive and would falter in the absence of governmental support. While use of adult cells and cord cells are non-controversial and already in use, the use of totipotent stem cells from the very early human embryos will continue till such time as methods to harvest these cells without destroying the embryo are established (from recent reports it appears that this is currently almost achieved.) Unfortunately, even though the potentiality of successful treatment of human diseases is as yet limited, some physicians, either independently or on behalf of commercial concerns are already "selling" stem cell therapy to currently incurable diseases [19]. As our knowledge and control of human stem cells improves, one hopes that many of the diseases now untreatable will become amenable to successful therapy.

References

1. J M. Hawkins Oxford English Dictionary, vol. III D-E. Oxford, Clarendon Press, 1970. p. 312 c 2.
2. Monier Monier-Williams. A Sanskrit Dictionary (Searchable Digital Edition). Bhaktivedanta Book Trust, Mayapur, West Bengal, India 2002, p. 510.
3. V S Apte. The Practical Sanskrit-English Dictionary, 4th ed. Delhi, Motilal Banarsidass, 1965. p. 522–4, 7.
4. A McLaren. Ethical and social considerations of stem cell research. Nature 2001;414 (6859): 129–31. Review.
5. Google search on the term "Stem cell Research", www.google.com, January 7, 2006.
6. Pubmed (National Library of Medicine) search on the term "Ethics", www.pubmed.com, January 7, 2006.
7. S Smith, W Neaves, S Teitelbaum. Adult stem cell treatment for diseases? Science 2006;313 (5786): 439. Epub 2006 Jul 13.
8. http://search.yahoo.com/bin/search?fr=ybr_vzn&p=New%20Advent, accessed on 1/31/2006 10:50:22 a.m.
9. E F M Wijdicks. Determining brain-death in adults. Neurology 1995;45:1003–1011.
10. Langman's Medical Embryology, ed. T W Sadler, 5th edn. Baltimore, William & Wilkins, 1985.
11. A T Hertig. The overall problem in man. In Benirschke K (ed.) Comparative Aspects of Reproductive Failure. New York, Springer-Verlag, 1967, p. 11.
12. M B Mahowald. The President's Council on Bioethics, 2002–2004, an overview. Perspectives in Biology and Medicine 2005;48(2):159–71. This article has a significant bibliography and also gives the URLS of a number of related sites as well as the site from which the Report of the Council can be downloaded.
13. R Dresser. Stem cell research, the bigger picture. Perspectives in Biology and Medicine 2005;48(2):181–94; W B Hurlbut. Altered nuclear transfer as a morally acceptable means for the procurement of human embryonic stem cells. Perspectives in Biology and Medicine 2005;48(2):211–28.
14. The complete resolution is at :http://urj.us/cgibin/resodisp.pl?file=stemcell&year=2003 N. Accessed 2/1/2006 5:40 p.m.
15. Kathoponishad 1, ii, Eds. and Trans., A. C. Sen, Sitanath Tattyabhusan, M. C. Ghosh (Bengali trans.), Haraf Prakshani, Calcutta, January 1994, pp. 83–101.
16. American Association for the Advancement of Science's article is available at http://www.aas.org/docs/resolution.
17. The map is available at http://mbbnet.umn.edu/scmap.html, accessed on Feb 2, 2006.
18. The publication of the Indian council of Medical Research is available at http://www.icmr.nic.in/bioethics/guidelines, stemcell.pdf, accessed on Feb 2, 2006.
19. See S. Smith, n.7.

Index

MIX
Papier aus verantwortungsvollen Quellen
Paper from responsible sources
FSC® C105338

FSC
www.fsc.org

If you have any concerns about our products,
you can contact us on
ProductSafety@springernature.com

In case Publisher is established outside the EU,
the EU authorized representative is:
Springer Nature Customer Service Center GmbH
Europaplatz 3, 69115 Heidelberg, Germany

Printed by Libri Plureos GmbH
in Hamburg, Germany